Hans-Martin Sass

Cultures in Bioethics

Ethik in der Praxis/Practical Ethics

Studien/Studies

herausgegeben von

Hans-Martin Sass
Ruhr-Universität Bochum,
Georgetown University Washington DC

Schriftleitung: Arnd T. May

Band 40

LIT

Hans-Martin Sass

Cultures in Bioethics

LIT

Cover image: Erwin J. Löhr

This book is printed on acid-free paper.

Bibliographic information published by the Deutsche Nationalbibliothek
The Deutsche Nationalbibliothek lists this publication in the Deutsche Nationalbibliografie; detailed bibliographic data are available on the Internet at http://dnb.d-nb.de.

ISBN 978-3-643-90755-4

A catalogue record for this book is available from the British Library

Klosbachstr. 107
CH-8032 Zürich
Tel. +41 (0) 44-251 75 05
E-Mail: zuerich@lit-verlag.ch http://www.lit-verlag.ch
Distribution:
In the UK: Global Book Marketing, e-mail: mo@centralbooks.com
In North America: International Specialized Book Services, e-mail: orders@isbs.com
In Germany: LIT Verlag Fresnostr. 2, D-48159 Münster
Tel. +49 (0) 2 51-620 32 22, Fax +49 (0) 2 51-922 60 99, e-mail: vertrieb@lit-verlag.de
In Austria: Medienlogistik Pichler-ÖBZ, e-mail: mlo@medien-logistik.at
e-books are available at www.litwebshop.de

I. CULTIVATING BIOETHICS CULTURES
1. Bioethics: The World and the Vision
Bioethics and the Bioethical Imperative *11*
1.1. The Bioethical Imperative 11
1.2. Conceptual Modifications of the Term Bioethics 14
1.3. Biotopes Interconnecting Individuals and Communities 19
1.4. Integrating Visions and Cultures of Global Bioethics 21
We have to make choices *24*

2. Cultural Harmonies and Moral Cultures
A merchant fell under the robbers 25
2.1. Love Your Neighbor 25
2.2. What are the Golden Rules? 26
2.3. Nature: Cruel or Harmonious? 28
2.4. Cultures: Suppressing, Liberating, Harmonizing? 30
2.5. Did Socrates Give the Answer? 32
Bioethics Statements: Chennai, Eubios, Rijeka *36*

3. The Properties of Bios in Human Specification
The special human heritage 41
3.1. Is our Human Bios Deficient or Incomplete? 41
3.2. Human Properties in Successful Cultivation Practice 45
3.3. Integrating and Cultivating the Eight C Properties and Virtues 51
The little town by the river *53*

II. RISKS AND REWARDS IN MANIPULATION
4. Manipulating and cultivating Non-Human and Human Bios
Risks and rewards in manipulation *59*
4.1. How to Integrate Expertise and Ethics? 59
4.2. From Indirect Breeding to Direct Manipulation 60
4.3. Patenting Non-human Life? 63
4.4. Creating In-Vitro Flesh 66
4.5. Manipulating and Cultivating Biotopes 68
4.6. Transgenic Animals and Enhanced Humans 71
Ethics towards bios has no borders 75

5. Research on animals for human health benefit
Limits to animal manipulation? 77
5.1. Who should be the 'Guinea Pig'? 77
5.2. The Seven-R Principles in Animal Research 81
5.3. Research Ethics, Bioethics, Corporate Ethics 84
5.4. Risk Reduction Outline in Animal Research 84
Animal research risk reduction scheme 85

6. Human subjects in research
Research and knowledge, a gift from heaven 87
6.1. Medical Research and Care Are Moral Obligations 87
6.2. Managing Risk by Regulation? 89
6.3. Professional Ethics and Corporate Governance 91
6.4. Learning from Research Tribunals in Nuremberg and Japan 93
6.5. Human Experimentation and the Limits of Regulation 96
6.6. New Partnerships, Public Discourse, Informed Choice 97
Embryo talks on embryoid constructs 102

III. CARING FOR HUMAN BIOS
7. Beginnings and ends of individual human life
Stages in human bios? 107
7.1. Interpreting and Protecting Individual Human Life 107
7.2. Bioethical Interpretations of Biological Facts 108
7.3. Animation: Brain Life and Brain Death 111
7.4. Consensus on Symmetry between Brain Life and Brain Death? 114
7.6. Shortcomings of the Potentiality Argument 119
7.7. Subsidiarity: Dignity of the Individual Conscience 123
A universal life protection act *126*

8. Competent care for personal health
We people are different 129
8.1. Individual Health Profiles and Global Health Governance 129
8.2. Health Information and Carrier Ethics 131
8.2. Individual Choice and Informed Contract 134
8.3. Personal Health Care Cards 138
Stakeholders in caring for personal health 141

9. Citizen-expert partnership in caring for health and happiness
The little prince and his jewel 143
9.1. Partnerships in Caring for Health and Happiness 144
9.2. Competence in Professional Ethics 148
9.3. Principles and Guides in Health Care Ethics 149
9.4. Partnership Covenants 152
A covenant for interactive virtues in the care for health 155

IV. COMPETENCE IN BIOETHICS

10. Cultivating Cyberspace Territories

This is no game, it is the real world! *159*
10.1. Populating new Territories in Cyberspace 159
10.2. Instant Equal Access to Previously Privileged Knowledge 162
10.3. Promoting New Cultures in the Care for Health 164
10.4. Meeting Places for Health Communities 166
10.5. Should Cyber Territories Be Regulated? 169
Action guide for E-Health netizens and health care surfers *171*

11. Solidarity and Subsidiarity in Healthy Markets

Subsidarity and solidarity build stable communities *173*
11.1. Vested Interests in Modern Health Repair Shops 173
11.2. Replacing Health Repair with Health Care 175
11.3. Basic Health Care Is a Moral and Cultural Obligation 179
11.4. Supplementary Care, Individual Preferences and Finances 180
11.5. Charitable Care for Controversial Services and the Needy 181
11.6. Competent Compassion in Solidarity and Subsidiarity 182
Stakeholders action guides in subsidarity and solidarity 183

12. Training and Learning in Biocultures

The great way of learning 187
12.1. We learn and train for Life, not for School 187
12.2. Integrated Training for successful Decision Making 189
12.3. Integrating Technology Assessment and Value Assessment 191
12.4. An Alternative Checklist in Health Care Ethics 196
12.5. Preparing for yet Unknown Situations 198
12.6. Conflicts unsolvable in Training and Discourse 202
A Case of professionally unsuccessful service *205*

V. BIOPOLITICS AND COLLECTIVE BIOS

13. Companies and Corporations are Living Beings

Corporations are complex adaptable systems of bios 209
13.1. Corporate Bios in integrated Biotopes 209
13.2. The many Faces and Personalities of Corporate Bios 211
13.3. Clinics and Health Care Institutions as Living Beings 213
13.4. Building Healthy and Happy Corporate Bodies 216
Action guides for corporate and political bodies: the clinic *220*

14. Diversity and survivability of political bodies
Promoting great harmony *221*
14.1. Political Bodies, Similar but not Identical 221
14.2 Diversity and Adaptability of Political Bodies 224
14.3. Social Bios Changing and Adapting 225
14.4. Diseases and Disorders of Political Bodies 226
14.5. Political Struggles and Gross Happiness Products (GHP's) 230
Societal strength and diversity in political bodies 234

15. Risks to political bodies
Risky roads, rooms, territories *235*
15.1. Bios is not without Risk 235
15.2. 21th Century Risk to Cultures of Human Bios 238
15.3. Open Future for Human Biocultures and Political Bodies 246
15.4. Bioethics in Cultivating the Leviathan–Behemoth Struggles 247
Towards a bioethical manifesto? 249

Index of Names 251

INTRODUCTION

The Greek word *bios* means *life*; it is unspecific and includes all forms of life. The Latin word *culture* directs at *cultivating*, improving, manipulating, nourishing, refining, and humanizing something that originally was given naturally. Digging into natural soil and planting vegetables for human consumption, improving hunting skills or shelters, refining personal and clan behavior are early form of cultivation. Individual life and species life are interconnected and have multiple perspectives and roles in those interactions. Individual life is more or less adapted and integrated into various complex and modular biotopes, which themselves modify as complex organisms over time, together with their constituent bios. In discussing life as *complex, highly adaptable, pluriperspective and integrated bios*, we focus on a broad concept of bios, which includes individual bios, species bios, cosmic bios, natural bios, environmental bios, social bios, cultural bios, corporate bios, political bios, technology-integrating bios, and geography-and-cyberspace-integrating bios.

Individual bios is terminal, but species bios and biotopes have longer lifespans, depending on changing environments and their own adaptability. Some species integrate tightly and inflexibly into their very specific biotope and thus become extinct, as they cannot adapt to new climates or otherwise changing conditions. The woolly mammoth is now extinct because of naturally occurring changes in climate and the Siberian biotope, to which it could not adjust. Human culture today alters the environment of the Northwest Coast of the United States by logging traditional woodlands and using timber for houses, infrastructure, and energy, thus threatening the spotted owl with extinction.

In order to survive and to adapt, bios is endowed with properties of communication and cooperation, competence and competition, contemplation and calculation, compassion and cultivation in different mixtures and degrees in plants and animals, fungi and bacteria, archaea and humans, but also in communities and corporations, and in religious and political bodies. Species-specific endowments with each of these properties have enabled the *élan vital* and supported a more or less successful s*truggle for life* of individuals, species, communities, and biotopes. Most species are hard-wired to survive healthy and happy in their specific biotope, but within limits, they have complex powers of adapting to new conditions. In comparison to other species, humans seem to be rather soft-wired, highly adaptable and capable of manipulating and cultivating our biotopes as no other species has ever done. Once upon a time, our predecessors left the trees of central Africa and ventured into other biotopes by foot, camel, donkey, horse, wagon, and later by ship, bicycle, train, airplane, and internet.

We have manipulated uninhabitable ecosystems and made them habitable by constructing tools, houses, farms, factories, walls, and fences. We have applied our properties of competence and competition by developing expertise in science and technology, government, and commerce. We have demonstrated our communicative, cooperative, and compassionate endowments in developing a multitude of different, but similar human-specific cultures. *Social connectedness* rather than *theoretical correctness* seems to have been the most successful vehicle in promoting health and happiness of human individuals and communities. Nevertheless, as cultural anthropology and the history of cultures show, the history of human cultivation was seldom a one-way street to *emancipation of freedom*, as Hegel had envisioned. Quite often, extreme examples of some of our properties resulted in destruction of nature, communities, and cities, in torture, robbery, theft, murder, and the exploitation of fellow humans. As Jacob Burkhardt noted, *human rights* and *civil rights* had and have to be defended and developed against the fashion trends in human history.

It is here, that *ethics* comes into play. Ethics call for actions that promise the health, success, survival, and happiness of my clan, my biotope, and myself. Human history is full of commandments, laws, regulations, rules, and suggestions – issued by kind and unkind rulers, by healthy and unhealthy religions, by contracts and constitutions, by progress and regress, and by revolt, revolution, reform. Other species do not seem to have our species-specific wiring to be *right or wrong*, cruel or kind, just or unjust; neither do they learn the way we humans do: by manipulating, modifying, and cultivating our biotopes and ourselves. Other species live successful or unsuccessful lives depending on their bios and their ecosystem; our human species lives successful or unsuccessful depending on our ethics in cultivating our own bios and our biotopes.

Therefore, this book is not about the *cultures in bios*, of which we do not know as much as we might want to know. Rather, it concerns our human *cultures in bioethics*, namely a human-specific challenge, vision, and capacity to survive and to prosper, – and to live in a healthy and happy way. We, thus, will have to address more specifically this integrated and integrating interaction and connectedness in our cultures. We find bio-ethics in personal and communal ethics, in health care and medical ethics, in the ethics of manipulation and cultivation in business, agriculture, environment, commerce and production, in science and technology, in geography and in cyberspace, and in the ethics and cultures of social and political health, happiness, and survival.

Life and lives are interconnected; I would not exist without my mother and my father. Our human bodies cannot survive without interacting with trillions of different microbes in our gut, throat, mouth, nose, and throughout the body. Outnumbering human genes 100:1, microbes co-digest our food, protect us from unfriendly microbial invaders, and synthesize vitamins and nutrients. Human bios, as does all other bios, depends on and integrates with the seasons, day and night, oxygen, foods, and liquids. All of these elements are essential to keep our organisms, communities and ecosystems alive and flourishing. In light of such a pluri-perspective and complex interconnectedness of bios, we must transform traditional biological, philosophical, and *political concepts of autonomy and self-determination* into the realities of *interconnected bios* and the challenges and visions of bioethics. Who am 'I' and who are 'they'? Who are 'we' and who are 'them'? Old Vedic wisdom gives an answer '*tat tvam asi*' - they are also you. *This is you as well*: the plants and flowers, the mice and crocodiles, the invisible worlds and spirits, the biotopes in geography and cyberspace, the hungry and suffering fellow creatures and fellow humans, my friends and foes, the disappearing and the prospering biotopes of countless shapes and shades.

Plurality and diversity, interconnectedness and integration seem to be basic constructive elements of bios and biotopes. Therefore *bioethics* as a practice and a theory is the most appropriate, most prudent, and most advantageous way and tool for humans to survive and to live well within our natural and cultural biotopes. Cultural traditions have stabilized the principles of a good bioethical life, and they have come in forms as diverse as bios itself. Devoted Jewish Rabbi and enlightened philosopher Moses Mendelsohn suggests as follows: '*Brethren, if you want true peacefulness in God, let us not lie about consensus when plurality seems to have been the plan and the goal of providence. No one among us reasons and feels precisely the same way the fellow human does. Why do we hide from each other in masquerades in the most important issues of our lives, as God not without reason has given each of us his/her own image and face*?' The Qur'an earlier already extended Mendelsohn's insight into the diversity of systems of orientation and belief: '*If the Lord would have wanted, then all on this earth have the same faith together. Now, will you enforce the people to do so?*' Jesus, when tricked into a doctrinal dispute about Mosaic Law, came up with a basic and unassuming bioethical response *'go lowly under your God and love your neighbor as you love yourself'*, an answer not too different from the Vedic *tat tvam asi*.

The term *bioethics* was coined in 1926 by German pastor and educator Fritz Jahr in a teacher's journal article entitled *Life Sciences and the Teaching of Ethics* with an honest and most humble subtitle *Old Wisdom in New Clothing*. Here he also presents the *Bioethical Imperative*: '*Respect every living being as an end in itself and treat it, if possible, as such.*' I use bioethics in Jahr's comprehensive, inclusive and integrating understanding and definition and not in the narrower concept of being synonymous with medical ethics. Bioethics is primarily a practice and an attitude. Only secondarily, it is a theory and an academic and cultural reflection towards bios as integrated, interacting, self-modifying, and self-organizing and accessible to manipulation and cultivation. Individuals, species, cultures, nations and other competitively connected biotopes self-organize and thus modify each other in biology and society. Therefore, medical ethics, together with other fields of professional and communal applied ethics, have to review and translate their specific challenges from within the broader integrating perspectives and fields in bioethics.

I first discuss the word *bioethics* and the vision associated with it (chapter 1), various conceptual religious and philosophical traditions in bioethics (chapter 2), and the eight basic bios properties, as they are specifically confirmed and expressed in human bios, human history, and in day-to-day human action (chapter 3). Then I review benefits and risks in manipulating bios (chapter 4), in particular in animal research (chapter 5) and in human experimentation (chapter 6). The beginnings and ends of individual human life (chapter 7), individual health care risk and benefit (chapter 8), and new opportunities and challenges for cultivating cyberspace territories (chapter 9) lead into a discussion of special issues in lay-expert partnerships (chapter 10), caring for each other's health (chapter 11), and examples in training and educating in applied bioethics (chapter 12). The analysis of corporate bios, corporate profile and mission, using the clinic as an example (chapter 13), and an evaluation of the diversity, dynamics, and strength of political bodies (chapter 14) are followed by political and social risk assessment and the avoidance of disaster, death, and disease by national and international bodies (chapter 15). The narratives, quotes, and action guides, opening and ending the chapters, invite the reader to reflections and dialogues beyond those specific topics and arguments.

This book is dedicated to the memory of my wife Renate, to my parents and those in my family tree, and in gratitude to academic fellow travelers and friends: H. Tristram Engelhardt (Houston), Henk ten Have (Pittsburgh PA) Hou Cai (Bejing), Jingi Kanda (Tokyo), Rita Kielstein (Magdeburg), Rihito Kimura (Tokyo), Arnd T. May (Erfurt), Amir Muzur (Rijeka), Li Zhongshang (Beijing), Fernando Lolas-Stepke (Santiago), Irene M. Miller (Charlotte SC), Edmund M. Pellegrino† (Washington DC), Leo Pessini (Sao Paulo), Qiu Renzong (Beijing), Peter Schroeder-Baeck (Nijmegen) Tai Michael Cheng-tek (Taichung) Zhai Xiaomei (Beijing), Robert M. Veatch (Washington DC), Herbert Viefhues† (Bochum), Hanns-Peter Wolff† (Salzburg). I thank Arnd T. May for a critical review of the manuskript and Lit Publishers, in particular Dr. Hopf and Dr. Rainer, for the generous support of the three series of *Ethik in der Praxis / Practical Ethics*, all dealing in different ways and perspectives with cultures in bioethics.

Hans-Martin Sass

I. CULTIVATING BIOETHICS CULTURES

1. BIOETHICS – THE VISION AND THE WORD

'The Bio-Ethical Imperative: Respect every Living Being in general as an end in itself and treat it, if possible, as such!'

Fritz Jahr, 1926[1]

'Bioethics is an interdisciplinary subject including the study of environmental, ethical, legal and social issues raised by applications of biology, medicine and science. Wide interdisciplinary debate is encouraged.'

Chennai Statement on Bioethics, 1997[2]

'If these ideas are successful, bioethics will become a truly open field of meeting and dialogue of various sciences and professions, visions and worldviews, that have been gathered to articulate, to discuss, and to solve ethical issues related to life as a whole and each of its parts, life in all its forms, shapes, stages, and manifestations, as well as of life conditions in general.'

Rijeka Declaration on the Future of Bioethics, 2011[3]

1.1. The Bioethical Imperative

Bios is a Greek word for life; *ethika* is the Greek term for attitude or custom. The term *bioethics,* thus, means ethical behavior towards life. Ethics is a rule-based or learned set of respectful cultural practices, attitudes, and customs in relation to fellow humans that apply in most traditions in different ways and to non-human bios and biotopes as well. Today bioethics is also an academic discipline applying ideational or practical reasoning to the fields of human behavior. As such, ethics are represented in all cultures and religions; we can demonstrate in *biology* and *sociology* that ethics towards life has been and remains a genuine characteristic of human beings and their cultures. The term *bioethics* was first used in 1926 by Fritz Jahr, a Protestant pastor in Halle an der Saale, when he introduced his 'Bio-ethical Imperative' ('Respect every living being in general as an end in itself and treat it, if possible, as such!') in a small-circulation journal

---

[1] Jahr F 1926 Wissenschaft vom Leben und Sittenlehre in: Die Mittelschule, 1926, 40:604-605 (December 15, 1926); Jahr F 2013 Essays in Bioethics, Miller IM and Sass HM eds., Münster: Lit, 21; frequent presentation of the Bioethical Imperative pp. 21, 28, 40, 84; further references to and quotes from Jahr refer to this 2013 English-language edition.

[2] Chennai Statement on Bioethics, January 16-19, 1997, in: Bioethics in India. Proceedings of the International Bioethics Workshop in Madras: Bioethical Management of Biogeoresources, Azariah J, Azariah H, Macer D eds., Christchurch, New Zealand: Eubios Ethics Institute, XIf.

[3] Rijeka Declaration on the Future of Bioethics 2011, in: Fritz Jahr and the Foundations of Global Bioethics, Muzur A, Sass HM eds. Berlin: Lit, 380.

for teachers called *Die Mittelschule.*[4] Only a month later, in a 1927 editorial in the influential science journal *Kosmos. Handweiser für Naturfreunde und Zentralblatt für das naturwissenschaftliche Bildungs und Sammelwesen*, the theretofore unknown pastor and educator detailed his concept of bioethics under the headline *Bioethik. Eine Umschau über die ethischen Beziehungen des Menschen zu Tier und Pflanze* (*Bioethics. Reviewing the Relationships of Humans to Animal and Plants*).[5]

Jahr argues that progress in the natural sciences – in particular in physiology and the psychology of plants, animals, and humans – strongly suggests dismantling the traditional conceptual differentiation between non-human and human bios in European culture. Jahr refers to Rudolf Eisler's term *Bio-Psychik* (*Seelenkunde alles Lebendigen*)[6] in coining the term *Bio-Ethik*: 'From Bio-Psychik it is only a step to Bio-Ethics, i.e. the assumption of moral obligations not only towards humans, but towards all forms of life. In reality, bio-ethics is not just a discovery of modern times. An especially attractive example from the past is the figure of St. Francis of Assisi (1182–1226) with his great love towards all animals, his warm sympathy for all forms of life, centuries before Rousseau's romanticism for the entire nature.'[4] Jahr refers also to Buddha, Friedrich Schleiermacher, Arthur Schopenhauer, Richard Wagner, and Eduard von Hartmann. He closes the article of 1927 with the proposal that 'the guiding rule for our actions may be the bio-ethical demand: 'Respect every living being on principle as an end in itself and treat it, if possible, as such!'[6]

In his earlier article of 1926, he had referred indirectly to Immanuel Kant's Categorical Imperative in summing up his reflections: 'This results in the guiding principle for our actions in the Bio-ethical Imperative: Respect every living being in general as an end in itself and treat it, if possible, as such!'[6] For Kant, it was the Moral Law that gave authority to the 1785 Categorical Imperative: 'Act in such a way that you treat humanity, whether in your person or any other, never merely as a means to an end, but always at the same time as an end in itself.'[7] Jahr calls the Bioethics Imperative the 'Golden Rule' into which the Fifth Commandment ('Thou shall not kill') must be translated.[8] The old lady fattening her pet poodle 'in false love' and the teenager picking and then throwing away

---

[4] Jahr l.c. 21.

[5] Jahr l.c. 24; 'Bioethik. Eine Umschau über die ethischen Beziehungen des Menschen zu Tier und Pflanze, originally in: Kosmos, 24. Jg. (1927) 2-4. Aufsätze zur Bioethik 1924-1948. Werkausgabe, May AT and Sass HM eds., Münster: Lit 2013; Brazilian translation in: Revista BioEthiKos 5 (3) (2011) 2442-2268; Spanish translation of Life Sciences and the Teaching of Ethics (1926) and Bioethics (1927) in: Aesthethica 8 (2013) 12-23; Croatian translations in: Rincic I and Muzur A 2012 Fritz Jahr i radanje Europske Bioetike (Zagreb 2012) 187-292, an extensive bibliography on Jahr and Bioethics on pages 301-320.

[6] Jahr l.c. 28; for the term *Bio-Psychik* see Eisler R: Wörterbuch der philosophischen Begriffe, Berlin.

[7] I. Kant: Grundlegung zur Metphysik der Sitten. Akademie-Ausgabe vol. 4, 429.

flowers both violate the Bioethical Imperative: 'Respect every living being, including animals, as an end in itself, and treat it, if possible, as such! And if someone does not accept the validity of this principle, as far as it is concerned with animals and plants, then, in repeating what already was said, one nevertheless should follow in recognition of the moral obligation towards human society in general.'[8]

In respecting the other forms of bios, Jahr differentiates between the needs (*Beduerfnisse*) and destiny (*Bestimmung*) of non-human bios in reference to Herder and Krause. In farming corn and salad, the difference between harvesting them is that the individual corn plant has reached its destiny to produce the seed for the next generation of corn crops, but the green salad has not yet reached its destiny in producing seeds and still displays its will to live. Jahr also argues that there are higher responsibilities towards other fellow humans than to animals and plants. We humans need to use prudence and good judgment in all situations of our living together: 'At first hand, it might look like utopia to realize such moral obligations towards all living beings. But we may not overlook that such moral obligations toward a living being in practice are determined by its needs (Herder) respectively by its destiny (Krause). So the needs of animals seem to be lower in quantity and less complicated in content than those of humans. That is even more true for plants, so that practical moral obligations, which are already there towards animals (if not basically, but practically) create less difficulties. Additionally, we have to take into account the principle of struggle for life and existence, a principle which in some way also modifies our obligations towards fellow humans, even though we might feel unhappy about it. Our entire life and activity in politics, in business, in administration, in the laboratory, in the workshop, in the fields is ... in its reasoning and goals not focused on love in the first place, quite often rather focused on struggle with some sort of fellow competitors. Quite often we don't recognize it, as long as such a struggle is without hate and in a legally accepted way. As much as we cannot avoid the struggle with fellow humans, similarly the struggle for life with other living beings is unavoidable. Nevertheless, neither in the first nor in the second case, we will lose the idea of moral obligations as a principle.'[9]

Thus, contrary to Kant's Categorical Imperative, Jahr's Bioethical Imperative is *situational, not categorical.* Being a Protestant theologian, Jahr includes not only the integrated and integrating social and corporate bodies of bios into our human biotopes, but he includes unseen worlds in his bioethical reasoning as

---

[8] Jahr l.c. 40; Jahr l.c. 77-84; in *Three Studies on the 5th Commandment,* 1934, in three steps he refers (a) to the ' Golden Rule,' also expressed in Matth. 7:12, in Luke 6:31 and in Kant's Categorical Imperative, (b) to the 'duty of self-preservation,' i.e., personal health responsibility and responsibility for public health and the community's harmony, and (c) to the Bioethical Imperative to protect all life from harm, a commandment culminating in the Bioethical Imperative.

[9] Jahr l.c. 39f

well. In reference to Comenius, he differentiates between three 'dwelling places' for individual human life: 'the womb, the earth, the heavens.'[10] The first two stages always end with pain and feelings of destruction, while in reality they could be considered thoroughfares to stages of more freedom. Due to the turbulent times of the Weimar Republic and Nazi rule, Jahr's concept of a bioethical imperative to protect all different and integrated forms of bios and biotopes from harm lacked resonance, and he was forgotten for a long time.[11] The following chapters on cultures of bioethics for the integrated and integrating bios and the application of innate, human-specific properties in cultivating raw nature and in protecting and furthering human-specific culture and harmony are based on Jahr's original broad vision of a bioethics imperative and the integrated and integrating biotopes of bios.

1.2. Conceptual Modifications of the Term Bioethics

In 1970, Van Rensselaer Potter, an oncology researcher at McArdle Laboratory (University of Wisconsin Medical School, Madison), published an article titled *Bioethics: the Science of Survival*, concerned with the challenge to human survival of mushrooming sciences: 'Mankind is in urgent need of new wisdom that will provide the *knowledge of how to use knowledge* for man's survival and for improvement in the quality of life. This concept of wisdom as a guide for action – the knowledge of how to use knowledge for the social good – might be called 'the science of survival,' surely the prerequisite to improvement in the quality of life ... Science of survival must be more than science alone, and I therefore propose the term 'bioethics' in order to emphasize the two most important ingredients in achieving the new wisdom that is so desperately needed: biological knowledge, human values.... Biology is more than botany and zoology. It is the foundation on which we build *ecology*, which is the relation among plants, animals, man, and the physical environment.'[12]

---

[10] Jahr l.c. 73ff; 107ff.

[11] Jahr was rediscovered only in 1998: Löther R 1998 Evolution der Biosphäre und Ethik, in: Ethik in den Biowissenschaften. Berlin, 61-68; Engels EM: Article 'Bioethik,' in: Metzler Lexikon Religion (Stuttgart 1999) 159-164; Jose Roberto Goldim: Bioetica: origins e complexidade. In: Revista do Hospita de Clinicas de Porto Alegre 26 (2006) 86-92; Fereira Carvalho, Leo Pessini, Oswaldo Campos: Reflexoes sobre bioetica ambiental. In: O Mundo da Saúde 30 (2006) 614-618; H.-M. Sass: Fritz Jahr's Bioethischer Imperativ. Bochum: Zentrum für Medizinische Ethik (2007); id.: Fritz Jahr's 1927 Concept of Bioethics. In: Kennedy Institute of Ethics Journal 17 (2007) 279-295; see also many references to Jahr on the Internet, most of them probably by Lolas or Goldim. For a review of the recent history of rediscovering Jahr, cf. Amir Muzur and Iva Rincic: Fritz Jahr: on how he had discovered bioethics and how bioethicists have discovered him. In: Fritz Jahr and the Foundations of Global Bioethics, ed. by A. Muzur and H.-M. Sass (Münster 2012) 169-177.

[12] Van Rensselar Potter: Bioethics: The Science of Survival. In: Perspectives in Biology and Medicine 14 (1970) 127-153.

Without reference to Potter, the *Kennedy Institute of Bioethics* at Georgetown University in Washington, D.C., was founded on October 1, 1971, on the initiative of the Kennedy family. At that time, it had three sections: population ethics research, genetic ethics research, and bioethics. The name *bioethics*, however, was dropped soon thereafter, and the Institute was simply called the Kennedy Institute of Ethics.[13] Sections for population research and human genetics later closed due to conflicts with Roman Catholic teachings, and scholars went elsewhere. Initiated by Edmund Pellegrino, Georgetown University Medical School later founded a *Center for Clinical Bioethics* for teaching, consulting, and research in clinical ethics, which still keeps that name. But the term *bioethics* has been associated with the Kennedy Institute since those early days (its 42nd Intensive Bioethics Course, 'Teaching Medical Ethics,' was held in 2016). Warren Reich researched the story of the 'bilocated birth' of 'bioethics twins' in Madison, Wisconsin, and in Washington, D.C. A scholar at the Kennedy Institute himself, Reich became the editor of the *Encyclopedia of Bioethics* and defines bioethics there as 'the systematic study of human conduct in the area of the life sciences and health care, insofar as this conduct is examined in the light of moral values and principles.'[14] As to the unfortunate terminological confusion of discussing bioethics as simply being identical with medical ethics, Reich had already suggested in 1995 '…to make the following distinction in the title of this discipline: to use the term "bioethics" in its original, global sense, as referring to the ethics of life sciences and health care: and then use adjectives to specify particular areas in concern within bioethics. For example, one might speak of *medical* bioethics, *environmental* bioethics, *clinical* bioethics, or *nursing* bioethics without implying, with these terms, any particular approach. This terminology could serve both to draw clearer boundaries of interest and to foster

---

[13] I had been associated with the Kennedy Institute since 1980, and Sargent Shriver once told me that the term *bioethics* was dropped primarily because expectations to use a new fancy word in fundraising had not materialized as the traditional term *ethics* was more familiar to alumni and potential donors; cf. Reich WT, 1994: The word 'Bioethics': its birth and the legacies of those who shaped it, in: Kennedy Institute of Ethics Journal 4 (1994) 319-335; also Reich WT 1995 The word 'Bioethics': the struggle over its earliest meanings, in: Kennedy Institute of Ethics Journal 5 (1995) 19-34. In his presentation to the Bioethics Conference 2001 in Losinj, Croatia, Potter mentions the founding of the 'Kennedy Institute of Bioethics' in 1971, but recollects that they were 'apparently unaware of my four publications,' cf. Potter VR (2012) The Intellectual 'Last Will' of the First Global Bioethicist, in: Fritz Jahr and the Foundations of Global Bioethics, l.c. 149-157; the four publications mentioned by Potter were 'Bioethics, the Science of Survival' (1970); 'Biocybernetics and Survival' (1970); 'Disorder as a Built-in-Component in Biological Systems. The Survival Imperative' (1971), and his book 'Bioethics. Bridge to the Future'; the first intellectual biography and a complete list of Potter's works: Muzur A, Rincic I 2016 Van Rensselar Potter. Zagreb: Pergamena.

[14] Encyclopedia of Bioethics: Introduction, by W. Reich (New York, London) vol. 1, p. XIX.

disciplinary links between the global and the narrower uses of the term "bioethics.'[15]

Due to the influential bioethics courses at the Kennedy Institute of Ethics, the term nevertheless became more or less identical with 'medical ethics' in concentrating on promoting the four principles of autonomy, non-maleficence, beneficence, and justice, three of which had been suggested by the U.S. Belmont Report[16] as basic principles in a pluralistic society and which became globally prominent through Tom Beauchamp and Jim Childress's book *Principles of Biomedical Ethics.*[17] Sponsored by a grant from the European Union Commission, a group of European bioethicists issued a set of four principles (autonomy, dignity, integrity, and vulnerability[18]) as 'European principles' to contrast with the so-called 'Georgetown Mantra'.[19] Xiaomei Zhai recently used the principles of 'justice, responsibility, proportionality, respect, inclusiveness, urgent priority, and solidarity' to discuss no-fault compensation for HIV patients.[20]

Kimura broadened the concept of bioethics to include Asian traditions and suggested civil action: 'Bioethics is a totally new form of discipline which goes beyond the notion of interdisciplinary studies: it is suprainterdisciplinary; it is deprofessionalizing medicine; it is a civil action movement. A new form of solidarity with all forms of life (a traditional Confucian concept) will have to lead

---

[15] Reich WT 1995, l.c. 29f

[16] The Belmont Report 1978 by the US National Commission for the Protection of Human Subjects of Biomedical and Behavioral Research presented respect for persons, beneficence, and justice as three principles that could be accepted by everyone in a pluralistic society.

[17] Beauchamp TL, Childress JF: Principles of Biomedical Ethics (New York 1979, 7th ed. 2013) present the four principles (respect for autonomy, non-maleficence, beneficence, justice), due to the global recognition of this set of values associated with the teachings of the Kennedy Institute of Ethics, they are also called the 'Georgetown Mantra.'

[18] Rendtorff JD 2002 Basic ethical principles in European bioethics and biolaw: autonomy, dignity, integrity and vulnerability – towards a foundation of bioethics and biolaw. in: Medical Health Care Philosophy 5 (2002) 235-244, describing the results of the 1995-1998 EU project BIOMED, which included participants from 22 European countries.

[19] Two international programs at the Kennedy Institute of Ethics, one run by Rihito Kimura, who simultaneously worked at Waseda University in Japan, and the other by Hans-Martin Sass, who had a position at the Ruhr University in Bochum, Germany, made the 'Georgetown Mantra' model of the four bioethics principles globally known, introduced the 'informed consent' principle widely and helped to reduce a sometimes extreme professional medical paternalism in Asia and Europe towards a transition to physician–patient partnership.

[20] Zhai XM 2014 Can a No Fault Approach to Compensation for HIV Infection through Blood Transfusion be ethically justified?, in: Asian Bioethics Review 6(2)143-157. - As an alternative to the so-called Georgetown Mantra I have for discussing issues in medical research used the principles of risk-reward, precision, solidarity, minimax (minimal risk, maximum result), basket (reviewing a basket of widely accepted values), dignity, cf. Sass HM 2006 Bioethics and Biopolitics. Xian, 85-115 (Chinese), 302-338 (English).

us into the next millennium.'[21] Renzong Qiu, also called 'the father of bioethics in China,' wrote from a Chinese perspective: 'Bioethics is located in the intersection of Human Values and Public Policy. The most pressing issue is the just allocation of scarce medical resources. Medical and bioethical values in China are influenced by Confucianism and Marxism. Benevolence is the most basic Confucian value, it would have supported a just system of equal access to health if actual Confucian politics would not have practiced preferential treatment for people of social worth. During the Cultural Revolution there was a Marxist interpretation which favored and practiced preferential treatment. Competition between Chinese and Western medicine, various forms of organizational settings and shared responsibility for health by the citizens and the physicians might produce a most harmonious coordination of human values and public policy.'[22] Quite a number of academic journals in medical ethics today still carry the name *bioethics*[23]. The *International Association of Bioethics* (IAB) held its 13th International Conference in 2016 in Edinburgh; issues discussed were mostly related to medical ethics and public health.

The narrow concept of bioethics as being identical with a modern form of medical ethics did not go without critique. Jayapaul Azariah, the Founding President of the All Indian Bioethics Association, wrote a specifically harsh critique of the American approach.[24] An Asian vision of bioethics and a critical response to the 'Georgetown Mantra' was published by Michael Tai, presenting as Asian principles 'ahimsa or nonmaleficence, compassion, respect, righteousness, dharma or responsibility.'[25] A more recent concept of '*integrated bioethics*' was introduced by Ante Covic as a specific European heritage, defining bioethics as 'a pluriperspective area in which the interplay of heterogeneous perspectives establishes the footholds for orientation in the issues related to life or conditions of its sustainment.' *Jahr. European Journal of Bioethics*, founded in 2011 by Amir

---

[21] Kimura R 1986 Bioethik als metainterdisziplinäre Disziplin. in: Mensch Medizin Gesellschaft 11, 247-253.

[22] Qiu RZ 1986 Bioethik im Schnittpunkt zwischen politische Prioritäten und menschlichen Werte, in: Mensch Medizin Gesellschaft 11, 253-257.

[23] The journal 'Bioethics' published its 30th volume in 2015, other journals include 'Eubios. Journal for Asian and International Bioethics'; 'Asian Bioethics Review'; and 'International Journal for Feminist Approaches in Bioethics.' The American Society of Bioethics and Humanities (ASBH) held its 17th Annual Conference in 2016. The European Society for Philosophy of Medicine and Health Care and the journal edited by the ESPMH do not use the term *bioethics*. The Tuebingen International Center for Ethics in the Sciences, founded in 1985, and the Bochum Center for Medical Ethics, founded in 1986, avoid the term *bioethics*; so does the German medical ethics journal 'Zeitschrift fuer Ethik in der Medizin'; cf. 'Zentrum fuer Medizinische Ethik 1986-2006,' Brenscheidt, May A, May B et al. eds, Bochum 2006; 'Ethik in den Wissenschaften. 1 Konzept, 25 Jahre, 50 Perspektiven, Quinn RA and Potthast T eds., Tuebingen 2015.

[24] Azariah J 2012 Path-maker in Bioethics. In: Fritz Jahr and the Foundations of Global Bioethics, l. c. [note 4] 295-310.

[25] Tai MC: The Way of Asian Bioethics (Princeton 2008).

Muzur, represents the original broad understanding of the 'father of bioethics,' Fritz Jahr. Konstantin Khroutski and others founded the *International Society for Cosmobiology*, which focuses on methodological issues, also on climate change and its influence on human societies[26]. In 1987 I wrote a report on the development of bioethics in the USA for the Division of Ethics of Science and Technology, German Federal Ministry for Research and Technology (BMFT); it was published a year later under the title 'Bioethik in den USA'[27], not including the specific public policy recommendations to the BMFT. A similar report was written in 1991 by Noelle Lenoir for the Prime Minister of France, and the published version contained her public policy suggestions.[28] A small preparatory group from UNESCO that included Lenoir and myself was charged in 1991 with devising an *International Bioethics Committee* (IBC), which was established by UNESCO in 1993 to promote reflection on the ethical and legal issues raised by research in the life sciences and their applications. UNESCO since has issued a declaration on the human genome and on other issues of bioethical relevance[29]. UNESCO's education programs address the broad concept of bioethics including environmental and social bioethics.

Following Jahr, Kelsen, and Foucault, I include corporations and companies and religious, social, and cultural communities as living beings in integrated and integrating, symbiotic and complex, and highly adaptable interaction[30] using eight species-specific human properties. These can be called the virtues of 'communication and cooperation, competence and competition, contemplation and calculation, compassion and cultivation' and are discussed in detail later in Chapter 3.[31] Just as Pastor Jahr easily included the invisible worlds of angels and

---

[26] Internet: see Biocosmology – Neo-Aristotelism, an electronic journal.

[27] Sass H-M 1988 Bioethik in den USA. Methoden, Themen, Positionen (Berlin 1988).

[28] Lenoir N 1991 Au Frontiers de la Vie. Une Ethique Biomedicale à la Française. Rapport du Premier Ministre (Paris 1991).

[29] UNESCO 2008 Bioethics Core Curriculum. Paris: UNESCO; website UNESCO. Ethics Education Program, Division of Ethics of Science and Technology (Food for Thought. Thought for Action). For discussion on the interrelation between bioethics and biopolitics see Bishop JP, Jotterand F 2006 Bioethics and Biopolitics, in: J Medicine and Philosophy 31:205-212; Salter B 2004 Cultural Biopolitics, Bioethics, and the Moral Economy. www.globalbiopolitics.org: Working Paper 1.

[30] Kelsen H 1945 General Theory of Law and State, Clark, N.Y. 2009. Foucault M 2004 Naissance de la Biopolitique, English version: The Birth of Biopolitics (Basingstoke 2008); id.: Du Government des Vivants (Paris 2014); Sass H-M 1991 Professional Organizations and Professional Ethics, in: Ethics, Trust, and the Professions, ed. by Edmund D. Pellegrino et al. (Washington DC, 1991) 263-284; id.: The Clinic as a Good Corporate Neighbor. In: Croatian Medical Journal 54 (2013) 78-82. A 2014 International Symposium on Bioculturology, sponsored by the Guangdong Life Culture Association at Guangdong Medical College (Dongguan 2014.11.7-8) broadened this bioethics concept even more into the analysis of cultures as living phenomena of symbiotic communities.

[31] Sass H-M 2015 Integrative Bioethics in the New Epoch, in Synthesis Philosophica 8 (Zagreb 2015); Sass H-M 2011 Cultivating and Harmonizing Virtues and Principles, in Asian

spirits in his bioethical reflections, we are well advised to include traditional, non-visible biotopes and the new cyberspace-based biotopes and cultures in our bioethical reflections and actions as well; they have been and are more than ever before an essential element in the daily bios of us all.[32]

1.3. Biotopes Interconnecting Individuals and Communities

Other terms were used during the early 20th century to analyze and evaluate the new discoveries of interrelated forms of life in the natural sciences. After studying maritime flora and fauna in the Kieler Bucht, German zoologist Karl Moebius coined the term *biocenosis*, combining *bios* and *koinonia* to describe an ecosystem or biotope as an 'ecological community' or 'bionic community.' He described it as 'a self-sufficient community of naturally occurring organisms occupying and interacting within a specific biotope' containing 'mutually dependent species and individuals, the variety and number of which are determined by the average external living conditions and sustained in an appropriate area by means of reproduction.'[33] Moebius's approach to study

---

Bioethics Review 3 (2011) 36-47; Sass H-M 2008 Asian and other Ways of Bioethics: Community, Compassion, Competence, Cultivation, in Formosan Journal of Medical Humanities 9 (2008) 5-12; Sass H-M 2012 The 5 C Model, in: Synesis 2012, G52-59.

[32] Jahr F 1934 Vom Leben nach dem Tode; Jahr F 1938 Drei Abschnitte des Lebens, l.c. 73ff, 107ff [note 2] 73 ff. and 107 ff.; cf. H.-M. Sass: Ludwig Feuerbach über virtuelle Realität im Internet, in: Aufklärung und Kritik 19 (2012) 29-37; id.: An Early Hegelian Vision of the Internet. Ernst Kapp's 1845 Philosophy of Cultivating Space and Time. in: Jahrbuch für Hegelforschung 15-17 (2014) 11-34; id.: Earth, Universe and Multiverse are Living Beings. Fritz Jahr and the Foundations of Global Bioethics, in: Fritz Jahr and the foundations of global bioethics, Muzur A and Sass H-M eds., 2012, 345-357.

[33] Karl August Möbius: Die Auster und die Austernwirtschaft (Berlin 1877); English in: US Commission Fish and Fisheries Report (1880) 683-751. R. H. Francé, often called 'the father of sustainable agriculture,' used the term 'Biozoenose.' In: Die Welt als Erleben (Dresden 1923) 96 ff. in order to explain the phenomenon that ‚jedes „Ich" mit seiner Umwelt in gesetzmäßigen Beziehungen steht, welche nach einer Epharmonie tendieren', die biologische Biozönose also ‚eine Teilerscheinung der allgemeinen Gleichgewichtstendenz' des 'Bios' ist; cf. Eisler: Wörterbuch … l.c. [note 1], vol. 1, 226. Czar Nikolas I in 1852 used biomedical terminology when describing the moribund Ottoman Empire as the 'sick man at the Bosporus'; disintegrating, millennia-old societies such as Iraq and Syria might be infected by a sort of 'cancer' or 'auto-aggressive disease.' Societies unwilling to modify into the modern world have been called 'sclerotic'; the impact of coronary or infectious disease, dementia, hypertension, and diabetes but also 'preventive care,' fitness training, and the support of happiness can be translated into the worlds of economy and politics, describing clans, communities, healthy and growing countries, and weak and disintegrating societies; see chapters 14 and 15 below. Successful biocoenose can occur in a small pond of fish, plant, and algae and in a large socio-cultural lake or ocean of people, cultures, politics; using the terminologies of biology, biocoenose, or biomedicine thus might help us to better understand social and political developments of and in living cultural, social, and political bodies, business corporations, local clans and cyberspace communities.

intertwined collective communities of organisms and microorganisms, and it produced great early insight into the interaction of the entire world of bios in microbiome research. Actually, biotopes and habitats, in particular microbiomes, have been described as 'metaorganisms'[34] because neither the host nor the biome associated with it can live by itself (both have developed complex interspecies relationships, and their genomes, phenotypes, and ecosystems have evolved accordingly and in symbiosis). Potter mentions that neurologist Peter Whitehouse of Case Western Reserve Medical School had suggested using the term *Deep Bioethics*[35] to include environmental ethics centrally in bioethics (and in reference to the 'Deep Ecology' movement of those days and the followers of Aldo Leopold).

At the beginning of the 21st century, we have thus further broadened our understanding of bios and our challenges in the cultures and ethics of bios even more due to an extension in knowledge and the creation of new worlds of bios such as the following: (a) the zoonotic world of microbes, bacteria, viruses, parasites, and pathogens, in which more than 80% of organisms have not yet been discovered and could be manipulated or modified, just as we have cultivated plants and animals; (b) the new and expanding worlds of cyberspace; and (c) a combination and integration of the new biotopes of hardware and software in genetics and electrics. In his *Novum Organon* of 1670, Francis Bacon had already emphasized that nature is not only the free, natural bios untamed by humans, but, more expansively, bios as being bound, manipulated, pressed, and formed by man via science and technology. Where there is light, there is also shadow, and new technologies of various kinds can and will be used for cultivating purposes as well as for destruction in novel dimensions of our new and rapidly growing biotopes.

The powers of national and international governmental bodies might be shrinking, and the powers of businesses and the translation of biological knowledge into biotope modification and cultivation might be growing, together with the powers of individuals, clans, and groups to build their own biotopes and habitats in cyberspace. Along with the potential impact of uncivilized individuals and groups bent on destruction, the powers of governments simultaneously grow into new dimensions, as George Orwell sketched out in his novel *1984*.[36] Revolts and rebellions using new science and knowledge (including new powers

[34] Bosch TCB, McFall-Ngai 2011 Metaorganisms as the New Frontier, in: Zoology (Jena) (4):185-190; Doolittle W, Zhaxybayeva O (2010) Metagenomics and the units of biological organization. Bioscience 60:102–112; Nicholson JK, Holmes E, Wilson ID (2005) Gut microorganisms, mammalian metabolism and personalized health care. Nat Rev Microbiol 3:431–438; The Human Microbiome Project Consortium 2012 Structure, Function and Diversity of the Healthy Human Microbiome, in: Nature 486:207-214.

[35] Potter VR (2012) l.c., 156.

[36] Orwell G 1984 NY: Penguin 1948.

on the Internet) will be on the rise as well.[37] At the end of 2015, Facebook, launched in 2004, had more than 1.5 billion inhabitants – outnumbering the population of the People's Republic of China with its nearly 1.4 billion citizens and more than five millennia of history and culture.[38] Detailed and systematic research on our mutual biotopes with microbes in our houses, offices, hospitals, subways, and factories has only just begun. Such research should lead to a better understanding of this relationship and to improved services in public health, eventually fostering cultivation and breeding in the microbial world such as we have done with animals and plants in agriculture.[39] Work is underway to create biological drones for surveillance, stunning, and killing.[40] We will have to include these technical and cultural risks and the great opportunities of these newly created and newly studied worlds of bios in our reflections on the 'cultures of bioethics,' because this is 'our bios' in all of its integrations and interactions, fights and faults.

1.4. Integrating Visions and Cultures of Global Bioethics

Close to 100 years after its first use by Jahr, the terminology has been established and the field is alive: changing, integrating, and broadening. One thing seems to be clear already: bioethics is not identical with medical ethics as apples are not identical with oranges: apples and oranges are fruits, and fruits belong in the botanical kingdom. Together with microbes, animals, humans, teams, societies, and geographical and non-geographical biotopes of all sorts, they form the interactive and interacting community of life, the 'koinonia of bios.' In 1979, Peter Singer called for 'animal liberation' and argued that the potential to feel pain or pleasure and to have conscious experiences marks the difference between morally significant beings and those that are otherwise.[41] He points out that certain animal species have higher levels of understanding and intelligence than intellectually compromised humans, but that the respect animals are owed rests on their capability to experience pain and pleasure similar to us. Albert Schweitzer coined the phrase 'reverence for life' (*Ehrfurcht vor dem Leben*) to

[37] Blum G, Wittes G 2015 The Future of Violence, New York: Basic Books; Casti J 2012 X-Events. The Collapse of Everything. New York: Harper Collins.

[38] Cukier K 2015 Charting Change. The World in Transition, in: The Economist. The World in 2015, p. 94-96.

[39] Lajaunie C, Morand S, Tan Boon Huan 2014 Barcoding, biobanking, ebanking for 'One-Health' projects in South-East Asia, in: Eubios 24(4)129-131; Hotz RL 2015 Scientists in 18-Month Project Gather DNA Throughout Transit System to Identify Germs, Study Urban Microbiology, in: Wall Street Journal, Febr 6, pp. 1 and 10.

[40] Blum G, Wittes B 2015 New Threats Need New Laws, in: Wall Street Journal 04-18/19, C3: 'The old social contract has its roots in the security dilemmas of the Enlightment era. In our new era, everyone is simultaneously vulnerable to attack and menacing by others. That requires a different, more complex social contract – one that we are just starting to imagine.'

[41] Singer P 1975 Animal Liberation. Harper and Row.

include all human individuals, races, and cultures, but he also embraced animals and all other living beings: 'The farmer, who has moved thousands of flowers as food for his cows in the meadow, may never decapitate a flower on his way home just for fun; this would be a crime towards bios (*Leben*) as he would do such a thing without pressure or necessity.'[42] Still, contemporary society's small, misleading, and misplaced definitions of bioethics as being more or less identical with physicians' or medical ethics must be changed. These influential yet imprecise terminologies are rooted in unclear reasoning and will definitely lead to unclear and morally deficient actions in academics, science, society, and culture.

A broad definition of '*total bioethics*' as 'bioethics for enhanced sustainability' of all of bios and for different fields of human action and responsibility was developed at an international conference in Chennai, India. Jayapaul Azariah, who organized the conference with Darryl Macer, defines bioethics as a practical challenge to do the right thing: 'It refers to the right and wrong in life: the good and bad or simply the love of life … which makes us to seek after what is good and right and proper life. This makes life loveable and pleasant to live with people and in harmony with the environment. This is total Bioethics'. He argues further: 'Philosophers, Poets, Technologists, Scientists, Legal experts, Physicians, Public Administrators, Historians, Educationalists, Economists, Environmentalists, Marine Biologists, Theologians, Anthropologists, Non-Governmental Organizations, Sociologists and Chemists are thinking together under the one roof of Bioethics. In this important event we have the presentation of views from different religions too. Our concern is that in such a diversity in human thinking and thought process, there should be stability … To relate Bioethics with enhanced sustainability of bio-geo-resources we should endeavor *to develop systems of relationship among various approaches and views to basic issues in life and in death.* One such sure tool to reach the above goal is bioethics education. We should remember that human diversity in thinking produces sometimes conflicts and conflict drains energy. We should be the people who generate sound bioethical teaching. We should develop exercises in Bioethics Curriculum Development. Bioethics Education has come to stay and to improve the quality of human life. The way of life of human beings may change during the 21st century. Some of the changes may include the absence of agricultural fields if food (plant/meat) is grown biotechnologically. In a few years' time we may not use our conventional medical shops to sell bottled medicines and pads of tablets and pills. These will be replaced by gene therapy and disease targeted medical probes and many other changes. Our next generation must be educated to prepare themselves for such changes in lifestyle.'[43]

---

[42] Schweitzer A 1948 Kultur und Ethik, vol. 2, München: Biederstein, 249.

[43] Azariah J 1997 Preface, in: Bioethics in India, Azariah J, Azariah H, Macer D eds., Christchurch, New Zealand.

The Chennai Declaration calls for including the wisdom of indigenous people and of world religions into supporting sustainable bios[44] A 1993 parliament of world religions discussed the future role of religions in respecting and protecting bios. They agreed on four cultural directives that they found in all religions: non-violence and respect for life, solidarity and just economic order, tolerance and a life of truthfulness, and equal rights and partnership between men and women.[45] A United Nations 'World Charter for Nature' in 1982 argued as follows: 'Every form of life is unique, warranting respect regardless of its worth for man ... This type of valuation is intrinsic. We need to ask whether there is intrinsic value in nature and life. We could reconsider the term selfishness as the conservation of intrinsic value, but we are left with a fact that "The planet loves life and so do we.'[46]

It is not far from Jahr's first presentation of the term *bioethics* in 1926 to a summary by Luka Tomasevic in a 2008 book dedicated to Ivan Segota on the occasion of Segota's 70th birthday: 'Today we speak of bioethics from the medical, religious, cultural, philosophical, legal, sociological and even political standpoint. No matter how many perspectives, approaches, and standpoints bioethics has, they all are focused on one point we call *life*, and bioethics itself at the extreme is nothing else than *love for life*. At the same time, all men accept that *life must be respected* in all its forms, phases and circumstances of appearance. If we set off from this fact, then all of us, on different sides of the world, in different disciplines, cultures and traditions, can better understand and exchange thoughts and experiences.'[47] To this, I would merely add that we should not forget the protection of, cultivation of, and love for cyberspace-based bios and its interactions and integrations with geographical space and land cultures. Locally and on a global scale, virtual and real worlds have expanded and are used by good and bad people, by business, charity, terror, crime, care, construction, and destruction. Today, individual human lives and cultures are embedded not only in in natural and cultivated geographical spaces as biotopes and environments, but also in cyberspace-based biotopes and environments of communication and cooperation in information, commerce, and social websites; private, semiprivate, and public networks of all kinds; fields of supporting or educating; and fields of spying, exploiting, lying, and cheating. These multiple, integrated biotopes of the Internet have become an essential and foundational

---

[44] Chennai Declaration 1997, in: Bioethics in India, lc, XIf (13 and 14).

[45] Macer D 2012 Fritz Jahr and Love of Life, in: Fritz Jahr and the Foundations of Global Bioethics, lc., 258; Kueng H 1996 Yes to a Global Ethics. London: SCM Press.

[46] Quoted by Macer 2012 lc, 263; Rolston H 1994 Conserving Natural Value. New York: Columbia.

[47] Tomasevic L 2009 Foreword, in: From Medical Ethics to Integrative Bioethics. Dedicated to Ivan Segota in Occasion of his 70th Birthday. Zagreb, p. 15; cf. Sass H-M 2009 European Roots of Bioethics: Fritz Jahr's 1927 Definition and Vision of Bioethics. In honorem Ivan Segota, lc, 19-31.

part of our modern human world of bios, as much as clothing, houses, fences, tools, arms, agribusiness, and manufacturing have been for millennia. Synthetic biology and artificial intelligence have been introduced into the new biotopes of human and non-human forms of bios in the 21st century and will gain increasingly more moral recognition and political/cultural power. A systematic study and evaluation of the old and new zoonotic worlds of modern urban life and of the multitudes of uncounted microbial colonies has yet to begin.

In his 2001 address to the International Bioethics Symposium in Croatia, Potter reviewed the new term *bioethics* and the global mission it represents: '1. Survival in the long-term boils down to a matter of bio-ethics, not traditional ethics. 2. For the long-term future we will have to invent and develop a political ethics bioethics. *Traditional Bioethics* is about interaction between *people and people*; bioethics is about interaction between *people and biological systems*. Political bioethics is essential for healthy political decision-making and for the creation of sound policies. In other words, action will have to be constrained and guided by biological knowledge as bioethics emerges and is finally turned into voluntary agreements or into regulatory law in specific cases.'[48] He also mentions that he should have chosen the title *Bioethics, the Morality of Survival* for his 1970 book instead of *Bioethics, the Science of Survival*.[49] The last chapters of this book will discuss the properties and opportunities of the political bios to protect, support, and contribute to survival and happiness as well as the risks involved in political actions, for individual and collective bodies may do good or bad, succeed or fail. In his conclusion, Potter summarizes the choices as follows:[50]

WE HAVE TO MAKE CHOICES

'We need political action. We need to demand that our leadership achieve humane Global Bioethics aimed at global sustainability for the long-term. So, finally, I want to declare that as we face the future, we have two possibilities. The Third Millennium will be either be The Age of Global Bioethics or the Age of Anarchy. The choice is ours to make.'

---

[48] Potter VR (2012), l.c. 152
[49] Potter VR (2012), l.c. 151
[50] Potter VR (2012), l.c. 154f

2. CULTURAL HARMONIES AND MORAL CULTURES

A MERCHANT FELL UNDER THE ROBBERS

A traveling merchant fell under the robbers, was mugged, badly beaten, and left half-dead. Various people passed the scene thereafter, orthodox theologians, experts in ethics, also a moral and religious stranger in this area around the Jordan River, one of the people from Samaria, a not well educated and not well respected group among the neighboring cultures and communities of the eastern Mediterranean. When the others passed the crime scene and saw the helpless victim, none of them stopped to provide first aid and help; their reasons might have been (a) fear of the robbers still around, (b) not feeling a moral obligation to a stranger, or (c) a discrepancy between ethical theory and factual moral practice. Only that man from Samaria stopped and helped, brought the victim to the next hotel and paid for his care.

Narrative told by Jesus[1]

2.1. Love Your Neighbor

What did this travelling merchant from Samaria do? He compassionately cared for a fellow human in great need, while others did not. He competently brought this man out of danger and into a safe environment. He calculated and paid the cost of care, having little time for further contemplation in such an emergency situation. He did not have competitors or supporters in 'doing good'; others had sidestepped and dodged the opportunity to serve and to relieve. That man just applied basic human species-specific properties – communication, cooperation, competence, compassion, calculation, contemplation, competition, cultivation – in an urgent, concrete situation with emphasis on competence and compassion. Billions of people of different cultures and backgrounds have contemplated this narrative told by Jesus 2000 years ago and pondered what they would have done in such a dangerous situation and what their own religious or ethnic background would have called for.

When asked by his adversaries, fundamentalist Jewish theologians and experts in Mosaic Law and rules, how he would define principles of neighborly love, compassion, and the ethics of solidarity, Jesus refused to get involved in an academic doctrinal and dogmatic exchange by responding with moral and theoretical minimalism: 'You shall love the Lord your God with all your heart, and with all your soul, and with all your strength, and with all your mind; and your neighbor as yourself.'[2] Would Jesus have become angry if someone had said '*love and be good to all bios*, or *love and follow the way of Tao*?' We know of similar teachings of humaneness (*ren*) by authoritative masters in other cultures:

---

[1] Luke 10:25-37.

[2] Matth 5:43; Luke 10:27.

The Confucian rule 'do not do to others, what you would not desire yourself'[3] expresses the same vision as the Kantian Categorical Imperative. Hindu, Buddhist, Muslim, and Jewish cultures have similar traditions of neighborly love and compassion for the poor, sick, and needy. They all call for humaneness as a prime virtue and for moral principles beyond theological/ philosophical teachings and quarrels. Based on a 'Doctrine of the Mean,' Confucian ethics sets communication and cooperation in ethics within a conceptual framework of harmony among humans and their natural and social biotopes, to be accomplished through self-cultivation. In the narrative of the 'good Samaritan,' self-cultivation meant the personal internalization and the practical application of those principles by each individual. Religious and philosophical arguments in favor of 'neighborly love' or 'compassion' might have different backgrounds, but the 'product' (i.e., the practice of competent compassion) will be the same, and that is all that counts in a *global competition among worldviews and traditions.*

In telling a story rather than accepting the invitation to an intellectual academic debate on theories of universal ethics, solidarity, and community, three conceptual and moral insights are presented: (1) There is a difference between ideologies, religious dogmas, or academic theories on one side and actual care and the practice of solidarity on the other. Moral attitudes are not necessarily based on explicit ethical theories. Some edifices of moral theory even neglect to recognize the 'stranger' as a fellow human being of equal human dignity and therefore withhold solidarity and compassion; some have even been built for the purpose of exploitation and domination. (2) There are basic moral obligations and common moral principles so prevalent in cultural, ethical, and religious traditions that they can be called universal ethics. (3) As universal ethics, they need to be evident to each person in every moral community, in the words of Confucius 和而不同 (he er bu tong), diversified and in harmony, but not identical.[4] Deng Xiao Peng applied this goal-oriented insight of Jesus to the use and abuse of theories: 'it does not matter whether a cat is black or white, what is important is, that the cat catches mice.'[5]

2.2. What are the Golden Rules?

German philosopher Immanuel Kant made an epistemological distinction between *a priori* knowledge (i.e., what is evident to everyone without prior empirical experience) and *a posteriori* knowledge (i.e., what becomes evident only after experiments and various kinds of experiences. If we transport that dis-

---

[3] Analects 12:2.

[4] Zhai XM 2011 Diversified and in harmony, but not identical, in: Asian Bioethics Review 3(1):31-35.

[5] Quoted from a speech of Deng Xiao Peng to the Secretariat of the KPC; the slogan is actually a well-known proverb in the Szechuan Province.

tinction from the field of epistemology and metaphysics to the fields of ethics, culture, and education, we may define universal ethics as moral principles, contractual relations, values, and attitudes evident to all reasonable people and shared by individuals and communities independently of their particular system of belief or orientation. Kant holds that all humans are born with an inherent respect for the moral law (*sittengesetz*); that is, respect for humaneness (*ren*), the law of morality. In arguing that all humans are naturally endowed with properties to distinguish good and evil, virtues and vices independently from culture or experience, he follows the Western natural law tradition since Aristotle, who taught that the basic norms of ethics are inherently present in nature. He differs from that tradition, however, in questioning whether a particular custom or the moral rules of one particular community can be argued for by reference to nature and natural laws. Saint Paul argued similarly that those who believe in a God would have received the message of such a common universal morality by Divine command, but that others would have the opportunity to recognize the same common and natural moral principles in the rules of nature as 'original revelation.'

If a universal common morality does exist, then specific rules of moral communities must be evaluated in regard to whether or not they embody what was universal to all humans in Kant's vision: compassion, respect for human dignity, and respect for rules, contracts, and principles that support the respect for human dignity. Kant's approach to universal ethics has been called formalistic because he calls for no specific human rights or obligations beyond respecting human dignity and following rules that, if generalized, would be good and acceptable rules for everyone. This formalism had a mission and vision of content: maxims in ethics, moral attitudes, and moral communities and traditions always need to be assessed as to how far in a specific situation they support or suppress fellow humans and the respect for their dignity, liberty, and security — how far they treat people as ends in themselves and not merely as means to an end.

Humaneness and solidarity with fellow humans in extreme situations of danger and suffering are definitely such principles; in fact they are universally recognized in all moral communities based on respect for human dignity independently of religious belief, race, gender, social position, or specific personal properties, gifts, or handicaps. In the long list of cultural traditions and moral communities, a vast majority support the value and principles of humaneness as reflected in solidarity with the most vulnerable, the sick, the poor, and the dying; sincerity as in self-cultivation and honesty; and bravery as in determined and courageous action and in prudent risk-taking 'for the neighbor's good.'

Kantian, Christian, and Islamic understandings of universal ethics are matched by Confucian, Buddhist, and other traditions based on the vision of a natural respect for human dignity, and they challenge themselves to find the most agreeable and harmonious expression of such a vision in a particular situation or moral community. Therefore, all cultural traditions need to be highly critical of any principle or custom that does not support or is counterproductive to the recognition of solidarity and compassion found in the *Golden Rule*. The Taoist said 'the world is a sacred vessel, if you tamper with it, it will be ruined; if you treat it as an object, you will lose it. In fact, there is a time for going ahead, and a time for being behind, a time for being in motion, a time for being at rest.'[6]

There are limits to human intervention. We cannot change the seasons or cosmic movements, but we can build houses and produce clothes, tools, and food for us and for our neighbors. However, we also have destroyed biotopes, killed in wars, and tampered with more or less harmonious forms of bios. Overbearing theories may also harm common moral intuitions and harmonious relationships; some might lead to ideological extremism and terrorism. Some custom-based cultures hold on to outdated etiquette, while others are strong and vital enough to abandon old customs and cultivate new humaneness and solidarity. Systems of ethics, abstract rules, laws, or regulations are written on paper only, and the attitudes and actions of people in respectful moral behavior do not necessarily or directly depend on those maxims, doctrines, or regulations alone. Those rulings are powerless in themselves if not embodied in real-life behavior and action.

2.3. Nature: Cruel or Harmonious?

Many cultures have used heaven and earth as reference poles to picture physical and metaphysical landscapes for human orientation and action. While in most cultures heaven and earth complement and interact with each other, together they provide harmony and guidance in Chinese reasoning. Iranian and European traditions interpret this world as the great battleground between the sons of good against the sons of darkness and evil, a concept originally formed in Persia with long-lasting influence on the traditions of the Middle East and Europe. Whatever the structural differences in the architectural design of these houses, it seems that their goals were similar: narratives, role models, and theories to understand the world and oneself, to differentiate between good and evil, to position an individual within a community, to define humaneness, love, and nobleness, and to express visions and goals for individual and collective action.

A pre-established heavenly harmony (*daode* in early Chinese terms, *logos* in European Platonic reasoning) predetermines requirements for good human behavior and virtues (*de)*, such as *ren* (humaneness) and *lunli* (interpersonal relations) in Chinese, solidarity and respect for each other and for each other's position in society in European natural law tradition.[7] We find similar references

---

[6] Dao Te Ching 29.

[7] Sass HM 1986 The moral a priori and the diversity of cultures, in: Analecta Husserliana 20:407-422.

to pre-established, exemplary situational harmony in different shades of love: spousal love (*fuqi enai*), filial love (*xiao),* and neighborly and patriot love or loyalty (*zhong*). In more personal terms, monotheistic religions have encouraged people to 'love God and love your neighbor' or more precisely 'love God by doing good to your neighbor', in particular to the poor, sick, and frail. In European secular humanist terminology, the three principles of the French revolution (*égalité, liberté, fraternité*; equality, liberty, solidarity) express a similar request for kindness as humaneness (*ren*) to each human being, including the kindness to tolerate other people's visions and principles while enjoying one's own.

Of course, emphasis on individual autonomy or family/community is different in many traditions and may change over time within traditions. But we find the principle of solidarity in worldviews as different as Jewish, Christian, and Islamic religion, Buddhist, Confucian, and Taoist reasoning, socialist *Weltanschauung*, and even Kropotkin's anarchism.[8] It is worth mentioning that references to pre-established, exemplary heavenly or natural harmony occur in eras of social and cultural turmoil and insecurity, such as that of Confucius or of late Hellenism, when Greek authors used the relationship between the sun, moon, and stars as a model for forming a harmonious human society. While these references support diversity in human cultures, they have also been used to defend inequality among fellow humans and between genders, races, and classes, big fish and small fish, big stars and small stars. Those fighting for humaneness, compassion, personal liberty, and security against oppressive powers can interpret actual situations as an aberration from nature or define culture as a means to overcome raw nature. Both strategies can be found in either of the traditions of European thinking: cultivating or dominating raw nature in various levels of intensity. In contrast, Asian traditions try to orient themselves in a pre-existing harmony of heaven and earth, within which people have to find their rightful position. Buddhist views on the relationship of the individual to the world are centered in a personal challenge of individual heritage and responsibility for oneself and one's biotope. The precise percentage of inherited and lifestyle challenge cannot be known to the individual; therefore, in a model of interrelated forces of 'dependent origination,' failure and sickness cannot be blamed fatalistically on genetic or social heritage. To live a good and liberating life and to be as healthy as the *kamma* allows, one needs to practice morality (*sila*), mental discipline (*samadhi*), and wisdom (*panna*).[9] Extreme forms of misguided compassion and false, situational love do exist. Jahr refers to the old lady who fattens her poodle with unhealthy meats and sweets, not calculating the implications for the dog's health and life expectancy; at the same time she lets her employees go hungry.[10] In one of his former lives, Buddha is said to have of-

---

[8] Kropotkin A 1902 Mutual Aid.

[9] Ratanakul P 1999 Buddhism, health, disease and Thai culture, in: A cross-cultural dialogue on health care ethics, ed. Coward H, Ratanakul P, Waterloo Ont.: Laurier 19.

[10] Jahr, l.c. 36.

fered himself for food to a hungry tigress and her cubs, an extreme form of compassionate love associated with the prospect of a gratifying re-incarnation in the cycle of bios.

2.4. Cultures: Suppressing, Liberating, Harmonizing?

As it would be wrong not to differentiate between different ethics teachings and practices within large cultural traditions, we must also be aware that traditions can become ceremonial and lacking in the power to guide real-life actions. Cultural history is full of contrasting references to nature, understanding it either as an exemplary model of harmony or as cruel and needing to be overcome and cultivated. Similarly, the protection of 'culture' has been used both for suppression and exploitation and as a tool for promoting and doing good. The fight against the suppressive powers of tradition and the liberating experience of being empowered by it are the two eternal aspects of culture.

Applications of cultural and moral traditions in moral conflict resolution can be strongly authoritative and exhortative to individuals and communities; regulative and informative in drafting rules and advising legislation; educative, discursive, and adjuvant in case management and scenario assessment. Traditions never provide ready-made recipes to be used inflexibly without careful assessment of the technical, cultural, and ethical variables in a situation and without identifying the responsibilities, values, and wishes of priority stakeholders. Some traditions are older, more metaphysically elaborate, shinier in appearance and ceremony, and supported by more people than others. As far as the transfer from orientation to action is concerned, the only thing that counts is the motivation and real-life application of theories, beliefs, and principles in concrete situations, as exemplified in the parable of the Good Samaritan. As Jesus suggested, religions sometimes make ethical problems more complicated instead of helping solve them. In the encyclical '*Veritatis Splendor,*' Pope John Paul used the 'subsidiarity' principle in arguing that the gifts of an individual conscience and of personal morality are based on natural law: 'Like the natural law itself and all practical knowledge, the judgment of the conscience also has an imperative character: man must act in accordance with it. If man acts against this judgment or, in cases where he lacks certainty about the rightness and goodness of a determined act, he stands condemned by his own conscience, *the proximate norm of personal morality.*'[11]

In the developing 21st century of globalization and migration, a traditional challenge in all cultures becomes even more pressing: the moral recognition and treatment of the ethnic or moral 'stranger' as a fellow human. Tribal societies and ones that are ethnically or culturally closed have particular problems in recognizing the 'other' as being of equal dignity and as deserving of equal rights.

---

[11] John Paul II 1993 Veritatis Splendor, Vatican City, art. 60; cf. Hoeffner J 1983 Christliche Gesellschaftsehre. Kevelaer.

Jesus, Deng Xiao Ping, Confucius, Lao Zi, Kropotkin, Spinoza, and Locke all present strong arguments for the view that respect for human dignity includes respect for diversity, for personal abilities and disabilities, and for conceptual differences and dissenting positions on deep philosophical and religious issues. They also hold that actions count independently of how shiny, golden, bizarre, strange, or crude one finds the ideas, convictions, or visions of others. After centuries of ideological battles (including the slaughter of 'infidels,' torture of Christian believers by other Christians with different dogmas, and persecution or exclusion of ethnic or moral outsiders from society), European thinkers like Spinoza, Locke, and Voltaire proposed *tolerance* as a supreme moral and cultural principle as regards the dignity of an individual's moral values and religious vision.

Similarly, respect for an individual's fate and personal challenges (*kamma*) in Indian tradition and for compassion and humaneness (*ren*) in most Asian traditions was a strong force for tolerance in accepting differences in orientation and lifestyle. Daoist, Buddhist, and Hinduist models of harmony, compassion, and personal moral challenges do not seem to differ much from the mainstream of monotheism, even though they anchor themselves on different pillars of thought. The various foundations for orientation make it culturally and morally mandatory to serve the poor and sick, to be pious by being compassionate, and to respect the many forms of non-human bios and biotopes. Terrorism and political or economic domination by dictators have always abused religious and philosophical tools and teachings to exploit and destroy the 'stranger,' the 'other,' the 'infidel.' The concepts of humaneness, compassion, and nobility would fail if we even began thinking about applying them only to selected groups such as our own moral communities and inner circle of friends and family. Appealing not only to his Jewish fellow-believers, but to an already religiously pluralistic European cultural scene, enlightened Jewish rabbi and philosopher Moses Mendelsohn put it this way in the 18th century: 'Brethren, if you want true peacefulness in God, let us not lie about consensus when plurality seems to have been the plan and the goal of providence. No one among us reasons and feels precisely the same way the fellow-human does. Why do we hide from each other in masquerades in the most important issues of our lives, as God not without reason has given each of us his/her own image and face.'[12]

Cultural diversity, debate, and competition are signs of a rich life; so is dissent in moral intuitions, values, and visions. Uniformity is boring, non-creative, and uncivilized. Spinoza, a European philosopher of Jewish tradition who was discriminated against by his hometown synagogue, called for religious and cultural diversity and for the promotion of individual culture and morality in the midst of cultural and religious transitions and modifications in Europe at the end of the 17th century. Spinoza believed that the ultimate test of solidarity and

[12] Mendelsohn M 1819 Jerusalem oder über religiöse Macht und Judentum, Ofen: Burian 201.

compassion is the fair and dignified treatment of one's enemy. In his *Tractato Theologico-Politicus* of 1670, he suggested that the fabric of society would not fall apart when individual freedom and liberty were granted; rather peace, respect for persons, and civilized life would fall apart if individuals were not allowed to be prime moral agents. Long before Mendelsohn and Spinoza, Lao Zi expressed it this way: 'the more taboos and inhibitions there are in the world, the poorer the people become' and 'the more articulate the laws and ordinances, the more thieves and robbers arise,'[13] circumventing or exploiting these rules.

2.5. Did Socrates Give the Answer?

What is the role of bioethics within the many religious and philosophical traditions? Is ethics just an application of specific religious or philosophical worldviews or of public law and governmental regulation? How can civil rebellions against existing laws be understood? I suggest a different perspective: worldviews stabilize and support cultural and moral behavior; they do not invent it. In his dialogue with Euthyphron 2,600 years ago, Socrates argued that the Gods favor good deeds not because they are based on divine laws and rules, but because they are good in themselves and are therefore loved by the Gods and by good people.[14] Would Socrates' insight allow us to review the wide cosmos of worldviews from the point of the innate properties of human bios in living and surviving happily and in good health? In following Socrates, we might speak of an *ethos spermatikos* as a human-specific biological property inherited and applied by all of us and documented in human history. This inherent propensity toward ethical behavior has likely been supported by the generative principle of the universe, a *logos spermatikos* of integrated bios, distributed and alive in various quantities and intensities over the centuries and in different individual and collective cultures. Respect for bios and compassionate cultivation may be rooted and well supported in a particular religious revelations, but empirical evidence in cultural and religious history, together with similar teachings in different traditions, suggests a strong biological grounding in being good. Montesquieu discussed moral theology and religion, in the words of Althusser as 'no more than elements internal to given societies which govern their forms and their nature'[15]. Writes theologian and bioethicist Richard McCormick, S.J.: 'One need not to be a Christian to be concerned with the poor, with health, with food problems, with justice and rights. But if one is a Christian and is not so concerned, something is wrong with that Christianity. It has been ceased to be Christian because it has ceased to what his founder was – human.'[16] Can we say

[13] Tao Te Ching 57.

[14] Socrates, Euthyphron 9b.

[15] Althuser L 1972 Politics and History. London: NLB, 23.

[16] McCormick R 1980 Does religious faith add to ethical perception? in: The Distinctiveness of Christian Ethics, Curran CE, McCormick RM eds., New York; Ramsey, 156f.

the same about Buddhists, Muslims, Hindus, Secular Humanists, Animists, Marxists, or Capitalists of today?

In the drama *Nathan the Wise*,[17] German poet Gotthold Ephraim Lessing presents the narrative of a miraculous ring that gave his owner much wealth, friends, success, and happiness. When the owner died, he handed each of his three sons one identical ring and challenged each to prove he had the genuine one. This is precisely the situation of the religious bios and vision within our social and political bodies and our individual faith and commitment: traditional religions and systems of belief together with secular value systems compete to prove that they are productive and supportive for all happy, harmonious societal bodies. A Sikh boy wearing a turban or a Muslim girl wearing a headscarf in an open, pluralistic, harmonious society exercise the same right to self-expression as a girl wearing a trendy miniskirt, a boy the most modern fashion of blue jeans, or people sporting body tattoos: they all exercise their human and civil right of personal identity. Whether belonging to conservative or trendy communities, all of them are in development and are part of an open society.[18] The moral and cultural contribution of either one of these individuals and their communities or groups cannot be judged by their atttire, but by their deeds; '*judge them by their fruits'* (erkenne sie an ihren Fruechten*)* argues a German slogan.

Jesus avoided inflexible, dogmatic rhetoric in saying: 'love God and love your neighbor' (i.e., give respect to the highest integrating bios and help your fellow living being as your next neighbor). Jesus was well versed in Mosaic Law and religion, but he refused to go into the specifics of law and order. He focused rather on respect and recognition of the 'higher order' (the God as understood in Rabbinic tradition), requesting the recognition of all and other forms of bios (i.e., the 'neighbor'). The Vedic slogan *tat tvam asi* and Jesus's *love your neighbor* are just different expressions of Jahr's Bioethics Imperative. They are the results of contemplation and calculation for the purpose of protecting and furthering cultures in teaching competence and competition, communication and cooperation.

For centuries, Christians persecuted, tortured, and killed each other over doctrines such as the essence of the Holy Trinity and the transubstantiation of wine and bread in the Last Supper. Today we recognize dogmatic fights within Islam and from Islam towards 'infidels' in association with geopolitical visions. Injustice in economic distribution and exploitation have been reduced in some countries; however, metabolic disturbances in cultures and infections from the outside can happen any time in contemporary societies, just as they have occurred over the millennia everywhere. Moses Mendelsohn has observed rightly that not only religions, but also secular movements violate human and civil rights: 'the without-God movements (*Ohnegoetterei*) as we unfortunately expe-

[17] Lessing GE 1779 Nathan der Weise.
[18] Hochschild M 2008 Biopiraterie. Ueber die Gesellschaft der Natur. Muenster: Lit, 79.

rience, have their own fanaticism.'[19] Today, Christians rarely fight about dogmatic differences. Would Jesus have fought for a position regarding the dogmatic teachings of the Holy Trinity, the Last Supper, or for details in the Nicaean Creed of 325 A.D., which condemned the teachings of Arianism and other Christian groups and was strongly supported by Emperor Constantine for geopolitical motives? Would Buddha have been interested in the different interpretations of spiritual and bodily reincarnation and transition, or how many unseen worlds, gods, goddesses, and spirits might exist and their character and relevance for us? Would Confucius be concerned if the 'Son of Heaven' might be represented today not by one person, but rather by a central committee, a senate, a corporate body, or a parliament? Could Jesus, Buddha, or Confucius have agreed with Deng Xiao Peng's observation that a good cat catches mice independent of the color of its hair? Can we say the same about religions and worldviews, that good religions, dogmas, and ethics can promote and stabilize good deeds, cultural harmony, and moral cultures, independent of the nuances of their conceptual teachings?

If invited today to an international body such as the United Nations, would Jesus replace the Good Samaritan in his narrative by a Muslim woman, a Buddhist monk, or another fellow human of a different religious or philosophical background? Socrates would definitely have supported Jesus in doing so. The Chinese concept of 'effortless effort' 无为 (wuwei), representing the highest form of human cultivation in following the way of the Dao in spiritual life and in every-day practice, refers to a biocosmological harmony which is symbolized in the harmonious movements of sun, moon and stars. Following are two prayers, one by a Confucian scholar and the other by Jesus, demonstrating the support of moral actions and cultures, each surrounded by cultural and conceptual harmony – 'similar but different' 和而不同, (*he er bu tong*), as Confucius would have said.[20] The 'Our Father' prayer by Jesus provides a wide orientational framework of bios/creation within which the human challenge for doing good is positioned.[21] The classical Confucian biocultural meditation on the Great Harmony of cosmological, individual, and communal bios expresses the same.[22] Do they represent true, healthy religion and moral theology in contrast to false, sick religions and theological teachings? Can we translate both of them

---

[19] Mendelsohn l.c., 199.

[20] Lun Yu 13:23, quoted by Zhai XM 2011 Diversified and in harmony, but not identical, in: Asian Review of Bioethics 3(1)31-35.

[21] Matth 6:9.

[22] Chang Tsai (1020-1077) The Western Inscription, in: A Source in Chinese Philosophy, Chan WT ed., Princeton University Press, p. 497-498, 1972; for the role of ritual in 'recovering' the original property of the 'Great Harmony' of bios in Confucian reasoning cf. Chow KW 1993 Ritual, Cosmology and Ontology, in Philosophy East and West 43(2)201-228.

into our common future of human bios and biotopes in the globalized, high-tech, and Internet-pervaded world of the 21st century and beyond?

'Our Father in Heavens, hallowed be your Name. Your Kingdom come, your Will be done, on Earth as it is in Heavens. Give us today our daily bread. Forgive us our sins, as we forgive those, who sin against us. Lead us not into temptation, but deliver us from the Evil. The Kingdom, the Power and the Glory are yours, now and forever. Amen.' (Jesus)

'Heaven is my father and Earth is my mother, and even such a small creature as I find an intimate place in their midst. Therefore, that which fills the universe I regard as my body and that which directs the universe I consider as my nature. All people are my brothers and sisters, and all things are my companions. The great ruler (the Emperor) is the eldest son of my parents (Heaven and Earth), and the great ministers are his stewards. Respect the aged; this is the way to treat them as elders should be treated. Show deep love toward the orphaned and the weak, this is the way to treat them as the young should be treated. The sage identifies his character with that of Heaven and Earth, and the worthy is the most outstanding man. Even those who are tired, infirm, crippled, or sick, those who have no brothers or children, wives or husbands, are all my brothers who are in distress and have no one to turn to. When the time comes, to keep him from harm, this is the care of a son. To rejoice in Heaven and to have no anxiety, this is filial piety at its purest. He who disobeys [*the rule of bios*] violates virtue. He who destroys humanity is a robber. He who promotes evil lacks (ethical) capacity. But he, who puts his moral nature into practice and brings his physical existence into complete fulfillment, can match (Heaven and Earth). One who knows the rules of transformation will skillfully carry forward the undertakings (of Heaven and Earth), and one who penetrates spirit to the highest degree will skillfully carry out their will. Do nothing shameful in the recesses of your own house and thus bring no dishonor to them. Preserve your mind and nourish your nature and thus (serve them) with untiring effort. Wealth, honor, blessing, and benefits are meant for the enrichment of my life, while poverty, humble station, and sorrow are meant to help me to fulfillment. In life I follow and serve (Heaven and Earth); in death I will be at peace.' (Chang Tsai)

Fritz Jahr gave his 1926 article 'Life Sciences and Teaching of Ethics' the subtitle 'Old Wisdom in New Clothing.' As examples in *translating* old wisdom into modern times[23], I mention three recent statements with Asian and European perspectives on the future of integrated bioethics, presenting different viewpoints but seem akin to the biocosmological and bioethical visions of Jesus and Chang Tsai.

---

[23] Sass HM 2012 Jahr's Translational Ethics. How to translate Traditions into the Present and Future. Muenster: Lit, 365-377

CHENNAI STATEMENT ON BIOETHICS, JANUARY 16–19, 1997[24]

1. Bioethics is an interdisciplinary subject including the study of environmental, ethical, legal and social issues raised by applications of biology, medicine and science. Wide interdisciplinary debate is to be encouraged. 2. We request that funding agencies be more liberal, rational and equitable in the allocation of resources. 3. In all government recognized applied science, technology and humanities departments, ethics committees should be formed which would meet at least twice a year to review all ethical issues. Hospitals should also form ethics committees to foster the process by which ethical issues will be recognized and addressed within the ordinary operation of the hospital and the community it serves. These Ethics Committees will have four functions: (a) to provide education on ethics for the hospital; (b) to facilitate communication between all persons involved in the care and treatment process; (c) to be available for consultation on difficult cases; and (d) to provide policy recommendations to the hospital. 4. An oath should be taken by the Ph.D. research scholars at the entry to, and graduation from, all Ph.D. programs. The Oath could read: "I accept this award of the Degree of Doctor of Philosophy of ... University in recognition of my academic endeavors in the subject of ... proudly conscious that with this I become privileged to enter and join the group of intellectuals around the world having similar distinction. I am fully conscious and aware of, and take a solemn oath in the presence of my alma mater, peers and colleagues to discharge in every way the responsibility for exemplary moral standards, ethical conduct and unimpeachable integrity, which I shall always uphold and exhibit for scrutiny and emulation by all in society to be worthy of the honor bestowed on me by this degree and of the responsibility which comes from the possession of expert knowledge. Sd/In the presence of [place, date etc. can be filled up as desired]. 5. Bioethics should be taught at all educational institutions starting from primary level. 6. An Indian Society of Bioethics is to be formed with an executive committee consisting of a Chair and nine members elected by the membership. The executive committee should include members from diverse specialties and departments. 7. This Society will publish a journal in bioethics. 8. The participants resolved to seek government support and publicity for an annual "Ethics Awareness Day". The date and month to be decided by the committee for the Bioethics Society. 9. The Medical Council of India may be approached for the evaluation of Health Care Ethics and teaching of Ethics in Medical Schools. 10. The Hippocratic Oath or a similar Oath is to be administered to students at the time of joining and passing out (graduation) a Medical School Institution so that the real spirit of the oath can be understood and observed by medical students and staff. 11. Nursing should be recognized as a profession. Nursing Council of India to be approached for evaluation of teaching and practice of patient care ethics in Nursing Profession. 12. In animal experimentation the judicious mini-

[24] Eubios Journal of Asian and International Bioethics 7 (1997), 34.

mum and humane use of animals is to be practiced. Formulation of guidelines for schools and college teachers is to be undertaken. 13. The rights of indigenous people, the ecology of rural areas, bioethical management of the coastal zones, and knowledge of indigenous fisherpeople and farmers of their ecosystems must be respected, protected and documented. 14. A comparative study of religions with special reference to values is basic to developing ethics at the grass root level and when this can grow steadily, shall help in eliminating unethical acts by human beings. 15. Annual seminars with wide national publicity and rigorous selection of papers will be conducted. In January 1998 these are planned at Salem, Mangalore, Ahmednager and New Delhi. 16. It was resolved to hold the next International Conference on Bioethics during early 1999 at the University of Madras, Chennai.

EUBIOS DECLARATION FOR INTERNATIONAL BIOETHICS 2002 [25]

1. Bioethics is an interdisciplinary field that needs to be nourished by debate among all disciplines and people, not limited an academic specialty or professionals.

2. There is a variety of definitions of bioethics, and this variety is part of the intrinsic value of the field of bioethics. We consider bioethics to be the process of reflection over ethical issues raised in our relationships with other living organisms; the consideration of the ethical issues in spheres including environmental ethics, health care ethics, social ethics, and the use of technologies that effect life; and the love of life.

7. Every person has a lifelong responsibility to develop his or her bioethical maturity and values. We could define bioethical maturity as the ability to balance the benefits and risks of ethical choices, considering the parties involved and the consequences. At the social level, public policy and laws need to be developed, which requires a social mechanism for balancing conflicting ethical principles.

8. International cross-cultural bioethics should be developed, including studies and discussions, which respect individual cultures as long as they do not conflict with fundamental human rights... Honest reflection on the bioethical lessons of the past should be encouraged together with efforts to promote reconciliation on all levels.

9. Research and thinking and reasoning of all people should be more emphasized in order to understand the diversity of people's thinking. This is necessary for determining the degree of universality that is possible, and should be used to complement other research approaches in bioethics. There is no inherent reason to belief a priori that the views of one person is intrinsically more valuable than another, based on gender, age, educational background, physical, mental, or psychological condition or life experience.

---

[25] www.eubios.info/eeidec.htm

RIJEKA DECLARATION ON THE FUTURE OF BIOETHICS, MARCH 12, 2011[26]

Fritz Jahr used the term "bioethics" ("Bio-Ethik") as early as 1927. His "bioethical imperative" (Respect every living being as an end in itself, and treat it, if possible, as such!) should guide personal, professional, cultural, social, and political life, as well as the development and application of science and technology. In order to promote the Bioethical Imperative and the future of integrative bioethics, the participants of the Rijeka symposium "Fritz Jahr and European roots of bioethics: Establishing an international scholars' network (EuroBioNethics)", wish to highlight the following: 1. Contemporary bioethics quite often has been narrowed down to issues of informed consent and liability in medical ethics, whereas the practical impact of general ethical principles has been minimal. 2. It is necessary that bioethics be substantially broadened and conceptually and methodologically transformed so that it may consider different cultural, scientific, philosophical, and ethical perspectives (pluriperspective approach), integrating those perspectives into orientational knowledge and practical action (integrative approach). 3. Such Integrative Bioethics will have to harmonize, respect, and learn from the rich plurality of individual and communal perspectives and cultures of the global community. 4. Recognizing the inexhaustible source of relevant perspectives for Integrative Bioethics in the works of authors and teachings using the term and the concept of bioethics, but also of the other "precursors" of integrative bioethical and deontological ideas since antiquity, we strongly call upon the study of classical works and teachings. 5. Respect for life, the considerate treatment of all life forms, need to be supported by all citizens, public discourse and the media, and by educational programs at all levels. 6. If these ideas are successful, bioethics will become a truly open field of meeting and dialogue of various sciences and professions, visions and worldviews, that have been gathered to articulate, to discuss, and to solve ethical issues related to life as a whole and each of its parts, life in all its forms, shapes, stages, and manifestations, as well as to life conditions in general. 7. If these ideas are successful, bioethics will become the basis for the development and implementation of law, nationally and internationally. 8. If these ideas are successful, the recognition and implementation of bioethics will become the "bridge to the future", a "science of survival", and wisdom as "knowledge of how to use knowledge" (as Van Rensselaer Potter defined it in the 1970s) of modern medicine and technology.

The EuroBioNethics International Scholars' Network, promoting the above ideas, will organise further conferences and establish a website to improve global intercultural communication and cooperation. A Fritz-Jahr Award for the Research and Promotion of European Roots of Bioethics will soon be

[26] Fritz Jahr and the Foundations of Global Bioethics, Muzur A, Sass HM eds. Berlin: Lit 2012, 379-381.

announced. The Network invites scientists and ethicists for communication and cooperation in implementing these ideas of the Rijeka Declaration. Signed in Rijeka/Opatija (Croatia), on March 12, 2011, by Christian Byk, Ante Covic, Eva-Marie Engels, Igor Eterovic, Marcia Sanatana Fernandes, Jose Roberto Goldim, Nada Gosic, Hrvoje Juric, Dleni Kalokairinou, Tomaislav Krznar, Natache Salome Lima, Mair Mujzur, Iva Rincic, Ricardo Adres Roa-Castellanos, Hans-Martin Sass, Marija Selak, Ivana Zagorac.

3. THE PROPERTIES OF BIOS IN HUMAN SPECIFICATION

THE SPECIAL HUMAN HERITAGE

With the animal and plant, Nature did not only specify their disposition but she also carried these out herself. With man, however, she merely provided the disposition and left its execution up to him.... Among all beings known, man alone as a person has the privilege of breaking the bonds of necessity, to which all creatures of nature are subject, with his Will and can begin in himself a completely new series of phenomena. The act, through which he accomplishes this, preferentially is called action (Handlung), *the executions deriving from it are exclusively his own doings* (Taten). *He thus can prove that he is a Person already by his doings.... Because nature gives man his destination, but leaves the fulfillment of it to his Will, the actual situation of his being and its destination cannot be a work of nature but must be of His own.*

Friedrich Schiller, 1793[1]

3.1. Is our Human Bios Deficient or Incomplete?

Different species have different species-specific properties that allow them to survive in their respective environments within their specific sym-biosis with other forms of life. Dogs have highly developed olfactory senses; they can smell where I went yesterday or a few days before, even when I have already forgotten. After I educate their noses with the smell of a personal item, they can even locate strangers or drugs. I cannot compete with dogs or with bats, who use their acoustic senses to orient themselves in the dark of night. Eagles and other predatory birds use their eyesight to recognize prey far away, and birds migrating in summer and winter use other special senses and the magnetic field as their own global positioning system. These activities are also far beyond my genetic makeup or capacity to learn. Elephants and tigers have much more powerful bodies than I, while camels can travel without water for over a week. Warm-blooded animals can lower their blood temperature and metabolism to hibernate for months in cold, adverse climates, yet I cannot.

We human beings are not biologically 'finished.' We are incomplete, or as Arnold Gehlen defined us, deficient beings (*Maengelwesen*): 'Let us consider this strange and incomparable being who lacks the conditioning for survival which animals possess ... What clearly is at stake here is nothing less than the whole spectrum of man's inner life – his thought and language, imagination, unique structure of drives, unique motor skills, and mobility ... A higher complex, marvelous array of skills is necessary for a being with this particular physical constitution to survive until tomorrow, next week, next year ... Man is

---

[1] Schiller F 1783 Über Anmut und Würde, in: Neue Thalia, Schiller F ed., Vol. 3, Leipzig, 157f.

the not yet determined animal; he is somehow not *firmly established* ... He finds his existence a challenge and therefore needs to develop an interpretation of himself – a matter that has always been of crucial importance.' The answer we humans have found to compensate for deficiencies in our raw and unfinished nature was culture: 'The human being is incapable of surviving in truly natural and primitive conditions because of his organic primitiveness and lack of mental means. He must make up for this loss of means on his own by actively transforming the world to suit his own ends ... He acts because he is unspecialized and deprived of a natural environment to which he is adopted. The epitome of nature restructured to serve his needs is *culture* and the culture world is his world ... There is no human society without weapons, without fire, without prepared artificial food, without shelter, and without systems of cooperation. Culture therefore is the "second nature" in man's restructured nature within which he can survive.'[2] As Friedrich Schiller discussed with verve, vigor, and appreciation, the 'deficient' nature of humans is a benefit and a blessing. It is also a challenge for us to grow even stronger by cultivating our natural abilities into new and broader cultural properties, assets, and treasures.

A few hundred thousand years ago, our biological ancestors left their life in the trees for the savannahs, fields, rivers, and oceans of other continents, using their feet and legs for walking, running, and migrating. They used their hands and fingers for making tools, shelters, clothing, arts, and writing, and they used their brains for calculating, devising, envisioning, and dreaming. Since then, our dormant and non-dormant DNA has modified as well, and now it supports our human cultures and cultivated biotopes better than before. But we, as all other forms of bios, are still an integrated co-bios as a part of our universe and globe, with their seasons and cycles that change both predictably and unpredictably. We cannot change the universe or multiverse, but we use mathematics to envision and describe interacting or parallel multiverses that range from extremely minute to extremely vast.[3] We have also built our own universes of religious transcendence and of mythical and spiritual contemplation and teaching. We have also created applications ('apps') and networks for social interaction, friendship, commerce, competition, production, and trade by globally integrated muscles of online bios such as Facebook, Google, Amazon, Alibaba, and others.

Most recently we have broadened our personal social networks and capabilities with new wearables that monitor our bodily health, communicate with digital health care networks, compete and cooperate in work and business, access information from digital archives, and make our own skills available in these integrated digital multiverses. Multiple implantable devices extend our bi-

---

[2] Gehlen A 1940 Der Mensch. Seine Natur und Stellung in der Welt; transl by C Mcmillan, K Pillmer 1988 Man, His Nature and Place in the World,10; 29.

[3] Tegmark M 2003 in: Scientific American 288(5)40-51; Randell L 2005 Warped Passages. Unraveling the Mysteries of the Universe's Hidden Dimensions, NY: Harper Collins.

ological properties, from artificial hips, joints, limbs, heart valves, and pacemakers to hearing aids, eyeglasses, and neuro-stimulators. We have built transgenic, 'sentient' animals for research on human diseases and have, on the other hand, developed in-vitro flesh or 'cultured meat' for hamburgers and other food products. In neuroscience and digital software research, we discuss redefining the terms *sentient* and *free will* in regard to robots, computers, and human–machine hybrids.[4] This array of inventions shows that humans are not a 'deficient' form of bios at all; rather, we survive most successfully by manipulating bios and biotopes and by cultivating a natural world that had been both raw and cruel.

These new human-made biotopes are as fragile as the traditional, natural ones. Newly created biotopes resulting from human cultivation are threatened by war, exploitation, distortion, and willful or accidental manipulation (or simply by the failure of hardware or software). We will discuss the parameters of these catastrophic risks to our contemporary cultivated biotopes in more detail later. Traditionally, stabilizing features such as clans, states, systems of law, cultural traditions, and religious orientation are challenged by the emancipation of the individual 'person' as described by Schiller. The individual is newly empowered with immense control over digital and other high-tech biotopes – including evildoers, people with crazy, sick hallucinations, and fellow humans living primarily in cyberworlds and virtual realities. Where are we going from here? An old Chinese saying holds that 'Heaven and Man are an integral One. As a result, they are in constant pursuit of harmony between humanity and nature.'[5] We can read this slogan as a challenge to the 'will to action' described by Schiller. Similar models of harmonized spirit and matter, imagination and nature, bios and bioethics do exist, as the Confucian meditation and Jesus' prayer quoted at the end of the previous chapter demonstrate. In Mediterranean and Western traditions, Jesus, probably one of the first bioculturelogists, explained failures and success in bios and culture in the parable of a farmer who sowed seed onto the land. Some fell on the road and was eaten by birds; some fell on dry, stony land and grew initially but died from a lack of water and soil; and some fell under the bushes and failed to develop. Some seed fell on good land, however, leading to multiple harvests. When his disciples asked him why he did not speak directly to the people about the interaction between heaven and humans, about

---

[4] Fits N, Howlader D, Giordano J 2012 The Self and Personhood. Neuroethical Implications of a Shifting Paradigm, in: AJOB Neuroscience 3(3)37f. A conference on the ethics of in-vitro-flesh was held on September 2014; see a preliminary report www.new-harvest.org/.../conference-report-ethics-vitro-flesh-enhanced-animals. As to transgenic animals in research see chapters 4 and 5 below; also Sass HM 1996 Verantwortung und ethische Herausforderung. Transgene Tiere, in: genethik, Basel:Ciba.

[5] Quoted by Pan Yue, Chinese Vice-Minister of State Environmental Protection in: China Daily, July 27, 2006.

futile and successful 'action,' Jesus answered that the people would not understand those kinds of abstract sermons.[6]

Not since the French Revolution unlocked the conceptual powers of centuries of European enlightenment had the world experienced something like the unleashing of greater personal powers through new hardware and software. What became enabled were totally new, extremely high levels of communication and cooperation, competition and competence, and calculating and contemplating in nearly unlimited areas of politics, society, religion, and networking. Within traditional states, religions, and social classes, as well as among persons traditionally bound by clan, cultural, or blood loyalties, we see new forms of engagement and disengagement; upheaval and commitment; destruction and rebuilding; and reformation, restoration, and creation. Political, corporate, and social life will not be what it was for thousands of years, nor even what it was for the last generation. Here is where we face the new challenges, risks, and rewards regarding the cultivation of our mutual, integrated human bios. These involve both a new and expanded challenge to the ethics of bios in the new millennium and a quest and a call for the cultivation of the human bios in all of the fields of bioethics.[7]

Humans cannot live under water, but we have built submarines to cross underneath the oceans. We cannot fly, but we have airplanes to soar around the globe and rockets to take us to the moon. We cannot see as well as other species, but we offset our limitations with eyeglasses, microscopes, telescopes, x-ray machines, and tomography. We cannot smell as well as other species, but we have built machines to compensate for this and our other 'deficiencies.' Rather than being deficient, we humans are highly gifted! Yet these precious gifts come with special responsibilities to avoid using them for terror, exploitation, war, and destruction. We must protect our human bios and the integrated bios of our natural and cultivated biotopes. In broadening Fritz Jahr's 'Bioethical Imperative' and following Van Rensselaer Potter into a more comprehensive 'Call for Action,' we can say: This earth and the multitudes of integrated and interacting bios are the only ones we have. We must respect them for what they are, our houses and homes, and protect and cultivate old and new forms of natural and cultivated bios and biotopes for our own sake and for the well-being of the many other integrated and integrating forms of bios and biotopes.

---

[6] Matth. 13:1-13; Jesus' biocultural view fits well to the Daoist insight 'there is a time for being ahead, there is a time for being behind, there is a time for being in motion, there is a time for being calm, there is a time for being vigorous, there is a time for being exhausted, there is a time for being safe, there is a time for being in danger.' Dao Te Ching 29.

[7] See Sass HM 2012 The Earth and the Multiverse Are Living Beings. Let's Treat Them as Such! in: Fritz Jahr and the Foundations of Global Bioethics, ed. A Muzur, HM Sass, Muenster: Lit, 345-357; also Sass HM, Jahr's Translational Ethics: How to Translate Traditions into the Presence and Future, ibid, 367-377.

3.2. Human Properties in Successful Cultivation Practice

In Schiller's Kantian understanding of free will, the 'deficiency' of humans is viewed as a special, precious, gift and property. We are not bound by instinctive behavior. We lack many natural properties that make other forms of bios successful in interacting and integrating with their natural habitats. We humans have superior biological properties that allow us not only to survive in many different biotopes but to manipulate them into the cultivated human biotopes and habitats we call culture. As already mentioned, we can identify, eight human species–specific biological endowments that make us unique in what we can build or destroy. We are unique in our capacity to survive and to live good, healthy lives as individuals and as communities. I call these eight biological gifts or properties *'the eight Cs': communication, cooperation, competence, competition, contemplation, calculation, compassion, and cultivation.* Although we find them in all forms of bios, from quantum physics to algae, microbes, plants, animals, and human cultures, we will concentrate here on the specific human talents of distributing and interconnecting these eight Cs as highly complex, adaptable properties.[8]

These properties have been documented in cultural, social, and political contexts throughout our political and cultural history. They are value neutral and have been used in exploitation, corruption, and war for the short-term benefit of individuals and groups. They can be implemented with much better long-term benefits, however, by cultivating healthy and harmonious communities and biotopes. Detailed studies in cultural anthropology and history provide ample additional material to support the essential role of these eight Cs for doing good or bad, for building or for harming the individual bios and the integrated bios of biotopes. It is this '*openness*' to the world and this '*building of our own worlds'* (Schiller) that makes humans not only different from other species but also highly adaptable: sprawling, living well, and enduring in many forms of biotopes,

[8] The Chinese 'I Ching' (Book of Changes), known for over 3,000 years and ascribed to Fu Xi (the mythological dragon and ruler with a human face), offered eight times eight hexagrams based on the eight simple trigrams of 'earth, mountain, water, wind, thunder, fire, lake, heaven.' For thousands of years it has been interpreted and consulted in Asia and beyond by emperors and mandarins as well as providing oracles for everyone. It was most prominent and successful in explaining the essential taxonomy of the bios; G.F. Leibniz was informed by missionary Joachim Bouvet about the 64 hexagrams and the similarity to Leibniz's binary mathematical system. Bouvet described the I Ching as a 'métaphysique numeraire' and a 'methode générale de Sciences: 'ce system de Fo-hii, et le ancienne Philosophie de la Chine, prise selon les principles légitimes et solides, étant si conforme à la Philosophie du divin Plato, et a celles ex anciens Hebreux, c'est-à-dire de Moise et des anciens Patriarchs' (G.F. Leibniz 2006 Gesammelte Schriften und Briefe. Berlin: Akademie Verlag, Reihe 1, Bd 20, p. 574, in: Le Gobain letter to Leibniz, November 10, 1701, l.c 569ff. Cf. I Ching (Yijing) The Book of Change 2016 Minford J transl. Viking Press; I Ching. The book of Change 2016 Hinton D transl. Farrar, Strauss, Giroux Publ.

both natural and cultural. Although expressed differently, human bios shares the same properties as all bios; hence we need education and ethics to inform and form us as we attempt to use these properties in a productive, happy, and healthy way. Secular humanists and religious believers will understand the bioethical challenge in the bio-cosmological framework of creation presented by Iranian poet and Sufi mystic Rumi: 'Allah the Most High created the angels and placed within them intellect. He created the beasts and placed within them sensuality. And He created the children of Adam and placed within them both intellect and sensuality. So, he whose intellect dominates sensuality is higher than the angels, and he whose sensuality dominates his intellect, is lower than the beasts.'[9] Microbes, mice, flowers, and fungi need not make those ethical decisions regarding doing good or evil; they are hard-wired for survival and have limited flexibility in adapting or in making mistakes.

In 1781, Immanuel Kant described the operating systems for human reasoning and for recognizing the natural world. He claimed that time and space, together with other intuited concepts such as causality, precede all experience. In his view, they are specific properties that humans and other forms of life use to orient themselves. Kant's transcendental argument seems to find support in anthropology and comparative biology. He presents 'God, Free Will, and Immortality' as '*regulative ideas*,' and because he could neither prove nor disapprove their existence, he simply calls them 'regulative.' All three concepts are evident in cultural history as well, serving for millennia as guiding visions and commandments for doing good and building human cultures. Kant based his moral philosophy on a view of the Categorical Imperative as an obligation independent from will, preference, or nature as moral law: 'Act as if your maxims should serve at the same time as the universal law (of all rational beings).'[10] Voltaire cynically remarked that these and other regulative ideas were invented to encourage civilized and cultivated behavior.[11] Rudolf Otto described an apprehension of the 'holy' as an innate biological human property, not just an idea for regulating and guiding human behavior.[12] For our purposes in describing the

[9] Rumi (1207-1273) also was called *Mawlana*, the Master; see: Chittick W 1983 The Sufi Path of Love, The Spiritual Teachings of Rumi. Albany: SUNY.

[10] Kant I, Foundations of the Metaphysics of Morals, transl Beck WL, Indianapolis: Bobbs-Merrill 1959, 436-439, pagination following Kant Akademie Edition, vol 28. Berlin 1902.

[11] Voltaire 1764 Dictionaire philosophique; Schopenhauer, influenced by Hindu and Buddhist philosophy, in criticizing Kant, made 'compassion' the essential moral intuition; Schiller once complained that in serving his friend, he unfortunately did it out of friendship and not because the Kantian 'moral law' had called for it. Schiller F (1909) Philosophische Schriften und Gedichte, Kuehnemann E ed.; Jahr recognizes 'compassion' as an essential property in ethics, but did not use the term in the 'Bioethical Imperative,' calling in a more general fashion for 'respect.'

[12] Otto R 1917 Das Heilige (Engl. Edition 1923 The Idea of the Holy), recalls Origines 'the human soul originally is religious' (*anima humana originaliter religiosa*), as 'naturally' being bound back to something more superior, powerful, demanding, almighty and merci-

various challenges of cultures in bioethics, we can replace the Kantian, duty-based Moral Law with the following 'Reasonable Practice Imperative': Act based on your natural capacities for communication and cooperation, competence and competition, contemplation and calculation, compassion and cultivation, which in their integrated forms will serve as a universal challenge for all human beings.

Cultivating raw nature will change the object and the subject, the human person and the biotope. Confucian tradition compares people to pearls: both are naturally precious, but need polishing to shine and become most valuable.[13] Hebrew king David used a comparable narrative: 'Iron sharpens iron and one man sharpens another; he who tends a fig tree will eat fruit; and he who guards his master will be honored.' [14] The Latin term *cultivare* originally meant working untilled ground by seeding, weeding, fertilizing, watering, and protecting crops, bushes, and trees. We thus can view cultivation as a means of working the fertile soil of natural human capability: guiding towards flourishing in ways that eradicate the overgrowth of our more deleterious features.

Communication is essential for all life–life interaction and integration, and it is done in multifold ways by all species. We humans interact in many different ways with the microbes in our intestines, with the seasons of the year, with plants and animals, with fellow humans, and with corporate persons. Our communication includes facial expressions and body language, as well as spoken and written language. The vocabularies of general and expert languages and those shared by families, clans, and other communities display the richness, goals, and purposes of these different languages. When situations become complex, terminology becomes more detailed and accurate. In addition, social harmony and cultural interactions are often violated by exploitative, misleading rhetoric used to attract or tempt people. We also communicate with ourselves in contemplation and calculation and in reviewing our actions and those of others.

Opening the dimensions of communication far beyond our own direct experience are books, letters, and digital media; various fields of occupational and general education; and art, music, and theatre. These all allow for human understanding, weighing, pondering, and calculating in drawing on the experiences and mistakes of multitudes of generations and cultures. Communications in military, business, politics, production, trade, and research have their own terminologies, including specific modes in which information is shared or pro-

---

ful, both terrifying (*tremendum*) and fascinating (*fascinans*), an original numinous (*numinosum*) human understanding of a bios reality beyond rational and sensory experience. He gives plenty of evidence that these powers are found in monotheistic and polytheistic systems, in animism, in the withdrawal from earthly practice into meditation, and in cultural visions of final liberation from the wheels of karma and life.

[13] Legge J ed. 1963 Confucian Analects, the Great Learning and the Doctrine of the Mean, Oxford.

[14] Proverbs 27:17f.

tected. Rarely an end in itself, communication serves various individual, collective, and interactive goals and is part of nearly all human practices. Teams, joint production, mutual aid, and military or medical services are impossible without specific means and ends in communication. Just as all human capacities have limits, however, communication can be limited or unsuccessful, counterproductive or destructive. Heidegger called language 'the house of Being,' indicating that various languages, terminologies, and traditions express similar but differently expressed worldviews about our own bios and the integrated cosmic bios.[15] Persian philosopher Mulla Sadra argued that 'communicating is creating' because some concepts go beyond the words available to express them. This insight is shared by Taoist wisdom, which posits that 'the Tao is only a term.'[16] In addition to languages, books, music, and art, social and digital networks, hugging and smiling, and shouting and crying are among the different forms of communication in cultures of human bios.

Cooperation, just like communication, is a two-way street between individuals and within biotopes. For example, we are rarely aware of the many ongoing levels of cooperation and interaction within our microbiome, in our responses to the seasons, or within our neighborhoods. Cooperation in sharing information, services, and products is the goal of most forms of communication. Cooperation cannot work without competence and skills. To meet practical expectations and situational challenges, stakeholders contribute specific skills in competence, communication, or compassion. Cooperation must be trust-based, even in the most technical activities. In many settings, it is guided by training, quality norms, and/or contracts that spell out mutual responsibilities and rights. Evildoers, torturers, or robbers also cooperate, but such cooperation does not lead to harmony, health, and happiness.

Competence makes communication and cooperation successful. There are two sides of competence, technical and ethical. A dull knife will not cut, but a sharp one will; when not competently and compassionately handled, a sharp knife can also harm. Action requires expertise and training in cooperation and in improving, protecting, and cultivating the personal and professional competence of individual and corporate persons. Incompetent actions are dangerous in science, technology, medicine, and politics, as well as in personal and social matters.[17] The best intentions are fruitless if their application and realization are not executed competently. Leadership and teamwork competence integrate not only technical skills but social, interpersonal, and moral ones. Unfortunately, some fellow humans and groups have developed expertise in deception, robbery, and harming others.

---

[15] Heidegger M (1978) Letter on Humanism, Krell DF ed., Basic Writing, London: Routledge.

[16] Lao Zi (2008) Die Bambustäfelchen Lao Zi, Hou Cai ed., Münster: Lit, 123.

[17] Sass HM 1997 Moral Aspects of Risk and Innovation, in: Artificial Organs 21(11)1217-1221.

Competition between individuals and groups seems to have been a driving motor for millennia for fostering and improving levels of expertise, products, services, and commerce, as well as living conditions and social biotopes. The variety of baking products is a result of bakers' competing in a food market driven by the need to eat, by taste, and by social expectations. Patent laws protect both the inventor and the public; certain patents come with an obligation to monitor risk and to provide for compensation if necessary. When conditions in certain cultures and states become unlivable, people may leave their homes and migrate to other societies. When working conditions and pay are more attractive in other corporations, people will move and accept new challenges.

Contemplation is a human talent for withdrawing occasionally to reflect on our position within the larger cosmos of bios and within our own biotopes. We withdraw from the routines of interactions, but pondering both them and our relationship with higher or larger orders of bios plays an essential role in our understanding of ourselves and in preparing potential changes in our involvements. It is in contemplation that worldviews, concepts of myself and of 'the other,' perspectives on fellow humans, and attitudes toward other forms of bios and biotopes evolve. Most cultures have developed different styles of meditating. Some orient themselves in a large, harmonious, integrating bios, whereas others see combatting forces such as the Sons and Daughters of Light versus the Sons and Daughters of Darkness. Contemplation is not separate from other human activities. It is a special form of communication with oneself and the world that reviews and refines the goals and forms of our compassionate and other activities, while preparing our calculations and involvements in protecting, broadening, and cultivating our individual bios and our biotopes.

Calculation is action oriented in that it protects and promotes existing levels of personal, communal, and corporate life. Individuals, corporations, and groups all develop and implement strategies for survival and for a healthier, more successful life. Success is measured by different criteria, from simple survival to social recognition and fame. Other aspects might include making money, being healthy, enjoying pleasures such as music, sex, and fine arts, inventing machines, creating good hardware and software, building large, potent companies, forming powerful political parties or pressure groups, or helping the weak and needy.[18]

Compassion, as mentioned, is a central capacity for morally successful actions. Some goals cannot be achieved without it, such as caring for the elderly, frail, and weak. All cultural and moral goals need refined forms of situational compassion. Practice without compassion is blind and morally ineffective, and compassion without competence and cooperation is blunt and useless. Some

[18] Gross National Product, GNP, measures just some economic figures of a nation, while Gross Happiness Product, GHP, measures the overall health, strength, and happiness of a society; see the Internet for both terms.

technical activities may use other qualities as their prime point of orientation, but even constructing kitchen machines mandates a compassionate consideration of operational risk regarding the shortcomings of machines and humans. Compassion with the non-human environment is not just useful for future human cultures: it surpasses and refines the simple anthropocentric interest in the protection and cultivation of nature. Jahr, the 'father of bioethics,' called fashionable flower luxury 'murder' and quoted Eduard von Hartmann: 'Whenever I see a rose in a glass of water tied into a bouquet, I cannot fight the unpleasant thought that a human being has murdered a flower life for the sole purpose to enjoy his/her eyes, heartless enough to not sense the unnatural death under the appearance of life.'[19] Corporate persons use compassionate language and deeds to integrate themselves into their specific corporate biotopes.

Cultivation has been a landmark and a goal throughout human cultural history. Improving the status quo and not slipping back into less safe, less enjoyable, or less harmonious social and cultivated natural environments has always been a goal of making good things, attitudes, and morals more permanent. We can regard in the same way the cultivating effect of educating young people to avoid the mistakes of past generations and to improve on what their elders achieved. The road of morality and culture is not a one-way street. As did our forefathers and other cultures, we must acknowledge those heading in opposite directions, develop 'rules of the road,' and take detours. To proceed more comfortably, individuals, operational teams, and cultures in development should refine their practices and enhance cooperation by trial-and-error learning and by setting step-by-step rules. Cultivation is a process, not a fixed state; so is what we call culture. As Jacob Burckhardt[20] pointed out, the cultivation and progress of humankind had to be defended against the fashions and fads of history more often than not.

Cultivation also includes acknowledging limits to manipulation and cultivation but recognizing that such limits vary over time and cultures. Roman philosopher Epictetus defined a cultivated person 'not by the full possession of the things which are desired, but by removing the desire.' Such a person 'does not require a fig in the winter.'[21] Famous Native American Chief Seattle argued against selling and buying land for agriculture because it would ruin the harmony as given by the Great Manitou, for no one of sober mind would forbid others to enjoy the light of the sun or the moon. Similar to the settlers in Seattle's lands, cultivated and fair property laws have a different view at selling land and taking responsibility for its cultivation. We see limits to the 'cultivation' of nonhuman

[19] Jahr F, l.c. (1926), 19; cf. Hartmann E v 1885 Der Blumenluxus; Schnehen W v 1908 Eduard von Hartman und die Pflanzenphysiologie, Stuttgart.

[20] Burckhardt J 1905 World-Historical Reflections (Welthistorische Betrahtungen), Introduction.

[21] Cf. Epiktet, Handbuechlein der Moral; Capelle W ed. Jena: Reclam 1906; similar Tao Te Ching 29.

bios, however, when those 'products' have a miserable life – such as highly nervous and anxious pigs bred for human consumption or dachshunds suffering spinal cord pain from staircase use in private homes. As to 'cultivating' other humans, most cultures have supported using medical and other procedures to reduce pain and suffering and to train and educate. We are highly suspicious, however, in regard to 'enhancing' human bios by pharmacological or other interventions. We are particularly wary of potential extremes such as robots or software being empowered with 'free will' or fellow humans being manipulated by neuronal implantation into being obedient slaves or soldiers.[22]

Cultivation is a process; when culture becomes static, we call it 'etiquette' or 'protocol.' Etiquette expresses accepted virtues and values, but it can become so sterile and resistant to change that it loses its capacity to model the good life and to promote successful survival. The hairstyles of former days and antiquated garments need to make room for new lives, fashions, and cultures. Cultivation is a means and end in the self-development and autonomy of the individual, but it is also important thereafter for building communities of culture, compassion, and competence in matters of life and health. The Indian term *dharma*, 'living right,' describes a never-ending process of cultivation. Although cultivation involves the self (using a prudent personal mix of the eight Cs), it influences the cultivation of teams, workplaces, service centers, and neighbors. While presenting a role model and encouraging reciprocal behavior, cultivation thus creates harmonious, cultivated societies. Therefore, we may speak of the cultivation of persons, communities, corporations, lands, and biotopes.

3.3. Integrating and Cultivating the Eight C Properties and Virtues

Contemporary Confucian scholars have described a natural human propensity for *interactive dynamics*.[23] This heritage is not engendered by religions or philosophical teachings; rather, successful religions and philosophies have always built on it: 'What distinguishes human nature from animal nature is that human beings are disposed to enchant the ordinary, turning eating into cuisine; transforming warning cries and howls of pain into poetry and song; deepening and expanding uterine groupings into the growing of families, communities and nations; and transmuting procreative sex into romantic love and spiritual merger. Humans differ distinctively from other animals in respect of their capacities-for and apparent commitment-to qualitatively transforming every day. From a Confucian perspective, our distinctively human nature is to express remarkably

---

[22] Cf. Wilson D 2013 Amped. NY: *Vintage* is a science fiction novel describing the use of neural implants, originally developed to treat brain dysfunctions, for creating 'amplified' humans in military service, who then break free and cause severe social and political upheaval and social distress in the U.S.

[23] Hershock PD 2012 Valuing Diversity. Buddhist Reflection on Realizing a More Equitable Global Future. SUNY Press.

strong propensities for appreciating – that is, progressively enriching and being enriched – our constitutive relational dynamics.'[24] The eight-C model details some of the 'constitutional relational dynamics' described by Hershock and can serve as a tool for further biological, neuronal, anthropological, theological, and cultural research into a methodological and conceptual grounding of successful, harmonious attitudes and ethics regarding the worlds of bios.

Jahr predicted that moral principles such as egoism and altruism would not be successful or healthy when applied in their extremes.[24] Philosopher and bioethicist Tom L. Beauchamp asked whether ethical theory is actually 'foundational to the field and determinative in practice,' arguing that quite often moral practice is disconnected to 'the stumbling and confusing manner in which philosophers have attempted to link theory to practice.' Looking into the variety of theories and practices in cultural history, it seems that *social connectedness* rather than *theoretical correctness* has been more successful in building and preserving happy and healthy communities[25]. In sectarian traditions of many cultures, ontological and other types of arguments in encyclicals, metaphysical and theological theories, and philosophical or pseudo-scientific statements justify slavery, torture, and human rights violations on the basis of 'Divine Law,' nature, or science. Giordano calls for a closer interaction between the sciences of neurology, psychology, politics, and sociology.[26] Gabriel Marcel defined humans as *homines viatores*, 'itinerate people on the walk.'[27] The Chinese term *Dao* is most often translated as *the way*. Indeed, cultivation is a process of moving ahead by developing ourselves in tandem with our social and biological environments and it sometimes involves moving back or getting lost. As already mentioned, Socrates suggested that although doing good and living harmoniously might not be based on Divine commandments, the Gods will approve simply because these things are intrinsically beneficial. In the marketplace of Athens, where Socrates once taught, the apostle Paul later stressed that the Creator fashioned 'out of one blood all nations' and that He should be worshipped accordingly.[28]

---

[24] Beauchamp TL 2004 Does Ethical Theory have a Future in Bioethics, in: Law Medicine Ethics 32: 209-217.

[25] Lewis E, Cantor N eds. 2016 Our Compelling Interests: The Value of Diversity for Democracy and a Prosperous Society. Princeton U Press.

[26] Giordano J 2010 The mechanistic paradox: on the need for reciprocity of science, technology, ethics and policy. Synesis 1:1-3; Giordano J, Benedikter R 2012 An early – and necessary – flight of the Owl of Minerva: neuroscience, neurotechnology, human sociocultural boundaries, and the importance of neuroethics. J. Evolution and Technology 22(1):14-25; cf. Cacioppo J 2008 Loneliness: Human Nature and the Need for Social Connection. W.W. Norton & Co.

[27] Marcel G 1945 Homo Viator, Paris.

[28] Acts of the Apostles 17:26. It was Emperor Constantine, who 250 years later supported the preaching of a 'one for all' Christian dogmatism in the Nicaean Creed (e.g., in regard to the Holy Trinity and Holy Supper), hoping to build and to rule an empire of peace and

Close to the Jewish philosopher Mendelsohn, who praised the diversity among people and cultures as God's original plan of creation, is the Muslim lawyer and scholar Abu Hanifa, founder of the influential Muslim Hanafi Law School. Hanifa quotes a *hadith* by Mohamed recommending that communication and dialogue be used to solve social and religious controversies: 'Differences of opinion in the congregation must be considered as a special grace of Allah.'[29] The prophets Micah and Jesus are not far away from Hanafi's legal assessment of controversy in religious and cultural matters: 'You shall love the Lord your God with all your heart, and with all your soul, and with all your mind. This is the great and first commandment. And the second is like it, you shall love your neighbor as yourself. On these two commandments depend all the law and the prophets'[30].

The following narrative about a little town by the river was inspired by the Prophet Mohamed's *Contract of Medina*, drafted and implemented after his escape from Mecca to Medina. This story contemplates a successfully integrated use of our eight-C properties in building harmonious communities and biotopes for happy people and healthy social and natural environments, both in geography and in cyberspace.

THE LITTLE TOWN BY THE RIVER

Measured by the long river and the surrounding hills, this town is quite small, like a drop on a bucket. But it happens to be the only town beside the river, and the people are proud of their town, the river, and their great wealth. This wealth they see in the dignity and nobility of their citizens, their different city quarters, their cultivated lands and waters, and the wide connections in all forms of networking. The freedom and security of the citizens is cherished above all. They help each other and encourage the young generation to respect others, even if they do not share their opinions. They loathe lies, theft, murder, injustice, egotism, arrogance, and intolerance. Those who lie, steal, or kill are punished, even when thieves and murderers pretend to act in the name of God or out of a higher insight. They do not all believe in God, yet nonbelievers agree that, if there were a God, he would forbid these actions. This viewpoint is expressed by those living

harmony. However, centuries of denominational infighting and religious wars and suppression among Christians prove otherwise.

[29] Paret R 1979. "Innerislamischer Pluralismus." In *Die islamische Welt zwischen Mittelalter und Neuzeit. Festschrift Hans Robert Roemer*, Haarmann U, Bachmann pp. 523-529. Beirut/Wiesbaden: Steiner, p. 523. The oral hadith tradition in Islam displays a broad traditional and contemporary variety of fatwas, suggestions, and instructions by religious authorities; the Quran criticizes the ideational fighting primarily among the Jews and Christians and holds 'And if the Lord truly had wanted, he would have made humankind one single community (*umma wahida*); but they are still arguing (*muhtalifun*), except those in the grace of God (*rahima*); this is, why he has created them' (Sura 11:118f).

[30] Micah 6:8

in Atheist, Jewish, Christian, and Moslem houses. Those who believe in God are aware of the power of Satan; all know of the evil in mankind and about evil persons they feel obliged to fight against. They detest intolerance and spare no effort to create a culture of communication and cooperation through listening and arguments based on trust.

Each of them has a special competence and competes with others in improving and protecting the common goods of their integrated city bios. Of course, they are free to contemplate bios, biotopes, and creation individually or with networks of friends and to draw conclusions from their insights and intuitions in reflecting on their own position and contemplating how to improve their service to the town. Respect for each other and the world around them and compassion (in particular for the weak, desperate, sick, and needy) form the basis of their harmony and their wealth in values and valuables. Communication and cooperation, competence and competition, contemplation and calculation, compassion and cultivation are the pillars on which their culture is based. They are all aware that these eight Cs need to be defended against evildoers from the inside and aggressors from the outside.

They believe that human dignity finds expression mainly in respecting the individual conscience. They honor as inviolable their fellow citizens' religious or philosophical convictions. Overall, they respect and request the individual conscience's responsibility; they never accuse each other of immorality or of being uncultured when their own judgments in these matters differ. Even if they cannot accept the convictions of their fellow citizens or regard them as abstruse, they never force them to act against their convictions. For example, foods are labeled as kosher, halal, vegetarian, or organically grown. No one must take medication or abort unborn life, donate or accept organs, or take on work that violates personal values or religious/humanist beliefs. If someone proposes putting pressure on the conscience of others, they all become angry because they see this as a violation of the dignity of the little town and of the wealth of values held by its citizens. Most city laws contain a 'sunset clause' indicating that a law will lose its force after a specific number of years unless it has been extended or modified. They also include a 'conscience clause' allowing citizens to be conscientious objectors if no one else is harmed.

The citizens of this town live in harmony with their natural biotopes and the many other forms of cultivated bios (microbes, plants, animals, colonies, etc.), which they respect as 'brothers and sisters' within and around the bios of their city. They take pride in having their own healthy, personal microbiome and in creating probiotic biotopes in their houses, hospitals, schools, offices, factories, assembly halls, parks, and agricultural spaces. They enjoy reaching out to other people and cities, making prudent use of their eight C properties globally through their waterways, roads, and airways, digital networks of commerce and manufacturing, social networks of communication and cooperation, and friendships and partnerships inside and outside their geographical locality.

A look at the architecture of the houses shows clearly the cultural and ethical structure of this city by the water. As different as they appear, these houses are built on the eight-C pillars in the basements and first floors, which are connected to protect the population from hunger, murder, and torture, as well as for the care of all who cannot help themselves. The layout and furnishings in the upper floors show the rich variety in values and visions of their inhabitants. Debates take place in one of the houses on whether a human fetus has moral or legal rights or is part of the body of the mother, whose personal dignity and preferences should be paramount. In another house we hear debates on whether religious rules for fasting may be broken in case of illness to give patients medicine and nutrition. The century-old debate on whether a terminally ill person hoping for life after death should ask for a 'poisoned drink' has been toned down. There are adamant calls for physicians to make better use of palliative medicine in easing pain and suffering, however, thus making discussions about euthanasia and its potential abuse unnecessary. On the rooftops, we hear the loud, exhaustive, and sometimes confounding debates on complex questions such as whether God is one person in three, three in one, or a person at all; whether there is one primary prophet or even a representative of God on earth; whether all things in nature are divine and require respect or not; and whether invisible spirits or demons exist and whether they have power over us and the world of bios. Are human zygotes ensouled and can they be reincarnated or resurrected in Paradise? Do individual souls transmigrate; do animals or plants have souls; do transgenic animals having human DNA therefore have part of a human soul or spirit? Must one believe in a higher spiritual authority to be a decent person and a good fellow citizen?

Debates like these have gone on for a long time and most likely will never stop. In their own way, these quarrels represent the great richness of values and visions of this little town by the river. In some of the houses, people are sympathetic to such eccentric palaver, but others are not and sometimes judge it as silly, absurd, and unnecessary for being a valued member of the community. Some regard these things as 'divine secrets' calling for modesty rather than righteousness. Nevertheless, everyone would go out of the way to preserve the disputing parties' right of convincing, discoursing, quarreling, and dissenting. There is an awareness and appreciation that reasoning in the upper floors rightly influences the deeds on the lower ones, as long as fellow humans are respected and supported and not hurt or belittled. But the community does not accept when individuals or clans violate the rules of civility. Whoever does not like the local rules and ways of life is free to move, and it goes without saying that as long as people live in the village as citizens or guests they must respect its rules regarding mutual respect and the dignity of their fellow humans.

The names of the streets and plazas remind the citizens of their common history and the roots of the town's culture. One of the squares is dedicated to the victims of murder, violence, and terrorism; to the burned residents of Jericho and Ai, and Dresden; to the victims of innumerable pogroms targeting Jews and Free-Thinkers; to the tortured and burned victims of the so-called Holy Inquisition; to the victims of the rape of Nanjing; and to the victims of global terrorism such as occurred at the World Trade Center in New York City. On 'Houses of Contemplation' are murals representing the integrated and integrating harmony of the bios of the city and its surroundings.

The running streams of water (in geography) and data (in cyberspace) provide for everyday life and for connection to the entire world. The old Roman saying 'e pluribus unum, in diversity we are one' and the Confucian slogan 'he er bu tong 和而不同, in harmony, but different' are engraved in many places. So have they built their town, and they will need to make every effort to preserve their community against enemies of culture and dignity, as they have no other home.

II. RISKS AND REWARDS IN CULTIVATING BIOS

4. MANIPULATING AND CULTIVATING NON-HUMAN AND HUMAN BIOS

RISKS AND REWARDS IN MANIPULATION

Breeding, cultivating, and manipulating the many forms of bios for human purposes such as food, housing, farming, services, commerce, power, and fun has been with humans since prehistoric times. Manipulation and modification of individual and collective bios and of species and biotopes characterizes human bios and culture, as the following ancient narrative illustrates. Jacob had served Laban for over 20 years as a herdsman without pay. Finally, Jacob made a contract with Laban that as compensation he would receive the crossbreeds in Laban's herds after a few years. To produce as many crossbreeds as possible from Laban's purebred herds, Jacob led the flocks to the watering holes and let them graze and mate together, which was against the rules of pure breeding. When Jacob walked away at the end of the contract, Laban's sons angrily complained 'Jacob has taken all that was our father's; and from what was our father's he has gotten all this wealth.' The Bible remarks without any further moral judgment: 'the man grew exceedingly rich, and had large flocks, maidservants and menservants, and camels and asses.'[1]

4.1. How to Integrate Expertise and Ethics?

Jacob reacted with his unusual breeding trick in response to many years of work without pay. Jacob had been in love with Laban's younger daughter and Laban had agreed to a marriage, but at the wedding Laban gave Jacob his older daughter, Leah. When Jacob complained, Laban gave him Rachel as a wife as well. The story demonstrates how closely moral and immoral behavior in their extremes can be interrelated, not only in our dealings with non-human life but also with our love affairs, our families, and our communities. The animals most likely had similar sexual fun in making crossbred babies instead of purebred ones. Jacob cheated on Laban, who had earlier cheated on Jacob in business. In giving him Leah instead of Rachel, Laban again treated Jacob unfairly, probably against an earlier mutual understanding. But as a result of further negotiation, Jacob ended up with two wives, Leah and his beloved Rachel.

We find no words of compassion or moral concern in this biblical story, neither in regard to dealing with animals and professional contracts, nor with people and their feelings. Did the mating animals have compassionate 'feelings' for each other? What about the role of compassion, sex and love, or mutual respect and trust between Leah, Rachel, and Jacob? Did the animal mothers 'love' their crossbred offspring as they would have their purebred ones, and did the young animals enjoy juvenile play and have a normal, 'compassionate' relation

---

[1] Genesis 30:43; 31:1.

with their mother? Are swine and other livestock today happier when routinely given antibiotics against infections and for more rapid growth? Rachel and Jacob were in love before they married; did Jacob, Leah, and Rachel nevertheless develop a balanced and harmonious love life? What about so-called 'patchwork' families today and other newly configured cultures of respect, tolerance, sympathy, and love? Some traditional cultures integrated polygamy into their communities; and young people who broke the culture of arranged marriages often had to leave those communities with or without the blessings of their clan.

4.2. From Indirect Breeding to Direct Manipulation via CRISPR/Cas9

Traditional breeding and genetic refinement was indirect, and it took hundreds or thousands of years to manipulate and to modify the natural DNA building blocks of bios. This cultivation of nature has made human lives and communities safer and more comfortable. This process was often uncivilized, ethically wrongheaded and uncompassionate, but so were (and still are) many of our interactions with fellow humans. Thoroughbred horses are bred using in vitro fertilization and surrogate motherhood, and so are certain types of 'super' milk cows. Specially bred varieties of hogs have more ribs and produce more plentiful, higher quality meat than others, but they are high-strung. When kept as family companions in small apartments with staircases, several types of hunting dogs develop painful spinal injuries. Who is concerned with the physical and emotional health of these manipulated forms of bios or about their impact on the balances and harmonies in existing biotopes? Who profits from their cultivation?

Of course, the DNA of all forms of bios changes also in direct response to biotical challenges, incentives, and threats. These changes improve survival, integration, and life condition. In addition, microbes show much more flexibility in adaptation than do 'higher' forms of life. Currently, new genetic knowledge and capabilities allow for direct intervention in and manipulation of bios. In-vitro fertilization of oocytes from different species results in transgenic life, whether animal–animal hybrids, human–animal hybrids, animal–human hybrids, or chimeras. After birth, they may be used in medical research, for the production of medicines, or for cells or organs to transplant into human patients. Cybrids are human–animal products resulting from transferring human nuclear DNA into the cytoplast of an animal, with subsequent formation of a blastocyst as material for research or for eventual implantation. These cybrid cells are assumed to be 99% human, with some animal mitochondrion remaining. Regulation of them is different worldwide, with the United Kingdom having relatively liberal guidelines. [2] The new technologies of manipulation via CRISPR/Cas9 (clustered regularly interspaced short palindromic repeats/Cas9 protein) go much further. Scientists directly break up DNA segments by editing

[2] McNamee SP 2015 Human–animal hybids and chimeras: What's in a name, in: Jahr 61(1), 11:45-66.

the genetic setup of humans, livestock, plants, and microbes directly (like a proofreader does in correcting text), thus avoiding the long, indirect processes of selecting and breeding.[3] CRISPRs are found in microbes and also as RNA interferences in higher forms of bios. Comparative genomics studies show how microbes change their genetic setup in response to modifications in their horizontal or vertical biotope in order to survive and flourish. We can compare this inborn natural creativity of the smallest and earliest forms of bios in adjusting and surviving via their innate biochemical properties of 'cultivation' to human species–specific forms of 'cultivation' via the eight-C properties. Even though we are unable to translate their basic biochemical modes of cultivation into specific forms of human cultivation (which involve 'free will'), it is fascinating to recognize non-sentient 'calculations' in these basic forms of bios and to compare their modes of operation with those of specific human cultures and traditions.

The capability of simple forms of bios to distinguish their own DNA from that of others and to react appropriately reveals a basic property of all bios: that of adaptation, modification, and cultivation as a basic building block of bios for survival and defense and for building harmonious but flexible biotopes. We might compare the defensive and cooperative biological properties of bacteria and archaea and their sequences to medieval cities surrounded with walls and towers while connecting with their outside environment via commerce, communication, and cooperation. Microbes freely use CRISPR mechanisms as an immune response to invading viruses by guiding and integrating some of the viral DNA into their own, thus acquiring specific immunity.[4] In learning the mechanisms of repair by spacer acquisition and integration from microbes, we humans may be able to cut out certain unwarranted sequences in our own DNA and replace them by pasting in warranted segments to check inheritable diseases, thus creating better forms of bios and better health. The term *better*, however, needs to be discussed using detailed and specific bioethical arguments regarding specific and well-defined applications for humans, cultured crops, and animals, and in terms of impact on existing biotopes[5].

Compassion for all forms of life is one of the eight basic human-species–specific properties, and it is demonstrated empirically in civilized societies. The virtue and principle of compassion extends beyond individual animals, plants, and living biotopes, even though we might not apprehend the level of harm or

[3] Mali P, Esvelt KM, Church GM 2013 Cas9 as a versatile tool for engineering biology, in: Nature Methods 10(10):957-963. Doi:10.1038/nmeth.2649; Ledford H 2015 CRISPER, the disruptor, in: Nature 522 (7554): 20-24.

[4] Horvath P, Barrangou R 2010 CRISPER/Cas, the immune system of bacteria and archaea, in: Science 327(5962):167-170; Jinek M et al., 2012 A programmable dual DNA-guided endonucleose in adoptive bacterial immunity, in: Science 337: 816-821.

[5] Specter M 2016 DNA Revolution. Scientists ow have a new Tool to alter the DNA of Living Organisms. Should they use it?, in: National Geographic 230(2) 30-55.

loss of potential fulfillment they experience.[6] The closer those non-human forms of bios are to our human neurological and emotional setup, the easier it will be to guess what forms of fearful anticipation, pain, or suffering they might experience. Contemporary discourse and laws focus primarily on the suffering of mammals closest to us, but their spectrum of concern should embrace all living beings.[7]

Human cultures strive to overcome the obstacles, dangers, risks, and cruelties of raw nature. We have manipulated wild plants and animals and have often cruelly killed or eradicated unwanted non-human life perceived as dangerous. Of course, mice and pathogens do not belong in our hospitals and houses, and we rightly eradicate them in those places, but why should we harm them for no reason? As Albert Schweitzer argues in regard to cruelty towards animals (including those in medical research): 'When helping an insect in need, I do nothing else than reducing a part of the ever increasing guilt of humans to creatures.'[8] Care for non-human life follows different intuitions and orientational instructions. Jahr reports that a boy from a small Muslim caste in Burma and India will not kill a highly poisonous snake because 'also the snakes are our brothers and sisters.' Jahr does not agree to such a strict concept: 'We actually hold it to be our duty to kill harmful animals, if we can. We have our farm animals killed by the butcher and the harmless prey by the hunter, because we want to eat meat, which in our areas some feel they cannot do without, while in tropical countries vegetarian food is abundantly available. Our animal production, thus, has a utilitarian aspect, which is boldly disregarded by the Indians, while we content ourselves with avoidance of unnecessary suffering.[9]

Veganism is currently a fashionable, widely followed means of avoiding killing or using animals.[10] But do today's various vegan movements differentiate between food prepared from plants or trees that have fulfilled their purpose in life (i.e., to produce fruit or seed, such as potatoes, wheat, corn, and apples) as compared to eating vegetables that are still full of life and growing (such as healthy fresh salad greens, legumes, and carrots, which have not yet reached

---

[6] Sass HM 2012 Earth, Universe and Multiverse as Living Beings: Let's Treat Them as Such, in: Fritz Jahr and the Foundations of Global Bioethics, Muzur A, Sass HM eds., Muenster: Lit, 345-357.

[7] Institute of Medicine of the National Academies 2012 International Animal Research Regulations. Impact on Neuroscience Research (Workshop Summary 05-29-2012), in: http://www.iom.edu/reports/2012.

[8] Schweitzer A 1948 Kultur und Ethik, vol. 2, München: Biederstein, 250.

[9] Jahr F 1927, in: Jahr F 2013 Essays in Bioethics. Muenster: Lit, p. 27; for contemporary animal right advocacy cf. Phelps N 2007 The Longest Struggle: Animal Advocacy from Pythagoras to PETA. New York: Lantern Books.

[10] Norman Phelps, an influential animal rights activist and founder of the Animal Liberation Front [ALF] sees some benefits to animals and the environment by in-vitro flesh; cf. Phelps N 2013 Changing the Game. Why the Battle for Animal Liberation Is so Hard and How We Can Win It. Kindle Book; cf. www.animal-welfare.org.

their biological 'destiny' as Krause calls it, i.e., producing seed or fruit)? We do not eat apple trees, but we collect apples and deprive seeds in a fresh apple of their limited destiny to be buried in supportive soil and grow into apple trees. But lettuce and spinach are cut while living, without having fulfilled their destiny to bear fruit. We bring them to market dying, killing the spinach in boiling water and keeping the lettuce alive until we eat it. What kind of harm do fresh salads or legumes feel during preparation and when crushed by our teeth, as Herder might ask?[11] Of course, hamburgers made from artificially grown in-vitro flesh would not involve killing chickens or pigs, nor would fresh salads. Pork hamburgers, which have more omega-3 fats, will be healthier for human consumption than ones made of beef and actually might also benefit the health of genetically modified pigs as well.[12]

Four different areas in which humans use non-human life exhibit challenges, risks, and benefits as regards cultivating the worlds of non-human bios: (1) patenting non-human life derived from direct or indirect genetic manipulation, (2) creating in-vitro life for human consumption or other uses, (3) manipulating and cultivating new biotopes, and (4) creating hybrid transgenic non-human life with human genetic properties. The following chapters will deal more extensively with the question of ethically responsible ways to use animals in experimentation for human benefit and with humans as subjects in research.

4.3. Patenting Non-human Life?

Selecting, breeding, crossbreeding, and genetically manipulating animals and other non-human bios comprise just one aspect of shaping non-human life to benefit humans. For millennia, we have bred animals for farming and grazing, transportation, hunting, and protecting communities. We have also been successful with selected interspecies breeding, such as breeding mules. Goldfish have been bred for fun and varieties of dogs for tasks and services such as dog-fighting and leading blind people. Some animals bred for human use have disappeared because breeding was discontinued (e.g., particular kinds of goats, cows, horses, cats, dogs, pigeons, pigs, and goldfish). Do we have a special obligation to protect them from extinction as 'endangered species' because we had a hand in their cultivation?

Do cultivated, highbred plants and animals have different experiences of suffering or enjoyment than their non-manipulated sisters and brothers? This question

---

[11] As already mentioned, for Karl Christian Friedrich Krause the natural 'destiny' [*Bestimmung*] of life and for Johann Georg Herder natural 'needs' [*Beduerfnisse*] were the points of reference from which to discuss moral obligations towards non-human forms of bios; see Jahr F 1927, in: Jahr F 2013 Essays, p. 38f.

[12] Fiester A 2006 Why the Omega-3 Piggy Should Not Go to Market, in: Nature Biotechnology 1472f; Kolata G 2006 Cloned Pigs Could Provide Meat That Benefits the Heart, in: New York Times 04-26-2006.

is impossible to answer because we lack a way to do so. Whether cultured or not, the more these forms of bios differ from ours, the farther away from us they are biologically and neurologically. Would our obligation to races and breeds we cultivate be higher than the preservation of other endangered species? Would they lose in life's lottery of genetic and environmental opportunities, as have millions of other species? Does the little girl playing with her hamster or guinea pig recognize that they are night animals and that daytime is their natural sleep time? We have created transgenic animals such as onco-mice or kidney rats for studying human cancer and kidney cyst disorders, along with related drug development. Some transgenic animal models have made good progress in preparation for cell or organ transplantation into suffering humans, or even for use in antiaging medicine. Cockfights, dogfights, bullfights, and horse races are examples of how we cause animals pain or allow them to be killed for fun and excitement. But the middle-class girl playing with her guinea pig all day is not different from a family keeping a dachshund in an upstairs apartment with stairs, over time ruining his spine; from families overfeeding bulldogs, destroying their vulnerable cardiovascular systems; or families choosing German shepherds with hip problems resulting from over-breeding as pets. Of course, for 'good reasons' we kill (and even eradicate) viral and bacterial pathogens; we kill insects who carry them; and we kill rats and mice – all for the benefit of human life and public health.

There have been long legal, political, and ethical discussions about patenting life. Among breeders of highbred household animals such as dogs and cats, an informal model of reciprocity has developed. Under 'breeder's privilege' contracts, the owner of a male animal has first pick of the litter The story of Laban and Jacob reminds us that breeding and property ownership have long roots in human culture. Can new forms of life be patented and thus become the intellectual and commercial property of individuals and businesses? Human creativity has been fundamental in the cultivation of human life, including music, lyrics, novels, hardware and software, machines and processes. Some inventions have been kept secret so that the inventor could benefit without disclosing substances or procedures.

Article 23 of the United Nation's Universal Declaration of Human Rights holds that 'everyone has the right to the protection of the moral and material interests resulting from any scientific, literary or artistic production of which he is the author'; therefore, in modern times those benefits are protected by various models of intellectual property rights.[13] The 'International Treaty on Plant Genetic Resources for Food and Agriculture' (ITPGRFA) includes a global information system for protecting benefits and diversity in the field of agricul-

---

[13] Marchant GE 2007 Genomics, Ethics, and Intellectual Property, in: Intellectual Property Management in Health and Agricultural Innovation. A Handbook of Best Practices 1.5:29-35.

tural breeding. If Monsanto or another company obtains a patent for a specific genetically modified crop, then the patent holder can and must be held liable for potential harm to the agricultural environment and for the health of consumers.[14] Patents have benefits, risks, liabilities, and obligations that should be placed not on society but with the patent owner. These obligations would pertain to new crops resulting from genetically modified organisms (GMOs) as well as to pesticides and their impact on biotopes and on human health.

Research and development in the field of antibiotics has been beneficial to individuals and communities in protecting human life from the uncountable billions of microbial pathogens. Their developers rightly recover their initial investment and enjoy the economic benefits for several years. Over time, however, bacterial pathogens have modified genetically and have become resistant to widely used antibiotics. To make matters worse, the latter are routinely fed to livestock, not just to prevent them from becoming sick but to increase meat production and profits. Today, more people in the United States and Europe are killed by so-called superbugs, such as methicillin-resistant *Staphylococcus aureus* (MRSA), than by AIDS. The introduction of new forms of manipulated bios – whether protected or not by intellectual property patents – changes the equation of existing integrated biotopes, adding new benefits and new risks. The end of antibiotic drug efficacy will be the end of modern medicine as we know it. It will cause catastrophic disasters in a globalized and interrelated world, particularly in large urban centers. Research in developing probiotic remedies to fight multiple resistant bacteria on the microbial level has yet to obtain enough support to become successful.[15] A regulated reduction in or avoidance of the most efficacious broadband antibiotics in individual cases to benefit public health and reduce hospital deaths will cause new debates about equal rights and equal access to health care for all.

Legal disputes in patenting also address the question of whether or not farmers may keep seeds from the previous harvest to use the next season. In the case of GMO seeds from Monsanto, farmers still need to buy specific insecticides produced by Monsanto that do not hurt those particular seeds. Naturally

[14] Recently, on 03-20-2015, IARC (WHO's International Agency for Research on Cancer) has classified Roundup (glyphosate) as a potential cause for cancer in humans; earlier IARC has issued similar warnings for smoking and drinking; cf. Bunge J 2015 For Monsanto a Season of Woes on the Farm, in: Wall Street Journal 03-30-15, B4.

[15] A Global Probiotics Council (GPC) was established in 2004 through a collaborative arrangement between DANONE and YAKULT HONSHA CO., LTD: ' The role of the GPC is to promote and/or advance probiotics in the world, through means such as: 1. Raising awareness of probiotics and their health benefits through science-based education and dissemination of information to health care professionals and the public; 2. Communicating with government bodies, and other relevant interest groups; and, 3. Building relationships with leading researchers and research institutions and supporting collaborative research in the area of probiotics and intestinal microbiota'; website probioticsresearch.com.

occurring bios cannot be patented, because legally and ethically it is considered a product of nature, an entity of non-human origin in the struggle of life. But a biological patent can cover biological and farming technologies and products that do not occur naturally. The European Patent Office allows for patenting of biological products and gene sequences as long as they are 'isolated from [their] natural environment or produced by means of a technical process.'[16] In the United States, forms of bios 'isolated' from their natural origins by human manipulation have been patented (e.g., insulin, vitamins, various genes, and adrenaline), but a landmark Supreme Court decision in 2013 declared naturally occurring DNA sequences ineligible for patenting.[17] The issue is not yet resolved legally; arguments will continue related to the ownership of specific forms of bios and to economic benefits and risks associated with cultivation and manipulation.

4.4. Creating In-Vitro Flesh

Only recently have we become capable of directly intervening in cell structures and recombining cell life – including manipulating somatic cells into pluripotent forms of life. One of the first successful experiments in in-vitro cultivation of muscle cells was reported in 1971 by Russell Ross.[18] Recent research in manipulating muscle cell life by cutting, slicing, and rearranging natural DNA and RNA has taken place to alter bacteria, to 'enhance' plants and animals, to develop designer microbes or enzymes for human medicine, and to create 'in-vitro flesh' or 'cultured meat' for hamburgers and other human food.[19] Arising from

---

[16] EU Directive 98/44EC; cf. Sharples A 2011 Gene Patents in Europe Relatively Stable Despite Uncertainty in the US, in: Genetic Engineering and Biotechnology New, 2011-03-23.

[17] US Supreme Court 2013 Association for Molecular Pathology vs Myriad Genetics, in: www.supremecourt.gov/opinions/12pdf/12-398_8njq.pdf; however an Australian Court ruled differently in favor of Myriad Genetics in 2014. According to a report by Andrew Pollack in the New York Times 01-27-15 Myriad genetics finally gave up on pursuing the patenting of their lucrative genetic test for inheritable BRCA1 and BRCA2 breast and ovarian cancer.

[18] Ross R 1971 Growth of Smooth Muscle in Culture and Formation of Elastic Fibers, in: Journal of Cell Biology, pp. 172-186; the abstract reads: 'Smooth muscle cell derived from the inner media and intima of immature guinea pig aorta were grown for up to eight weeks in cell culture. The cells remained the morphology of smooth muscle in all phases of their growth in culture. After growing to confluency, they grew in multiple overlapping layers of cells. Basement membrane-like material also appeared adjacent to the cells. Analysis of the microfibrils showed that they have an amino acid composition similar to that of the microfibrillar protein of the intact elastic fiber. These investigations coupled with radioaudiographic observations of the ability of aortic smooth muscle to synthesize and secrete extracellular proteins demonstrate that this cell is a connective tissue synthetic cell.'

[19] Results of a conference 'The ethics of in-vitro flesh and enhanced animals,' held Sept 18/19, 2014 and sponsored by the Welcome Trust, will open more new fields and methods of directly manipulating natural forms of life directly on the RNA and DNA level; cf. http://tinyurl.com/3cl13wf; Palmer M, Findlay 2012 Faith in Conservation. World Bank.

compassionate competence in reducing animal suffering in chicken and pig facilities, these results will doubtless find spin-off applications in devilish new technologies harmful to existing life, including humans. But the cultural and moral benefit of in-vitro meat grown in laboratories from cloned cells would avoid raising animals in questionable conditions and then killing them. It has also been suggested that in-vitro meat would greatly reduce the use of water, land, and other global resources compared to raising animals for slaughter.[20] To improve taste by including other cell material such as fat and nerve tissue, it will be necessary to develop bio-incubators for economically viable production of in-vitro meat. Also, major shifts in social and culinary cultures must occur to make in-vitro nutrition successful.[21] But good taste and gourmet support will not be enough to promote in-vitro meats (and eventually artificial vegetables), as long as millions of fellow humans go hungry or die because of malnutrition.

Modern Meadow Inc., a 2011 biofabrication start-up, multiplies bovine cells in a cell culture medium. Over 30 days, small sheets of tissue develop for use in processing leather or meat. Lab-grown leather can supply designers in an $80 billion global market, thus eliminating the slaughter of millions of animals. The technical process of cultivating biofabricated 'meat' is more complex and expensive at this time. Marketable results are expected within a few years, while in-vitro leather may introduce in-vitro production of materials and foods via fashion design as a gateway into many more modern customer cultures.[22] If pa-

[20] Tuamisto HM, Teixeira de Mattos HM 2011 Environmental Impacts of Cultivated Meat Production, in: Environment Science Technology 45(14)6117-61123.

[21] Catts O and Zurr I report 2003 in the Winter edition 2005/6 of gourmet journal 'Cabinet Magazine' under the headline 'Ingestion – Disembodied Cuisine' about meat grown from frog stem cells.

[22] Cf. www.reeis.usda.gov/web/.../0228895-engineered-comestible-meat, Non-technical Summary for a 2014 Grant: 'Present farm and industrial meat production methods and technologies have a number of associated problems including health risks (infectious animal diseases, nutrition-related diseases), resource intensity (land, water, energy), damage to environment (greenhouse gas emission, erosion, biodiversity loss) and ethical challenges (animal welfare). With increasing worldwide demand for meat, it is expected that some of these problems will become critical. The objective of this proposal is to develop a fundamentally new approach to edible meat production. The approach is based on bio-printing, a novel tissue engineering technology. In this technology, conveniently prepared multicellular aggregates (the bio-ink particles) are delivered into a biocompatible support structure according to a design template (compatible with the shape of the desired biological construct) by a computer-controlled delivery device (the bio-printer). Biological assemblies form after deposition of the discrete bio-ink particles, through morphogenetic processes akin to those evident in early embryonic development, such as cell sorting and tissue fusion. The resulting construct is transferred to special purpose bioreactor for further maintenance and maturation to make it suitable for use (e.g. implantation in medical applications). So far, bio-printing has been applied to build three-dimensional tissues and organ structures of specific architecture and functionality for purposes of regenerative medicine. Here we propose to adapt this technology to building meat products for consumption. The technology has several advantages in comparison to earlier attempts to engineer meat in

tents are issued for specific products of in-vitro meat research, the patent holder will be responsible for any unhealthy results in people who eat them as advised. Would in-vitro meat burgers made from reprogrammed cells of chicken, beef, deer, turkey, and swine be bioethically as acceptable to humankind (and to animal-right activists in particular) as veggie burgers made from fresh green salad, cabbage, carrots, broccoli, or other 'slaughtered' vegetables?

4.5. Manipulating and Cultivating Biotopes

Ever since nomads travelling in search of food and exploitable environments changed their habits and settled down, humans have manipulated particular pieces of territory. They cultivated (i.e., dug the soil with hands and shovels), built fences around garden plots for protection against wild animals, and fenced meadows to prevent farm animals from escaping. Oil paintings from the late 18th century to today romanticize family farms, showing farmers, cows, chicken, swine, fruit trees, vegetables, stables, and barns in an idealized setting. Yet these landscapes are just as much a product of human manipulation as modern landscapes in agribusiness, with their gigantic fields of crops and heavy machinery. Urbanites today take a break from city life and hike in rural areas, enjoying these 'natural' environments and appreciating what cultures in forestry, agriculture, and animal husbandry have produced. At the beginning of the 21st century, few non-manipulated biotopes remain worldwide.

Cultivated landscapes have been the dream of different cultures and religions for millennia, and a paradise in the afterlife is envisioned by many religions. Nomads carry their 'gardens' with them on their travels as flower-covered carpets. Zen Buddhist gardens for meditation are famed, as is the difference between French and English-style gardens. While the French garden demonstrates the dominance of humankind ('le roi c'est moi') with its geomet-

---

vitro. The bio-ink particles can be reproducibly prepared with mixtures of cells of different type. This allows for control in composition that enables the engineering of healthy products of great variety. Printing ensures consistent shape, while post-printing structure formation and maturation in the bioreactor facilitates conditioning. As meat is a post mortem tissue, the vascularization of the final product is less critical than in medical applications (although important for taste an objective to be further pursued in Phase II). Overall, this process allows for greater structural precision than other approaches and higher throughput for eventual scaling to industrial production. We anticipate that this Phase I application will result in a macroscopic size (~2 cm × 1 cm × 0.5 mm) edible prototype and will demonstrate that bio-printing-based in vitro meat production is feasible, economically viable and environmentally practical. Successful in vitro meat engineering addresses a number of societal needs, thus the commercialization of the method has high market potential. The consumer acceptance of such products may not be without challenges. We expect it will first appeal to culinary early-adopter consumers and the segment of the vegetarian community that rejects meat for ethical reasons. With reduction in price, it can reach the masses with religious restrictions on meat consumption (people restricted to Hindu, Kosher, or Halal diets) and finally populations with limited access to safe meat production.

rical designs, trimmed trees, and shear-pruned hedges, the English garden favors single trees, non-geometrical ponds, and walls and ruins of stone. In an English garden, one is not supposed to see or reflect on the cultivating human hand.[23]

In modern times, so-called natural biotopes have been set aside as natural reserves, with no human interference. But these biotopes themselves have developed as a result of normal shifts in climate, habitat, and, to a certain extent, human action. Only since the 1995 re-introduction of wolves into Yellowstone National Park has the biotope developed into a more livable harmony. Deer have retreated into safer areas, the tree population has blossomed, the soil has become more stable and rich, and devastating run-offs of water have been diminished. As trees and other vegetation have reduced erosion, beavers build dams, providing for even richer ecosystems. These transformations teach us that nature never stands still, for baselines permanently shift, while 'keeping landscapes in a state of arrested development' runs contrary to the bios of natural biotopes.[24] The same is true for social and cultural biotopes, as the history of humankind has shown and as the future of cultivation will confirm. In the case of the Yellowstone biotope, 'rewilding' was the solution to stagnant life and disaster, and it provided many naturally occurring, surprise examples of the rejuvenating powers of bios and biotopes.

Not well discussed yet are our manipulations to housing and urban biotopes. Mold, cockroaches, microbes, moths, and mice in homes, offices, hotels, and hospitals are co-bios in contemporary city cultures. We fight these unwarranted forms of co-bios with insecticides, antibiotics, and antiseptics, but some forms of bios are genetically flexible enough to develop into eradication-resistant superbugs that pervade modern life. Methicillin-resistant *Staphylococcus aureus*[25] is a prime example. Probably originating in hospitals, MRSA has the potential to kill more citizens than any other microbe, and it could eventually start a global pandemic. Actually, we have already changed our biotopes and those of our co-life forms by giving antibiotics to animals as well as using these human-made microbes for human health care. Antibiotics can legally be given to cattle, pigs, chickens, and other farm animals, thus widening the potential spread and uncontrollable DNA modification of these man-made forms of bios. Regulations against providing antibiotics to animals for better and quicker production of meat – and, of course, better profits – are

[23] Sass HM 1981 Mensch und Landschaft, in: Landschaft und Mensch, Höhl G ed., Mannheim: Humboldt Gesellschaft, 293-322; Jünger FG 1960 Gärten im Abend-und Morgenland. München: Bechte; Wright T, Katsuhiko M 2004 (12th ed.) Zen Gardens. Kyoto:Suiko Books.

[24] Monbiot G 2014 Nature's Way. Reintroducing Long-lost Species to our Environment Could Be the Key to Conserve Our Heritage, in: Royal Society of Arts Journal 2014(4)30-31.

[25] Reynolds LA, Tansey EM 2008 Superbugs and Superdrugs, in: Welcome Witnesses to 20th Century Medicine, No 33.

loosely worded and minimally enforced. On the other hand, modification by using CRISPR/Cas9 technology might have direct or indirect ecological affects as well, and it has been reported to modify non-targeted sequences indirectly so that they mutate as well.[26] Lima and Cicovacki[27] remind us that Prometheus, who stole fire from the Gods, had a brother named Epimetheus famed for his forethought, suggesting that both brothers' virtues should be combined in manipulating and cultivating.

Hospitals in particular experience unintended, dangerous alterations in microbial biotopes, which kill more people there annually than the flu. Recent studies on involuntary changes to urban microbial biotopes by humans used the New York subway to demonstrate severe, unexpected changes in urban human–microbial biotopes. Different subway stations host and breed varying germs, from bubonic plague in uptown to meningitis in midtown, stomach trouble in the financial district, and antibiotic-resistant infections throughout the system. 'Good' bacteria were also found eating hazardous chemicals and toxic waste, while the ubiquitous pizza-loving bacteria were particularly dense in areas with concentrations of pizza lovers.[28] What can we learn from one of these urban public health projects regarding future microbial studies on cities and from healthy and unhealthy biomes in our apartments, elevators, transportation systems, hotels, hospitals, kindergartens, and nursing homes? Will we eventually be able to devise and implement probiotic biotopes, so that we do not eradicate pathogens (more or less successfully) while burdening biotopes with pesticides and unhealthy cleaning materials? As we have done with large-scale agriculture, will we develop, plant, and farm powerful, small-scale, healthy bionomic environments that protect and improve human and environmental health? Will microbial research and farming focusing on cities be the next field in global biotechnology and bioethics? Will it lead to new public health initiatives for the prevention of infection and disease? Will this be a fascinating new area in the future of manipulating and cultivating bios ethically? Has the use of cleaning materials that kill microbes indiscriminately put living quarters and urban biotopes into 'a state of arrested development,' and should we rather search for

[26] Baltimore D et al., 2015 A prudent path forward for genomic engineering and germline modification, in: Science 348: 36-38; Lauphier E et al., 2015 Don't edit the human germline, in: Nature 519: 410-411.

[27] Lima NS, Cicovacki P 2015 Contemporary Ethics. The Promethean Challenges to Reprogenetics, in: Jahr 6(1)(11):29-44; they quote Nicolai Hartmann [Hartmann N 1931 Ethics, transl Coit S, vol. 2, p. 148] 'Foresight is the intuitive vision in man; in its highest power, it is prophecy. Prevision makes him move forward, conscious of his goal. Man does not live in the presence alone. He belongs to the future. And the future belongs to him—within the limits of his prevision'; foresight definitely is one of the combined products of well and successfully integrated eight-C properties.

[28] Hotz RL 2015 Big Data and Bacteria. Mapping the New York Subway's DNA, in: Wall Street Journal Febr 5.

more viable, healthy solutions with probiotic urban biotopes in our homes, offices, schools, hospitals, and factories?

4.6. Transgenic Animals and Enhanced Humans

Humans have always bred animals and plants across species lines for their own purposes. These include varieties of hybrid crops and trees, as well as animals such as mules (father a donkey, mother a horse) and hinnies (father a horse, mother a donkey). The latter are not considered a new species, as they are mostly sterile and cannot produce offspring. Crossbreeding between humans and animals is abundant in mythology, particularly among the gods and goddesses of various traditions. Lamassu, a figure with wings, a lion's body, and a human head and face, was a powerful mythological being of Assyria. Many such statues have been excavated in Nimrud, where they protected the Mesopotamian capital since the 10th Century B.C. They symbolize the human vision and drive to manipulate and cultivate properties of different species into human culture.[29] In Greek mythology, Daedalus made feathered wings for his son and himself, but Icarus flew so close to the sun that his wings burned (in medical talk, a spontaneous 'hyperacute rejection' occurred), and he fell down. Science fiction novels and movies have presented humanoids from other planets who share intelligence and walking upright with us, but differ in feelings, life span, and other properties. As such, they represent human visions of power, beauty, and intelligence that we perceive as lacking in ourselves.

Good scientific results and financial benefits have been achieved by producing transgenic animals in agriculture by embryonic stem cell transfer, DNA transfer from one cell into another, and the use of recombinant retroviruses. Benefits have been seen in improved food production (e.g., milk) and health in farm animals.[30] Also expanding the universe of bios are recent products of animal–machine hybrids such as crawling or flying insects, the muscles of which are stimulated and directed remotely by electrodes and which might be used for search-and-rescue missions in emergencies or for military attacks. Manufacturing is no longer solely a domain of science fiction.[31] The U.S. Defense

[29] Lamassu has been chosen as organizational logo by the International Xenotransplantation Association IXA and its journal 'Xenotransplantation.'

[30] Pursel VG et al. Dunham RA, Devilin RH 1999 Comparison of Traditional Breeding and Transgenesis in farmed fish with implications for growth enhancement and fitness, in: Transgenic Animals Agriculture, pp. 209-229; Lai L et al. 2006 Generation of cloned transgenic pigs rich in omega-3 fatty acids, in: Nature Biotechnology, p. 435f; Wheeler MB et al. 2003 Transgenic Animals in Biomedicine and Agriculture. Outlook for the Future, in: Animal Reproduction Science 79: 265-289.

[31] Wells HG 1869 The Island of Doctor Moreau, New York: Stone & Kimball; Wilson DH 2012 Robocalypse. New York: Random House; Wilson DH 2013 Amped. New York Random House.

Advanced Projects Agency (DARPA) studies animal–machine devices to be used in warfare or other situations[32] and has also sponsored research.

Recent successes in gene transfer and DNA manipulation have enabled a variety of techniques for the production of hybrids between humans and animals, such as rats and mice for research in medicines for humans. Examples include strategically designed onco-mice[33] and transgenic rats with human Autosomal Dominant Polycystic Kidney Disease (ADPKD).[34] Generations of pigs have been permanently modified to make their enzymatic and DNA setup more and more similar to human properties so that their kidneys, hearts, and other organs might be transplanted into humans. A European Biotechnology Directive of 1998[35] with minimal influence on patent law suggests in diplomatic terminology that 'modifying genetic properties of animals which are likely to cause them suffering without substantial medical benefit to man or animal … should not be patentable.' But the Directive fails to define the terms 'substantial benefit' and 'suffering' in regard to animals or humans. A 2005 empirical study among 511 diabetes patients in England (316) and Australia (195) asked about their willingness to accept transplants of organs, tissue, or cells. The positive answers were as follows: from humans 85% and 94%, from pigs 68% and 85%, and from non-human primates 67% and 82%.[36] Albert Schweitzer's 'reverence for life' and Fritz Jahr's 'respect every living being' can be used to interpret this 2005 review of patients' responses and the future progress of manipulating non-human bodies, tissues, and cells.

---

[32] www.darpa.mil; Michel Maharbiz, University of California, Berkeley, and his team have developed remote-controlled giant flower beetles in collaboration with Nanyang Technological University of Singapore; cf Yang S 2015 Cyborg Beetle Research Allows Free-flight Study of Insects, in: UC Berkeley, Media Relations 04-16-2015.

[33] The term *OncoMouse* and the genetic properties of this new cross-breed originally were patented to Harvard University in 1988 by the U.S. Patent and Trademark Office, Patent 4.736,866 as 'a transgenic non-human mammal whose germ cells and somatic cells contain a recombinant activated oncogene sequence introduced into said animal.' But in August 2004, a U.S. Patent, no. 6.781.030, on 'methods for cloning mammals using telophase oocytes (egg cells)' did not exclude human oocytes; the European Patent Convention, art. 53a, reserves the right not to issue a patent, using loosely worded language, if issuing such a patent would be contrary to the 'ordre public.'

[34] Koupepidou P et al. 2010 Cyst Formation in the PKD2 (1-703) Transgenic Rat precedes Deregulation of Proliferation-related Pathways, in: Nephrology 11:23; Gretz N, Kraenzlin B et al. 1996 Rat Models of Autosomal Dominant Kidney Disease, in: Nephrology, Dialysis, Transplantation 11(Suppl. 6):46-51; Sass HM 1997 Moral Aspects of Risk and Innovation, in: Artificial Organs 21(11): 1217-1221; Sass HM 1997 Ethics in the Application of Highly Advanced Medical Technologies, in: Artificial Organs 22(3):263-268.

[35] European Biotechnology Directive 1998, art. 6.

[36] Ellison T 2006 Ethics and Xenotransplantation, in: Xenotransplantation 13(6):505-509; for other public opinion polls see HFFA (Human Fertilization and Embryo Authority) 2007 Hybrids and Chimeras, London: HFFA; Jones DA 2009 What does the British public think about human-animal hybrid embryos, in: J Medical Ethics 35:168-170.

How would we describe the pain of mice suffering from human cancer and of rats with human Huntington's disease[37] or ADPKD who have been exposed to aggressive research for the benefit of humans? On the basis of comparative information from neuroscience and from individual expressions of pain, we must assume that the suffering of mammals is similar to that of humans, but a precise translation is difficult and becomes more so the more distant the animal bios (e.g., fish, plants, microbes, and other creatures) is from the human. It is surprising and unfortunate that scant research has been done to discern potentially changed patterns and properties of suffering in transgenic animals as compared with non-transgenic ones. The degree and specificity of pain would probably depend on the new transgenic properties and setup. The issue becomes even more pressing when making animals such as transgenic pigs more and more human-like in as many biological properties as possible, all of which are warranted for successful and safe transplantation of organs or tissues into humans.

Chimpanzees are high on the list of endangered species, so they are no longer candidates for transplanting their organs into humans.[38] Baboon–organs are too small for successful transplantation, and because as primates they are relatively close to us, the risk of transmitting diseases increases.[39] At the moment, pigs are the best candidates for step-by-step genetic modification towards more human-like properties in the setup of as many similar or equivalent properties as possible.[40] Because of the risk that diseases and pathogens virulent in animals but rarely so in humans might become a threat to us by means of xenografts, the U.S. Federal Drug Administration issued regulations a dozen years ago stating that all humans given xenografts must be monitored for the rest of their lives.[41] Also, various forms of rejection of organs, tissue, or cells may occur in individual cases, similar to hyperactive, acute vascular, or cellular rejections by transplantation of organs or cells from human to human. New models in manipulation of immunological properties in pigs raised for potential transplantation may promise progress in making transgenic pigs even more

[37] Underwood BR et al., 2006 Huntington disease patients and transgenic mice have similar pro-catabolic serum metabolic profiles, in: Brain 129(4):877-886.

[38] A small number of chimpanzees survived earlier research in a Texas facility; they now are living in an animal nursing home with a playground and swimming pool in Basel, Switzerland, on the campus of Novartis.

[39] Michler R 1996 Xenotransplantation: Risk, Clinical Potential and Future Prospects, in: Emerging Infectious Diseases 2(1):64-70.

[40] Dooldeniya MD, Warrens AN 2003 Xenotransplantation. Where are we today? in: Journal of the Royal Society of Medicine 96(3):111-117.

[41] USA, Federal Drug Administration 2001 Guidance for Industry: Source Animal Product, Preclinical, and Clinical Issues Concerning the Use of XT Products in Humans. Washington DC.

'human-like' than before, thereby becoming valuable donors of cells and organs for suffering or dying humans.[42]

However, even if these biological and medical problems related to the safety and survivability of the human body are reduced, remaining issues might become more pressing as progress in xenografting continues. Will better models of transgenic animal life feel pleasure and pain similar to that of non-transgenic pigs and other mammals while sharing some neurological properties with humans because of their new transgenic setup? Although they might not become sentient beings similar to us, their experiences of angst and their anticipation of risk, pain, and pain memory will doubtless change.

From neuroscience we know that measurable neuronal activity can be related and translated to feelings of despair, pain, and pleasure.[43] When considering a new breed of humanoids or trans-humans, neuroethics displays a truly humanistic concern about the genuinely human properties of liberty, angst, pain, and pleasure, but it has given little consideration to neuroscience issues in animals or in transgenic non-human life. In the words of a 2014 editorial in *Cambridge Quarterly*: 'The worry that cognitive enhancement poses a threat to authenticity presupposes that there is an authentic self, and authenticity is commonly understood in terms of psychological interaction. If this is correct, it is obvious why neuroethics has had little interest in non-human animals. For a common belief in regard to the minds of animals is that they lack such a sophisticated conscious mental life.'[44]

While little neuroethical research information is available for transgenic animals in comparison to non-transgenic ones, it has been suggested that animal research involving pain in animals is less acceptable if the goal of research is to improve human pleasure in comparison to the reduction of human pain and suffering.[45] Also, we need to learn more about xenotransplants into humans for neurological purposes. Partially successful experiments involving implanting neuronal cells from pigs into non-human primates with a Parkinson model significantly improved locomotor function. During the study, some monkeys also received genetically engineered human neural precursor cells and

[42] Li K, Kwon DN et al. 2014 Engraftment of human iPS cells and allogeneic porcine cells into pigs with inactivated RAG2 and accompanying severe combined immunodeficiciency, in: Proceedings of the National Academy of Science USA 111(20):7260-7265.

[43] Loveless SE, Giordano J 2014 Neuroethics, Painience and Neurocentric Criteria for the Moral Treatment of Animals, in: Cambridge Quarterly of Health Care Ethics 23(2):163-172; cf. also Buller T 2014 Animal Minds and Neuroimaging, in lc: 173-181.

[44] Editorial of a special issue 'Neuroethics and Animals' of the Cambridge Quarterly of Healthcare Ethics by Buller T, Shriver A, Farah M 2014:124-128.

[45] Shriver AJ 2014 The Asymmetrical Contribution of Pleasure and Pain in Animal Research, in: Cambridge Quarterly of Healthcare Ethics 23(2):152-162.

immunosuppressive therapy to prevent rejection, but with questionable success.[46]

I suggest that as long as neuroscientific and medical research options are in development, we should be careful with transgenic and xenograft research. We should be even more so with related applications as long we know so little about their implications on painience and sentience on both sides: (1) animals made more and more humanlike in certain properties and (2) humans enriched or compensated in properties of organs, tissue, and cells via CRISR/Cas9 or other processes.[47] Humane treatment of animals and other forms of bios cannot be based on reciprocity and mutual respect, but it should focus on human responsibility in bio-science and bio-ethics towards all forms of life, as discussed by Jahr and others. Even those who accept crossbreed animals such as mules and who support the eradication or mitigation of human diseases such as Chorea Huntington or ADPKD might on bio-ethical grounds perceive 'sentient' transgenic animals and biochemically 'enhanced' fellow humans as an eccentricity in human bios and an aberration in human culture. McNamee,[48] who discusses recent research on chimeras in Britain, criticizes sensational media reporting but expects that extended public discourse and sound public policy will affect future developments. Individuals in research and other fields of manipulation, as well as social and political bodies, would do well to act according to the old Roman slogan 'quidquid agis, prudenter agas, and respice finem': whatever you do, do it wisely and think about the outcome. Fritz Jahr put it this way[49]:

ETHICS TOWARDS BIOS HAS NO BORDERS

'This is the issue: when we have a compassionate heart towards animals, then we will not withhold our compassion and help towards suffering humans. If someone's love is great enough to go beyond the borders of human-only and sees the sanctity even in the most miserable creature, he or she will find this sanctity as well in the poorest and lowest fellow human, will hold it high and will not reduce it to class or society, interest group, one party or what else may be considered. On the other hand, senseless cruelty towards animals is an indi-

---

46 Ekser B, Cooper DKC, Starzl TE 2011 Clinical xenotransplantation; the next medical revolution, in The Lancet Oct 21, 2011doi:10.1016/S0140-6736(11)61091-X.

47 Sass HM 1996 Verantwortung und ethische Herausforderung, in: Transgene Tiere. Basel: Ciba.

48 McNamee SP 2015 Human-Animal Hybrids and Chimeras. What's in a Name? in: Jahr 6(1)(11):45-66 (this article also includes a valuable list of websites and blogs discussing issues of hybridization).

49 Jahr F 1928 Tierschutz und Ethik in ihren Beziehungen zueinander, in: Ethik. Sexual- und Gesellschaftsethik. Organ des Ethikbundes 4(6/7):101; Engl. transl., 'Animal Protection and Ethics,' in Jahr F 2013 l.c. 36.

cation of an unrefined character and is dangerous towards the human biotope (*Umgebung*) *as well.'*

5. RESEARCH ON ANIMALS FOR HUMAN HEALTH BENEFIT

LIMITS TO ANIMAL MANIPULATION?

'Those who do surgical and pharmaceutical research on animals or who inoculate them with diseases in order to help humans with potential results, never may feel comfortable that their gruesome action aims at a noble goal. In each individual case, they have to find out whether there really is a pressing urgency to make an animal sacrifice for humankind's good. And fearfully they must take great care to reduce their suffering as much as possible. How much harm is done in institutions of science by not giving anesthetics in order to save time and extra work! How much pain towards animals is produced in order to teach students basic and well-known phenomena! Especially since the animal has earned so much dignity in being an object in research for the benefit of suffering humans, a new and unique principle of solidarity has been developed for each of us between the animal and us. This results in a constraint for each of us to do all creatures as much good as possible. When helping an insect out of harm's way, I do nothing else than reduce some of the ever increasing guilt of us humans towards creatures. Whenever an animal is forced to be available to service us humans, we all have to be concerned with the pain associated with such a service.'

Albert Schweitzer, 1923[1]

5.1. Who should be the 'Guinea Pig'?

Albert Schweitzer kept the hospital in Lambarene free of lice, mice, and other unwanted creatures, but in his office he allowed an ant colony to establish a thoroughfare across his desk (he moved his files out of their way). Human cultivation of raw nature includes the cultivation (i.e., breeding and manipulating) of animals for different purposes, including research for the benefit of humans. In 1998, the official number of animals so used in the United States alone was estimated to be over 1.2 million. At that time, rats, mice, and birds were not included because they were not covered by the Animal Welfare Act, and the real number would have been tenfold (~12 million).[2] Today, approximately 50 to 100 million vertebrate animals are used worldwide in medical and cosmetic research; this number does not include microbes, insects and annelids, plants, fungi, and other forms of life.

---

[1] Schweitzer A 1948 Ethik in der Kultur, vol. 2 [2nd ed.], München: Biederstein, 249f.

[2] Bishop LJ, Nolen A 2001 Animals in Research and Education. Washington DC: National Reference Center for Bioethics, Scope Note 40; Animal Welfare Information Center, USDA http:/www.nal.usda.gov/awic.

Globally, animal experimentation is required as a central part in Controlled Clinical Trials (CCTs) to develop medicinal drugs for human health care.[3] Special toxicology tests are required to define the toxic dose necessary to kill 50% of a given animal cohort; it has been estimated that ~~at~~ about one-third of all animal toxicity tests are done for this LD50 (lethal dose 50%) scheme, which dates back to the 1920s. Approximately 5,000 animals are needed for each chemical tested in medicine and about 12,000 for testing agricultural products.[4] Testing is done orally; by intravenous, intramuscular, or subcutaneous injection; and by inhalation. Anesthesia in LD50 tests is not allowed, as it might interfere with testing results. Long-term tests of up to three or more months are required for studies of long-term harm to human organs. The Draize Test for eye irritancy is applied to test substances for cosmetics or in ophthalmology; if severe pain or distress occurs, the Organization for Economic Cooperation and Development (OECD) suggests that animals be killed.[5] The validity of efficacy tests in animals for use in humans is not more than a hint. According to regulations for placebo CCTs, studies in dosage increases and efficacy have to be done on human probands anyway.

---

[3] The website of DoSomething.Org, quoting PETA (People for the Ethical Treatment of Animals) lists the following 11 arguments against animal experimentation: '(1) Over 100 million animals are burned, crippled, poisoned, and abused in US labs every year. (2) 92% of experimental drugs that are safe and effective in animals fail in human clinical trials because they are too dangerous or don't work. (3) Labs that use mice, rats, birds, reptiles and amphibians are exempted from the minimal protections under the Animal Welfare Act (AWA). (4) Up to 90% of animals used in U.S. labs are not counted in the official statistics of animals tested. Take a stand by kidnapping your friends' products that were tested on animals (seriously!). (5) Europe, the world's largest cosmetic market, Israel and India have already banned animal testing for cosmetics, and the sale or import of newly animal-tested beauty products. (6) Even animals that are protected under the AWA can be abused and tortured. And the law doesn't require the use of valid alternatives to animals, even if they are available. (7) According to the Humane Society, registration of a single pesticide requires more than 50 experiments and the use of as many as 12,000 animals. (8) When used in cosmetic tests, mice, rats, rabbits, and guinea pigs are often subjected to skin and eye irritation tests where chemicals are rubbed on shaved skin or dripped into the eyes without any pain relief. (9) In tests of potential carcinogens, subjects are given a substance every day for 2 years. Other tests involve killing pregnant animals and testing their fetuses. (10) The real-life applications for some of the tested substances are as trivial as an 'improved' laundry detergent, new eye shadow, or copycat drugs to replace a profitable pharmaceutical whose patent expired. (11) Alternative tests achieve one or more of the "3 R's:" replaces a procedure that uses animals with a procedure that doesn't, reduces the number of animals used in a procedure, refines a procedure to alleviate or minimize potential animal pain.' Accessed April 15, 2015.

[4] Abbott A 2005 Animal Testing, in: Nature 438(7065)144-146; cf. Wikipedia: Animal Testing.

[5] OECD, Guideline 405; Secchi A, Deligianni V 2006 Ocular Toxicology. The Draize Test, in: Current Opinion in Allergy and Clinical Immunology 6(5)367-372.

Principled self-experiments in which doctors[6] tested new medicines and devices on themselves first have been reported over the centuries in many cultures of physicians' ethics. Unfortunately, even the most promising and life-saving results from self-sacrificing experimentation would not meet the criteria of modern bureaucracies in regulatory agencies today. Various species of vertebrate animals, frogs, and other animals are still used in medical education as required by curricula regulation, but the educational benefit has been questioned. Fortunately, vivisection of humans has long been outlawed. Different cultures represent different traditions and visions, but they share common concerns, intuitions, and visions regarding health, life, and environment, among them compassion for non-human beings. We have already seen that most cultures have a favorable understanding of the closeness of humanity to nature and its laws and limits, including respect and compassion for other living beings and plants. But moral concern is mostly about the use of sentient animals for the benefit of humans. Even the scientific validity and usefulness of using intact animal models for research in human medicine has been controversially debated, particularly for testing antibacterials.[7]

When Drosophila insects and non-human primates such as chimpanzees are both good models for the study of neurodegenerative diseases in humans, which animal model should be chosen? We would probably choose drosophila and restrict other unavoidable research issues to non-human primates rather than to patients with Alzheimer's disease. Such decisions are in line with millennia-old ethics that family and friends come first, but that we should not do harm to others without reason and judgment, as expressed in the Bioethical Imperative. Even though we cannot determine precisely how pain and harm differ between species, we might assume that bodily or psychological harm does differ between humans, non-human primates, mammals, fish, cephalopods, microbes, and so forth. But this is just an assumption because we lack the ability to translate neuronal or biochemical information from all of these beings into feeling pain, being under stress, calling for help, or screaming. Comparative neurology and biochemistry have been negligent in researching pain-and-suffering issues across the bios kingdom. We need more species-specific information on the well being of specific species in captivity. Aspects to be investigated might include normal life conditions, states of happiness and absence of harm, and the influences of environment, foods and drink, light, noise, smell, loneliness, and day-and-night cycles. Annelids primarily have both sectoral and somewhat interrelated nerve systems; how do we compare their nerve associations with pain as we feel it? Starfish have somewhat circular brain connections; depending on

---

[6] Altman LK 1987 Who Goes First. The Story of Self-Experimentation in Medicine. University of California Press; Boring M, Dendy L, Mordan CB 2005 Guinea Pig Scientists. Bold Self-Experimenters in Science and Medicine. NY: Henry Holt.

[7] Greek A, Hansen LA 2013 The Strengths and Limits of Animal Models as Illustrated by the Discovery and Development of Antibacterials, in: Biological Systems 2:109.

their neuronal wiring, do they feel pain separately or simultaneously? Vertebrates possess central nerve systems similar to those of humans, but what are the differences in their pain experience and how can research arrangements reduce it? Do we owe more compassion to dogs and cats, our cultural companions over thousands of years, and should we avoid using them in medical experiments? Berkeley[8] noted that each individual has his or her own feelings of pain, lust, and distress. He asserted that only from our own such experiences and by looking at fellow humans' behavior, facial expressions, and screams or laughter can we assume indirectly that they have similar feelings. We also know from our own experience that memories of pain and pleasure vary and are not identical with feelings we once had. Of course, intensities of comfort and discomfort appear in neuroscientific experiments, but as to their translation into subjective, existential feelings of pain and pleasure we still have no more knowledge than Berkeley did. How much more difficult will be the translation of neurochemical and other information from plants, microbes, and animals into bioethical regulation of research on bios.

Early regulations by the U.S. Department of Agriculture (USDA) did not include rats, mice, and birds. The U.S. District Court of the District of Columbia found that the definition 'animal' in the U.S. Animal Welfare Act was arbitrary and in violation of the Act itself. It ordered the USDA to change the rules, but a U.S. Court of Appeals overturned the verdict on the somewhat formal grounds that the plaintiffs 'did not demonstrate constitutional standing to sue and/or a statutory right to judicial review under the Administrative Procedure Act.[9] Later, in 2000, the USDA agreed to regulate rats, mice, and birds as well.[10] These legal quarrels demonstrate visibly our cultural uncertainties in dealing with different species – even vertebrates – in the moral and legal guidance of animal research. A European Commission Report on animal welfare committees called for replacing animal research by 'non-sentient material.'[11] Are Drosophila less sentient than guinea pigs or primates? Drosophila can learn and remember situations in which sugar makes them 'happy' and its absence 'unhappy'; how would one translate their 'happiness' and 'memory' into sentient language? What are the 'sentient' communication levels of viruses and bacteria within different tissue cells? What kind of information or 'cries for help' are sent out by green corn plants into the surrounding biotope via their roots when their stems are cut off? Is there a sort of stress, pain, or pleasure felt even in tissue research or cell and DNA segment manipulation? Research regulations routinely fail to define 'sentient' or 'non-sentient,' but they use those labels nevertheless. Buddhists and Hindi at least would support the widest possible definition of 'competent com-

[8] Berkeley G 1713 Dialogues between Hylas and Philonous, London.
[9] Animal Legal Defense Fund vs. Secretary of Agriculture; Decision May 20, 1994.
[10] http://www.labanimal.com/col/reg1100.htm.
[11] European Commission 2005 Animal welfare committees in the European research area. Luxemburg: EC: EUR 21786, p.13.

passion' with all forms of bios, which would include insects and microbes used as research subjects. The European Commission Community Research report suggests analyzing and assessing the 'ethical assumptions and frameworks of AWCs' (Animal Welfare Committees).[12] But confusion and inadequate understanding of terminology, rules, and regulations have been documented among AWC members.[13]

5.2. The Seven-R Principles in Animal Research

An indication of a sensitivity towards cruelty to animals in research across the lines of religions and traditions is the wide acceptance of the three-R principles of replace, reduce, and refine as presented in 1959 by W.M.S. Russell and R.L. Burch.[14] They called for the replacement of sentient living animals with no sentient animals or materials, reduction of the number of animals used in an experiment or procedure, and refinement of techniques to decrease the incidences or amount of animal distress. The Indian term for 'do not kill' (in the broader sense 'respect the stream of life') is *ahimsa,* based on the Hindu/Buddhist notion of seeing 'all living things as incarnation of a single life force.'[15] These three R's – *replace, reduce, refine* – are basic principles to improve the design and ethics of animal experimentation and they must guide research companies as well as national and international regulations and self-regulations. To these three principles, I add four more: *respect, review, rehabilitate, and relate.* They broaden the bioethical and cultural oversight and reduce the risk of using animals for the benefit of human health and society.

Replace: The use of conscious living beings should be replaced, if possible, by tissue cultures, perfused organs, tissue, or cells. Costs might be reduced thereby and research made more efficient. The original 1959 concept of 'sentience' was quite narrow and de facto has been applied primarily to primates and mammals. It should be extended and redefined based on specific new research for all forms of bios. New mathematical and heuristic models and overdue modifications in traditional four-phase trials (discussed in the next chapter) will also contribute to replacing the number of living beings in research.

---

[12] European Commission 2005, EUR 21786:39. 'Directive 2010/63/EU on the protection of animals used for scientific purposes,' which updates and replaces the 1986 Directive 86/609/EEC, was updated in 2010 and implemented in 2013.

[13] Schuppli CA, Fraser D 2005 The interpretation and application of the 3 R's by animal ethics committee members. ATLA 33:487-500.

[14] Russell WMS, Burch RL 1959 The Principles of Human Experimentation Techniques. London

[15] Pereira S, Tettamanti M 2005 Ahimsa and Alternatives. Aatex 22:3-6; Boo de J, Knight A 2008 Increasing the Implementation of Alternatives to Laboratory Animal Use. Aatex 13(3)109-117, quoting from a 2004 CPCSEA report to the Indian government on animals in research. Based on the Hinduist ahimsa principle, CPCSEA has recommended adding 'Rehabilitation' of research animals to the three-R principles: reduce, refine, replace.

Reduce: The number of animals involved should be reduced by using better statistics (not too few, not too many animals) and by avoiding overregulation and the unnecessary repetition of experiments.

Refine: Refine research strategies to minimize distress, harm, and pain, providing species-specific environments and treatment.

Respect: A 'respect for animals' principle will strengthen the introduction of the Bioethics Imperative into animal research ('Respect every living being as an end in itself and treat it, if possible, as such!'). It should not exclude non-mammals from being respected and must also take into account transcultural attitudes towards animals and their relationship with humans. Respect also includes honoring the involuntary contributions of research animals who suffered and died for humans. Ceremonies in disposing of tissue, organs, or animals used in research might be appropriate, to give thanks in a dignified way to victims of the search for remedies for human diseases.[16] Cosmetic research for human benefit associated with painful experiments on animals might not be acceptable in many cultures, and companies selling such products should provide relevant information to their customers. Research experiments using pigs to develop medicines often find reserved acceptance among Muslim or Jewish individuals; therefore, information about products based on or including substances derived from processed animal tissue should be labeled as such.

Review: Animal Welfare Committees are the instrument of choice to review and improve animal research on the local level and to reconcile different approaches and set standards on the national or transnational level. Corporate AWCs are indispensable, as only they can develop experience and set global standards, refine general corporate animal welfare policy for the local ethical and cultural environment, and relate their experiences and insights to regulatory bodies and the public. It is important that an open, internal discourse on methods, uncertainties, risks, shortcomings, and goals in animal research be held on the corporate level and continued without financial or other pressure. Equally important to communication and–cooperation with outside research partners are exchanging information and experiences, sharing basic guidelines and procedures, having a process of review and governance similar to the one practiced in-house, and having joint training sessions. Corporate AWCs must have access to all expertise within the corporation, preferably directly via members of AWCs or consultants. But corporate AWCs also need expert advice from the outside. Such advice can be provided by experts in ethics and culture and/or by members of moral communities (the so-called Institutional Review Boards [IRBs] reviewing CCTs in humans are well-established and well-received 'community representatives'). If necessary for internal corporate reasons, out-

[16] Japanese Medical Schools routinely hold annual memorial services for animals as victims of experimentation; a group of students at Keio University has started an empirical study on their content and rituals.

side consultants can also lend professional expertise in ethics and cultural attitudes. It is my experience that 'lay people' from the outside offer a useful service within the committee, as they introduce language and arguments that can be integrated directly into the reasoning and decision-making process. Also, lay people ask helpful questions based on ignorance that would never be formulated by purely professional experts.

Rehabilitate: Buddhist and Hindi interpretations of 'respect for the stream of life' have initiated regulation in some Indian states to honor animal survivors of medical experimentation and to allow them to end their lives naturally – and even find rehabilitation. Example of this noble and distinguished form of recognizing fellow living beings as partners in science include an Indian law that surviving research animals be send to rehabilitation centers and a pharmaceutical company in Basel that hosts surviving non-human primates in retirement quarters.

Relate: Animal research and its ethics are integral parts of medical and pharmacological research, including research in veterinary medicine. It is beneficial for animal research as well as for the company conducting it to relate issues, solutions, and even uncertainties as transparently, simply, and coherently as possible. Interrelating corporate policy, ethics, and profile with animal research labs from the top level throughout all sections and departments is the preferred design for developing a corporation's profile and accomplishing its mission. Such an integrated, well-supported corporate mission profile fosters: 1) internal leadership, encouragement, pride, and responsibility and 2) external respect, understanding, and support from the public and various moral communities; from the media, lawmakers, and regulators; and also from outspoken critics of medical experimentation (in particular foes of animal experimentation). Towards ideological enemies of animal research, only serious concentration on the corporation's core mission (of which animal research is for ethical and practical reasons one of the parts) will demonstrate persuasively the shortcomings of simplifications by critics and their disrespect for both suffering fellow humans and the great achievements and goals of modern medical research. The "relate" principle shares corporate profile and mission, research experience and design, corporate communication, cultural and ethical concerns, stakeholder relations, and public opinion and information — all in one integrated model. Following this principle not only benefits the corporation and its public image, but also improves future research design by integrating new input from internal and external sources into corporate research design and policy. National legislation and regulation also need to relate to cultural and moral traditions, fundamental rights issues, professional expertise, market rules, and public opinion and expectations. International governance bodies and professional organizations also have to find ways to relate and translate their recommendations and standards into global and local cultures, recognizing basic bioethical rights, market mechanisms, and their professional duties and possibilities.

5.3. Research Ethics, Bioethics, Corporate Ethics

Animal research and its attendant ethics are an integral part of the corporate mission of pharmaceutical companies, who act as good corporate neighbors by providing much-needed, efficacious medicines for fellow humans and for animals. It is important that this overall mission guides and governs animal research internally and externally. A global corporate neighbor needs to have a consistent global personality, set of corporate virtues, and moral and professional profile. Such a profile has to adjust to local sensitivities, cultures, and customs, but it also needs to withstand the test of global fundamentals in bioethics and governance. Individuals and corporations have to be open about their principles, visions, and actions, fairly and coherently. Regulatory compliance with national rules, customs, guidelines, regulations, and laws is important; so is the respect for international rules and guidelines. But regulatory and oversight bodies must also listen and learn from the hands-on experience of corporations and animal welfare officers[17]. No person should live by formally respecting rules and regulations alone. Similarly, corporate persons should, based on their specific character and special culture, translate and transform regulations and laws into their corporate profile to promote competent cooperation and compassion within the company and to present the corporate character profile in the local and global neighborhood. Communicative competence requires more than simply information, it includes personal involvement and compassion inside and outside the company. Much can be achieved by finding and applying a common mutual language in identifying technical and ethical issues, risks, goals, and concerns openly and fairly. Also important is dialog with critics and openness towards customers about bioethical issues they might be concerned with. Open discourse and communication/cooperation in trust with partners and stakeholders, not only with patients and prospective patients, will make the corporate person stronger. This strength will translate directly into the successful application and improvement of the seven R principles in dealing with animals in a dignified, compassionate way (i.e., in a more cultivated corporate policy than required by laws and regulations).

5.4. Risk Reduction Outline in Animal Research

The 2,500-year-old Taoist tradition says: 'We make doors and windows for a room; but it is these empty spaces that make the room livable. Thus, while the tangible has advantages, it is the intangible that makes it useful.'[18] In regard to research with animals for human benefit, we may paraphrase the Taoist insight

---

[17] I gratefully express thanks to corporate Animal Welfare Officers (AWO's) which I met at a global conference in Switzerland.

[18] Dao Te Ching 11.

this way: 'We make rules and regulations for animal research, but it is our personal, societal, and corporate competence, compassion, and cultivation that make animal research livable. While laws and regulations have advantages, it is our values and visions that make animal research useful.'

Below is a risk reduction strategy I have used successfully in corporate consultations for the biotechnical and bioethical improvement of CCTs, here adjusted for the implementation of the seven R's (replace, refine, reduce, respect, review, rehabilitate, and relate) with animals as stakeholders. In animal experimentation, they are not reciprocal partners in design and decision-making, but they are our most valuable and noble stakeholders.

ANIMAL RESEARCH RISK REDUCTION SCHEME

1. IDENTIFY DATA AND ISSUES
- *1.1. Collect technical (medical) data*
- *1.2. Collect animal data*
- *1.3. Collect value data*
- *1.4. Discuss interrelation with seven-R principles*

2. DEVELOP ALTERNATIVE OPTIONS
- *2.1. Establish reasonable options*
- *2.2. Refine options using seven-R principles*
- *2.3. Identify risk-and-harm features*
- *2.4. Fine-tune application discussion*

3. PRESENT PREFERRED OPTION
- *3.1. Present research risk/benefit in selection*
- *3.2. Present animal harm/risk feature*
- *3.3. Discuss with stakeholders using seven R's*
- *3.4. Discuss medical and moral uncertainties*

4. JUSTIFY YOUR SELECTION
- *4.1. Summarize reasons for selection*
- *4.2. Review AWC's input using seven R's*
- *4.3. Formulate objections to your selection*
- *4.4. Use seven R's in corporate profile and outreach*

6. HUMAN SUBJECTS IN RESEARCH

RESEARCH AND KNOWLEDGE, A GIFT FROM HEAVEN

When the wise man and prophet Moses was ill, the doctors offered him medicine. But Moses said: 'If God gave sickness to me, he will also take it away, when he decides to do so.' The next day, when Moses felt worse, the doctors argued: 'Your God created all the wonderful herbs and other sources for remedies, and he gave us doctors the intelligence for research and for producing medical remedies from nature.' Moses accepted that argument, that medical research and research results can be considered a 'gift from heaven'; he took the medicine and got well.

Narrative reported by Persian philosopher Al Ghazali, 1056–1111 AD

6.1. Medical Research and Care Are Moral Obligations

Medical research and drug development are not only justifiable; they are morally mandatory for reasons of solidarity with and support for fellow humans, in particular those who suffer, are sick, or are in pain. Compassion with other forms of bios, especially with close ones, has fostered cooperation and integration with other fundamental human C properties to develop medicines and promote healthy foods and lifestyles. The improvement of diagnosis and therapy to benefit patients, prevent disease, and alleviate suffering finds strong support in the religious and philosophical traditions of all major cultures. Progress in Hippocratic medicine resulted from expertise in the medicinal properties of herbs and foodstuffs, observation and modification of patients' lifestyles, and instruction in the so-called 'res non-naturales' (cultivating the harmony of sleeping and being awake, working and relaxing, balancing nutrition, and regulating emotions). Caring for health and improving knowledge in that field is predicated on trust-based communication and cooperation between experts and laypersons. Confucian scholar Mencius aptly observed that 'a person with good virtue will surely have longevity.'[1] In addition to traditional means of teaching and healing, self-experimentation and new innovative therapies have evolved over the centuries. We do not know whether doctors treated Moses with traditional interventions or in innovative, experimental ways. Systematic, extensive medical research began in academic hospitals and pharmaceutical companies only in the 19th century, again with the dual purpose of helping patients and improving clinical knowledge.[2]

---

[1] Cf. Sass HM 2006 Bioethics and Biopolitics, Xian, 362; when I asked an internationally recognized philosophy professor at Beijing University, who had studied with Husserl and Heidegger, about his age, Hsiung Wei smiled and proudly replied 'I am three years older than Confucius ever got.'

[2] Beecher HK 1958 Experimentation in Man. Springfield Ill.: CC Thomas; Foucault M 1973 The Birth of the Clinic, transl. AM Sheridan-Smith. London: Tavistock; Pappworth MH 1968 Human Guinea Pigs. Experimentation on Man. Boston MA: Beacon; Spicker SF, Alon I, de Vries a, HT Engelhard ed. 1988 The Use of Human Beings in Research. With Special Reference to Clinical Trials. Dordrecht: Kluwer.

Because patients and probands are fellow humans, it would be immoral to treat them like stones, dirt, or laboratory mice. It would violate the Bioethical Imperative to treat other forms of life simply as means and not respect them as ends in themselves, - also: lab mice or cut flowers in a vase cannot consent to their treatment. While animal research and manipulation for animal/human welfare are based on principles and regulations and are protected by animal welfare officers in research companies, as we have discussed, patients and probands are informed beforehand in general. This step depends on the researchers' own knowledge of medical facts and regulations and the intended procedures to reduce risk, gain insight, and seek treatments that improve or even save patients' lives – potentially helping many others in similar situations. This principle of *informed consent* seems to have been mentioned first in an official Prussian government directive of 1891 in regard to Robert Koch's experiments with tuberculin in Prussian prisons: 'The application of Professor Dr. Koch's remedy can according to a memorandum of the Minister of Religious, Educational and Medical Issues only be recommended when the prison doctor is familiar with the procedure and when there is a special hospital ward in the prison. Also, the prison doctor has to live in the facility, so he can provide the necessary surveillance to the patient. A condition is that the treatment with Koch's remedy occurs only in new cases and in similar situations and not against the will of the patient'.[3]

Traditionally, the goals of improving biomedical knowledge and health care services to everyone include not only better treatment of disease but also disease prevention and the enhancement of health. As far as medical research involving human subjects is concerned, a no-harm principle (*nonmaleficence, primum nil nocere*) must be balanced with the ethical goal of promoting health care knowledge. Yet research involving humans has been cruel and disrespectful to individuals subjected to pain, illness, and even death without their consent or knowledge. Because of this, only minimal risk to human subjects should be accepted, and clinical research requires the highest forms of quality assurance and control, including high ethical standards. The U.S. Presidential Commission for the Study of Bioethical Issues[4] names as a 'Common Rule' the necessity of '*informed consent, independent ethical review, and the minimization of avoidable risk.*'

---

[3] Quoted in Wienau R 1996 Medizin und Menschenversuch. Zur Geschichte des Informed Consent, in: Wiesemann C, Frewer A ed., Medizin und Ethik im Zeichen von Auschwitz. Erlangen: Enke, p. 20; the official Prussian Regulations for New Therapy and Scientific Research of 1900, in: Centralblatt fuer die gesamte Unterrichtsverwaltung in Preussen, 1901(2)189-190, made minimal harm and informed consent essential preconditions for using human subjects in clinical research.

[4] Presidential Commission for the Study of Bioethical Issues 2011 Moral Science. Protecting Participants in Human Subjects Research, Washington DC, p. 2

Partners and stakeholders in risk assessment and quality control are individuals as well as teams and corporations, oversight bodies, and regulatory agencies. In modern bioethics, the four principles of *autonomy non-maleficence, beneficence, and justice* form the core for developing and reviewing clinical research. Autonomy (respect for persons) translates into the informed consent principle, nonmaleficence (*primum nil nocere*) into risk–benefit-assessment and minimal risk principles, beneficence and justice into the fair selection of probands and patients. Sponsors of clinical research are essential stakeholders and need to have instruments in place for internal and external quality control and support: 'The ethical justification of biomedical research involving human subjects is the prospect of discovering new ways of benefiting people's health. Such research can be ethically justified only if it is carried out in ways that respect and protect, and are fair to, the subjects of that research and are morally acceptable within the communities in which the research is carried out.'[5] Central features in clinical research and drug development, supported by basic ethical reasoning and national and transnational guidelines and regulations, are as follows: (1) the free and informed consent of the patient or proband, (2) a research protocol with strong features of risk assessment and control, (3) the oversight, approval, and review and/or guidance of an ethics committee: 'A set of internationally recognized ethical and scientific quality requirements ... must be observed for designing, conducting, recording, and reporting clinical trials that involve the participation of human subjects.'[6] Thus, modern clinical research rests heavily on oversight and complex regulation, not on traditional physicians' ethics in caring for the patient. Actually, oversight bodies and committees not involved in direct care and treatment of research subjects are replacing the direct personal responsibility of the physician and the research and leadership teams. It might be time to move back towards less regulation and more professional responsibility and liability, thus regaining a true, lost partnership and a stakeholder model of all involved. Such a turnabout can be made more comfortable by new insurance schemes like worker's compensation and no-fault compensation in research and development, as well as by safeguarding the continuous assessment, distribution, and improvement of new medicines and devices.[7]

6.2. Managing Risk by Regulation?

Risk management in clinical research still follows the four-phase model in combination with animal and tissue research, mostly including randomization and

[5] CIOMS 2002 International Ethical Guidelines for Biomedical Research involving Human Subject. Geneva: CIOMS.

[6] WHO, Directive 2001/20/EC:1(2).

[7] Sass HM 1988 Comparative Models and Goals for the Regulation of Human Research, in: Spicker S et al. ed. The Use of Human Beings in Research. Dordrecht: Kluwer, 47-89; Sass HM 2004 Ethical Risk in Medical Research, in: Enabling Risk Assessment in Medicine. Farewell Symposium for Werner-Karl Raff. Muenster: Lit 83-93.

placebo control. But new coding methods (data protection plus data availability), biometrics, and pharmacogenomics will allow for more efficacious and safer drugs, including 'orphan drugs' for specific metabolizers, diseases, and indications, as well as improved research in 'blockbuster drugs' that involve a lower number of research subjects and feature individualized drug prescription. Bureaucratic regulatory procedures are slow to adapt to these new opportunities. Therefore, biomedical and bioethical openings for new methods of drug development and delivery will have to battle for quite some time with strong forces favoring routine, risk-averse oversight and regulation.

Contemporary regulatory and administrative procedures have reduced moral and professional burdens on researchers, shifting most of the responsibility to oversight or advisory bodies. But ethics committees or institutional review boards (IRBs) must not replace the ethical obligations of the researcher, the team, or the sponsor: the former review and advise only. Unfortunately, research ethics committees or IRBs rarely receive feedback or require immediate information during the protocol, and they rarely receive feedback at the end of the study on their own review quality. Sponsors would benefit by requesting feedback both during and at the end of a study. When multi-center studies have one leading IRB only, then a bioethics coordinator should guarantee that levels of ethics quality and internal bioethics discourse meet the standards of discussions in biometrics. If centers of different traditional cultures are involved in particular developing countries, then culturally sensitive, responsive features need to be designed and reviewed by local IRBs or by neighborhood involvement.

Xiaomei Zhai introduced the principles of '*family and community consent*' for situations in which European-style self-determination and individual autonomy principles are not the only cultural standards on which decisions are being made. Embracing them is important for other cultures as well as traditional ones: like individual humans, all cultures are 'diversified but not identical, harmonized as well as diversified.'[8] The prevailing 'one size fits all' approach of controlled clinical trials (CCTs) and IRBs needs to be reviewed and deregulated in light of the diversity of cultures and individuals, so that the eight C properties and responsibilities of individuals, teams, and corporations can prosper even better and provide for more favorable climates and social biotopes in clinical research. Whenever free, informed decision making by individuals is not part of the dominant local culture, then IRBs (and sponsors) are morally obliged to implement additional features to ensure that subjects, their families, and their communities are not harmed and that they receive educational and health benefits. It is time to re-activate and re-introduce the virtue of personal and

[8] Zhai XM 2011 Diversified and in Harmony, but not Identical. Harmonizing International Guidelines with Cultural Values and National Traditions, in: Asian Bioethics Review 3(1)31-35.

professional responsibility on the part of researchers, research facilities, and corporations.

6.3. Professional Ethics and Corporate Governance

The scope of corporate ethics extends far beyond the existing legal and regulatory requirements of good clinical practice (GCP) and CCTs. Yet in order to be formulated, maxims for ethical missions in drug research and development need to be defined and implemented that include teaching, training, and internal and external communication in support of such virtues and principles. For individuals and teams, the virtues of integrated communication and cooperation, of competence and compassion, of calculation and contemplation, of competition and cultivation will succeed in solidarity, prudence, cleverness, wisdom, and integrity. Hence, the advice of Confucian physician Yang Chuan 1,700 years ago is also true in the research situation when we replace 'physician' with 'researcher' or 'research corporation' and say: 'Trust only those research corporations who have the heart of humaneness and compassion, are clever and wise, sincere and honest.'[9] Comparable maxims for the profile and mission of a corporation or organization based on drug research and development would include *safety, reliability, trustworthiness, and sincerity*. All of these moral requirements for individual health care experts need to be translated into corporate ethics, corporate strategy, and the day-to-day bios of 'clever and wise, sincere and honest' corporate persons (i.e., drug companies and service providers in health care). Of particular importance for good corporate neighbors is the use of modern instruments of communication technology, including well-built web portals and interactive rooms for communication-in-trust and cooperation-in-trust with patients, consumers, and other partners. External risks pertinent to drug research and development include regulatory tendencies to (1) bureaucratization and regulatory support of outdated features and models, (2) powerful cultural and political trends of intellectual technophobia, and (3) changing public attitudes towards concepts of health and disease, health literacy, and the allocation of private and public resources. Because drug development, introduction, and public acceptance will depend on health-literate, competent citizens and fair, informed public discourse, research corporations should not be afraid to disclose risks and benefits and to open questions on drug research, availability, and delivery.

At the end of the 19th century (December 29, 1900), the Prussian government issued the aforementioned regulations on human experimentation. Its directives were printed in the official publication of the Prussian Ministry of Religious, Educational and Medical Affairs (which is similar to the U.S. Federal Register), and they are the first modern regulations by a state authority. Specifically and exclusively directed at medical research, they point out that 'medical

[9] Quoted by Qiu R 1988 Medicine, the Art of Humanness, in: Journal of Medicine and Philosophy 13(3)285f.

interventions for purposes other than diagnosis, therapy, and immunization are absolutely prohibited, even though all other legal and ethical requirements for performing such interventions are fulfilled if: (1) the person in question is a minor or is not fully competent on other grounds; (2) the person concerned has not declared unequivocally that he consents to the interventions; (3) the declaration has not been made on the basis of a proper explanation of the adverse consequences that might result from the intervention'.[10]

Other guidelines had been issued previously for purposes of diagnosis, therapy, and controversial immunization programs. Given the bureaucratic character of the Prussian state and culture, it would be unthinkable that these new ministerial directives would not have been treated with the utmost respect and scrupulously obeyed. Their rigidity is shown by the fact that research on children and incompetent persons was forbidden, and that bending those rules was prohibited. While the Prussian directive covered most of the northern part of the German Reich and the majority of the German population, the Reich Health Council (a central political body advising the Reich government and including representatives of the chambers of physicians, surgeons, and pharmacists; the Sickness Fund; and several central ministries) issued more detailed guidelines on new therapy and human experimentation in 1931.[11] Forms to be signed by all physicians seeking employment in open or closed health care facilities included these regulations; thus, they were part of the employment contract. Membership in medical professional organizations was mandatory, and health care institutions and professional organizations were required to implement these guidelines after they were published by the Reichsminister of the Interior. The 'Final Circular of the Reich Minister of the Interior concerning Guidelines for New Therapy and Human Experimentation,' dated February 28, 1931, was binding law throughout the existence of the Reich.[12] Thus, the Nazi experiments on prisoners, children, and other vulnerable populations violated the Reich's own regulations on legal grounds and on those of professional self-regulation. While they were more detailed than the Prussian instructions, they were somewhat easier on experimentation with children, not outlawing it altogether but calling it impermissible 'if it endangers the child or minor in the slightest degree.' They

[10] Preussisches Ministerium für Religion, Unterricht und Medizin (1900) Instruktionen für die Direktoren der Krankenanstalten und andere medizinische Einrichtungen. Centralblatt der gesamten Unterrichtsverwaltung in Preussen 1900, 188-189; Engl. transl. in: Annas GJ, Grodin MA (1992) The Nazi Doctors and the Nuremberg Code. New York NY: Oxford U Press, p.127.

[11] Sass HM 1983 Reichsrundschreiben 1931: Pre-Nuremberg regulations concerning new therapy and human experimentation, in: J Medicine and Philosophy 8:99-111.

[12] For unknown reasons, the Reich regulations were not included in the Omnibus Law (Ueberleitungsgesetz) passed by the German Bundestag after 1948, which transported hundreds of laws and regulations of the Reich into the Federal Republic's legal structure; see Sass HM 1997 The Nuremberg Code, German Law and Prominent Thinkers, in: J American Medical Association 277(9):709.

included another paragraph never repeated in subsequent regulations or guidelines: 'Experimentation with dying persons conflicts with the principles of medical ethics and therefore is impermissible.'[13] To my knowledge, no other national, international, legal, or professional guidelines on medical research have addressed the immorality of experimenting on dying fellow humans, even though ample anecdotal evidence proves that clinical trials, experimental surgery, and even teaching and hands-on medical training disrespect the dignity of the dying. Also, the Reich Regulations expressively address the importance of research ethics in medical education, an issue not mentioned in recent guidelines or regulations on medical research (§14). These and other groundbreaking features of the 1931 Reich Regulations were stricter than the Nuremberg Code of 1946, the Helsinki–Tokyo Declaration, and other regulations. As the Prussian directive did, they also unequivocally make the medical head of the institution personally and professionally responsible for the design, implementation, and review of human experimentation, a remarkable difference from regulations in force today. The approval of a committee or other collective body was not mandated. The Prussian instruction writes: 'interventions of this nature may be performed only by the director of the institution himself or with his special authorization.'[14]

6.4. Learning from Research Tribunals in Nuremberg and Japan

In October 1946, after the conclusion of the Nuremberg Military Tribunal, the other Allied powers (Britain, France, and the Soviet Union) gave the United States approval to begin prosecuting 23 German physicians who ordered or performed cruel and immoral human experimentation during the Third Reich ('United States vs. Karl Brand et al.'[15]). The court judges came exclusively from the United States, as did expert witnesses Andrew Ivy and Leo Alexander. They did not prosecute on the basis of the German laws and regulations governing human experimentation and criminal activity in force during the Third Reich, as the defendant physicians requested and legal experts and reasonable people might have expected. In the absence of specific laws or regulations within their own country, the judges referred instead to the 'Hippocratic Oath' and the principle of 'crime against humanity.' Ivy and Alexander elaborated at length on the Hippocratic principle of no harm. Alexander wrote a memorandum titled 'Ethical and Non-Ethical Experimentation on Human Beings.' It and sections of Ivy's statement were incorporated in the closing arguments in July 1947 by

---

[13] Sass 1983, l.c., p. 106; cf. Sass HM 2003 Ambiguities in Judging Cruel Human Experimentation. Arbitrary American Responses to German and Japanese Experiments, in: Eubios 13: 102-104.

[14] Reichsrundschreiben 1931: II.1.

[15] United States. Military Tribunal 1, Case 1 (1949) United States versus Karl Brand et al. Washington DC: US Governmental Printing Office, vol. I, 1004 pp; vol. II, 352 pp.

James McHaney, the chief prosecutor. McHaney mentioned the absence of animal experimentation, the lack of consent, poor design, and unproven expectations 'to yield results for the good of society.' He also held as follows: 'If there is a priori reason to believe that death or disabling injury might occur, the experimenters must serve as subjects themselves, along with the nonscientific personnel.... But important as these other considerations are, it is the most fundamental tenet of medical ethics and human decency that the subject volunteer for the experiment after being informed of its nature and hazards. This is the clear dividing line between the criminal and what may be noncriminal. If the experimental subjects cannot be said to have volunteered, then the inquiry need proceed not further. Such is the simplicity of the case'.[16] In their final judgment, the court used the language in Alexander's memorandum to summarize its position in what is now known as the 'Nuremberg Code.'[17] In its judgment, the court edited out of Alexander's memorandum the issues of proxy consent and of incompetent patients involved in research.

During the time of the Nuremberg trials, the U.S. military investigated similarly cruel experiments (primarily in regard to bacteriological and chemical warfare) by the infamous Japanese Unit 731 in China before and during the Second World War. The United States seemed to be interested in the results of those experiments, including methods and bacteria used, as well as protocols and results. In return for amnesty and immunity from further prosecution, Dr. Ishii, the notorious head of Unit 731, wrote an extensive account of his two decades of biological warfare experiments. Other experimenters produced thousands of slides and summaries of field tests, including a 600-page report on warfare experiments involving natural and artificial plague.[18] The U.S. War–Navy Coordinating Committee stated that these materials were 'of great value in confirming, supplementing and complementing several phases of U.S. research

[16] Annas GJ, Grodin MA 1992 The Nazi Doctors and the Nuremberg Code. New York NY: Oxford U Press, p. 135 and 137.

[17] United States, lc. 1949, vol 2:181-182; 1:2. In retrospect, the origins of the now-famous Nuremberg Code are associated with legal ambiguity and questionable legal and moral authority. The court proceedings violated essential principles of legal philosophy and conduct: (a) they did not prosecute on the basis of existing German law; (b) they arbitrarily and high-handedly wrote a 'code' and published that code on which they based their judgment only together with that judgment, (3) they thus violated the legal maxim 'nulla poena sine jus'; i.e., no punishment without a law established prior to the persecution based on that particular law. A court decision based on existing German law at the time when the Nazi crimes were performed would have been the correct and only legal remedy and most likely would have resulted in more and higher sentences. It is still a mystery why the Nuremberg Code has been eulogized as the most prominent cornerstone of modern research ethics.

[18] Harris S 1995 Factories of Death. Japanese Biological Warfare 1932-1945 and the American Cover-Up, New York: Routledge.

in biological warfare, and may suggest new fields for future research.'[19] The material and the 'business' dealings with the Japanese were kept secret. No one was prosecuted for those experiments, either by the Japanese or by the victorious U.S. authorities.

Open questions remain abundant: Why were German and Japanese physicians treated differently by the United States and its military? Did the United States have access to the results of the German experiments without having to grant immunity first, or were the Japanese experiments 'better' or more 'valuable' in design or results? In what kind of research into biological warfare was the United States involved to which the Japanese protocols were of such value in 'confirming, supplementing, and complementing'? The American Medical Association published its first guidelines on human experimentation in 1945; the Helsinki Declaration of 1964 was adopted in the United States in 1966. In 1974, 74 years after the 'Prussian Instruction,' the U.S. Department of Health Education, and Welfare finally published guidelines for the 'Protection of Human Subjects.'[20] While the Nuremberg trials made headlines all over the globe, particularly in Europe and the United States, the negotiations of U.S. authorities with the Japanese were conducted in secret and remained so. The only early source of information about the Japanese atrocities was a 1950 publication out of Moscow. It correctly described a few of the horrendously cruel Japanese experiments, but it was thought to be associated with propaganda at the beginning of the Cold War.[21] Local Chinese newspapers also reported tens of thousands of humans and animals infected with plague in Harbin province at the end of the Japanese occupation in China and beyond. It is still unknown why the United States recently returned the Japanese files, written in Japanese shorthand, after having paid the high price of complacency and of pardoning unpardonable crimes and cruelties against innocent people.

The publication of Henry K. Beecher's book on human experimentation in the United States documented the limited influence the Nuremberg Code and the publicity around it had – and how little those trials affected the attitude of many people in medical research. Radiation experiments in the United States seem to underscore the low impact of national or international guidelines or of the various revisions of the Helsinki Declaration.[22] In December 1990, the U.S. Food and Drug Administration published regulations permitting a waiver for military

---

[19] Chen YF 1997 Japanese death factories and the American cover-up, in: Cambridge Quarterly of Healthcare Ethics 6:240-242.

[20] United States. Department of Health, Education, and Welfare (1974) Protection of Human Subjects, in: Federal Register 39:18914ff.

[21] (Soviet Union) 1950 Documents on Trial Against the Former Military Personnel Prosecuted for the Preparation and Use of Bacteriological Warfare Weapon. Moscow: Foreign Books Publishing Press.

[22] United States Advisory Committee on Human Radiation Experiments 1995 Report. New York: The Free Press.

personnel participating in the Desert Storm battles of the requirement for obtaining informed consent from human subjects prior to the use of experimental drugs or vaccines. The U.S. Department of Defense had requested such a waiver[23] based on the argument that 'military combat is different.' We know that the vaccines or their combination were not tested prior to inoculation, thus resulting in diseases of a nature yet to be determined or publicly admitted and described. But in 1990, the courts refused to intervene to protect soldiers from unapproved drugs by declaring that 'the primary purpose of administering the drugs is military, not scientific…. The Department of Defense's decision to use unapproved drugs is precisely the type of military decision that the courts unfortunately have repeatedly refused to second-guess.'[24]

6.5. Human Experimentation and the Limits of Regulation

The history of regulating medical research during the last 50 years demonstrates that the ethics of human experimentation have lagged behind the progress of medical research. Anecdotal narratives tell that pharmaceutical companies or their subcontractors perform pilot studies without regulatory oversight or subject information/consent in countries with little or no regulatory structure prior to starting official clinical research procedures in the more strictly regulated countries in which they must finally seek approval. The U.S. government returned essential material that very likely could have documented crimes against humanity by Japanese physicians. The Japanese government, which previously called for those experiments, still harbors the experimenters and makes those files inaccessible. Both sides still seem to protect prospective war criminals and suppress access to the evidence of what really happened to the fellow humans who were unfortunate enough to be the victims of those crimes. In the 1940s, researchers at Johns Hopkins University inoculated non-consenting Guatemalans with sexually transmitted diseases to study penicillin and similar antibiotic medicines. In doing so, it had the support of the Rockefeller Foundation and Bristol-Myers, along with the awareness of the U.S. Public Health Service and Guatemalan public officials. After the information was disclosed in the aforementioned 2010 Report by the Presidential Commission for the Study of Bioethical Issues in Government, a one billion dollar lawsuit was filed in April 2015 against Johns Hopkins, the Rockefeller Foundation, and Bristol-Myers Squibb.[25] In a different case, lawyers of the Johns Hopkins–affiliated Kennedy Krieger Institute in Baltimore argued in 1991 that 'researchers have no legal obligations to those in their research studies.' Although two lower courts had

[23] Annas, l.c., 346-352.
[24] Annas, l.c., 216.
[25] Reverby SM 2015 Suing for Justice? More on the US STD Studies in Guatemala, in: Hastings Center Report 2015, 45(2), also bioethicsforum@hastingscenter.org 04-14-2015, accessed 04-14-15.

thrown out the complains of parents whose children were involved in hazardous lead exposure experiments and who claimed they had not been adequately informed of the health risk involved, the appeals judge rejected those arguments.[26]

6.6. New Partnerships, Public Discourse, Informed Choice

As in all fields of integrated and integrating bios, the promotion of better health care and medical knowledge should be done with closer communication and co-operation on the part of all parties involved. This means making the improvement of individual and public health a goal in trust-based partnerships of experts and laypersons and of corporate and oversight bodies. No doctor or pill can guarantee my full and enjoyable health. Doctors and other experts can, however, advise me in regard to beneficial living attitudes, sport, relaxation, and balancing work, fun, and sleep. Pills may help to reduce or even heal physical disease or depression, but I am ultimately responsible for my health. In discussing Confucian ethics and personal health, Ni Peimin holds that caring for health is 'not a matter of biology alone,' but 'a never ending journey towards the highest perfection of a human being.' [27] Similarly, prudence and personal responsibility in caring for one's health have characterized centuries of European dietetic traditions. These concepts of self-care and self-cultivation have often been lost under the influence of successful medical interventions in overhauling bodies and souls, much as cars are overhauled in repair shops.

Interactive, integrated biotopes on the Internet will soon support strong, promising lay–expert partnerships in drug monitoring and development. New apps in recent generations of smartphones allow patients to log into research-based sites for improving long-term efficacy of medicines and monitoring their side effects; such sites will probably be used later for new trials as well.[28] Recent developments in '*precision medicine*' (such as genomic cancer treatment) abjure outdated, four-phase CCTs. They are based, rather, on a partnership/stakeholder model among citizens informed about health risks and professionals with compassionate competence, both protected morally and legal-

---

[26] In second-guessing the Appeals Court judge's decision, the *Washington Post* chose the headline 'The judge went too far' (October 12, 1992). The lesson learned from the hypocritical complacency of governments in regard to criminal human experimentation, even to the extent of negotiating for its share of the results of those experiments and for keeping documents and evidence out of the public eye and scrutiny, are multifold.

[27] Ni Peimin 1999 Confucian virtues and personal health, in: Confucian Bioethics, Fan R ed., London: Kluwer, 27-44.

[28] See MyHeartCounts by Stanford for cardiovascular diseases, AsthmaHealth by Mount Sinai and AstraSeneca, GlucoSuccess by Stanford and University of Oxford for pre-diabetes and diabetes, ShareTheJourney supported by breastcancer.org for post-surgery breast cancer effects; cf. Winslow R 2015 Clinical Trials Find Patients Faster Using Smartphones, in: Wall Street Journal 04-14-2015, D1f.

ly. The U.S. Federal Drug Administration has published draft regulations[29] for new models of electronic interaction between researchers and human subjects, and this small step might lead to an interactive communication–cooperation model in clinical research, replacing informed consent with an informed contract. Hopefully, the new biotopes of improving health care will soon replace some of the outdated biotopes of bureaucratically regulated, four-phase, placebo-controlled trials with more harmonious and successful environments for improving health and well-being. We can identify many other fields of protecting and improving human health by new forms of partnership research: community involvement and consent, Internet-based partnerships in communication and cooperation, and public dialogue on goals and limits in repairing, improving, and enhancing individual and public health.

A few years ago, Chinese physicians and scientists began genetic and medical research in cooperation with the Harvard School of Public Health by sampling blood and DNA to study the impact of genetic and environmental risk factors. A disgruntled former employee and sensational, inaccurate media reports brought discredit to those studies, and a three-year investigation by the U.S. Office for Human Research Protections (OHRP) scrutinized the work of both Chinese and non-Chinese investigators. They found no wrongdoing, but they recommended a model of information that was more consonant with Chinese culture and expectations.[30] Zhai writes that 'family or community involvement should be promoted in a cultural and moral context, where family and community ties and traditional cultures are very strong; similarly, there might be families with these values also in predominantly individualistic cultures.... Such an approach does not mean that the family or community leader has the power to decide which member should participate in the research; the decision of consent must be made by the individual person herself or himself. So the term 'family consent' and 'community consent' is misleading. Actually this kind of informed consent may be coined as 'informed consent with the support and aid of family and community.'[31]

In 2002, the Nuffield Council of Bioethics recommended similar additional, culturally sensitive features for medical research in countries with less well developed medical and health care systems, saying that 'sponsors of research should require that the development of local expertise in healthcare is an integral component of research proposals. Consideration should be given to the extent to which any strengthening of local healthcare facilities can be done in such a way

[29] FDA, March 2015, Draft Guidelines for GCP, Use of Electronic Informed Consent in Clinical Investigations.

[30] Harvard School of Public Health 2003 Press Release: Conclusion of US Government's Inquiry into HSPH Genetic Research in China, May 30, 2003 (rherman@hsph.harvard.edu).

[31] Zhai XM 2011 l.c.:35.

that the changes are sustainable in the local context once the research is over.'[32] A few years ago, Taiwanese health care authorities prepared a public health project for the benefit of a genetic minority in the central part of the island, beginning with a broadly based and seemingly successful information-and-education campaign. They did not initiate the actual research, however, when community leaders expressed uneasiness and suggested that the community was not ready for this well-intended project.

Finally, however, we should not forget that individual conscience and the *freedom and right to choose* is one of the strongest values and virtues to be protected and supported. Here is Anita's story: At the age of 16, Anita was diagnosed with an inherited kidney disorder (ADPKD), which later in her life will cause the development kidney cysts and require hemodialysis or kidney transplants. At that time, she was a subject in a research project studying family histories. Her mother, 45 and divorced, is in dialysis treatment. When her grandmother died of liver complications related to many years of dialysis treatment, Anita decided that she never would have kids carrying the ADPKD disorder. Now Anita is 21, has a boyfriend, and has become pregnant against her will. A prenatal test confirms that the fetus is a carrier of ADPKD. Anita knows the complications of this disorder well and requests an abortion after two consultation sessions. Having evaluated issues of respect for life, self-determination, responsible parenting, and family planning, she schedules an abortion appointment, which she does not keep. Instead, she moves in with a relative in a different city and gives birth to a daughter, who has ADPKD but is otherwise healthy.[33] Anita is happy about her decision, one she never thought she would make.

New forms of partnership in biological and medical research are not restricted to traditional human communities. The Internet opens new avenues for including individuals of all cultures and ages directly in research while educating and motivating them; Anita's surprising decision might also have been influenced by information and communication on the internet. Not much is known yet about the dependencies and interactions between human beings and communities with their microbiomes. Each of us has billions of microbes, approximately two kilos, in and on our bodies. We cannot live without these colonies of fellow bios, which metabolize food for and with us, synthesize vitamins, and provide other essential services for our individual bios. We feel sick or even die when microbial invaders cause disharmony or when infighting within our microbiome disturbs our and their metabolisms. Constipation and diarrhea are two of the simpler results of such disharmonies, but they affect our bodily

[32] Nuffield Council on Bioethics 2002 The Ethics of Research Related to Healthcare in Developing Countries, London: Nuffield Council.

[33] For a detailed discussion of Anita's case, see Kielstein R, Sass HM 2001 Genetics: ethical issues and kidney disease, in: Ethics and the Kidney, Levinsky NG ed., Oxford University Press, 167-182.

functions, mood, and behavior as well. Antibiotics harm and kill good and bad microbes; patient rooms in hospitals and even surgical instruments are infected with antibiotic-resistant pathogens. Microbes with newly modified DNA regularly threaten individual humans, communities, and the bios in general. Research into the balances of harmony and new modifications of all forms of microbiome have just begun, and successful results will have immense implications for improving individual human life, human bios, and the many forms of integrated bios as well. The research corporation uBiome[34] provides sample kits globally for a small fee to use for swiping and submitting microbial specimens from my mouth, ears, nose, gut, and genitals. uBiome will then give me detailed information about my personal microbiome, its potential impact on my health, and how it relates to the microbiome of other people. Frequent email letters from uBiome provide interesting and helpful information about the impact on individual and public health of the individual microbiome of myself, family members, house animals, private rooms, offices, factories, mass transportation, and other surrounding microbial biotopes. Of course, uBiome does not collect specimens only to augment the public's limited knowledge. It will use the collected samples widely for their own and their partners' research and for potential breakthroughs in medicine and housing, for better use of probiotics and the avoidance of antibiotics in medicine and agriculture, and for cultivating better, more healthy, and more harmonious biotopes for humans and other forms of our integrated bios.

The future of research in medicine and most other areas will not be successful if we fail to cultivate more interaction between the academic halls of research, the factories and offices of research-based corporations, and the individuals and communities who will benefit from new hardware and software products, medicines, wearables, implants, and devices that allow for further manipulation and modification of bios and its most basic building blocks. It would bring more justice to participants in research if informed consent were to be replaced by informed contract, an issue discussed in regard to pharmacogenomics and personal health care in chapter eight.[35] *Informed contracts* outlining the risks, benefits, rights, and responsibilities of all stakeholders are the standard instrument of choice when venturing into risky and potentially harmful business.

---

[34] uBiome.com.

[35] We may differentiate between three forms of moral risk management — authoritative and regulative, educative and exhortative, discursive and adjuvantive. At the first conference of the UNESCO Bioethics Committee in 1995, I warned: 'The risks of the authoritative model include the suppression of the individual conscience and the promotion of double standards and the risk the authorities might change the course of fatherly instruction. The discursive model fits best into the scenarios of moral assessment by educated and risk competent individuals; it is the model of the future, but it needs to be careful to make good use of the treasures hidden in the moral history of many cultures'; Sass HM 1995 Some Cultural and ethical Reflections on Molecular Genetic Risk Assessment, in: International Bioethics Commission CIB, Actes 1995 Proceedings, vol. 2:64f

Unfortunately, that is not the case in medical research, where participants are quite often asked to consent on the basis of necessarily insufficient information.

Medical research for improving therapy and health care is a risk partnership in which probands and patients are the most vulnerable stakeholders.[36] They should be made equal partners by 'information and contract' and not only by 'information and consent.' Different religious and cultural evaluations of high-tech medical research and clinical applications will always exist. Therefore, probands and patients must be seen as responsible, morally concerned fellow-citizens capable of making their own decisions about risks in open, pluralistic societies rich in different moral visions.[37] The existing model of bureaucratic paternalism and tutelage can be replaced by various models that incorporate the integrated eight-C human culture properties in promoting the classical virtues of reducing risk and of promoting fairness, justice, and peace. We should also include the Confucian virtues of humaneness, compassion, cleverness, wisdom, sincerity, and honesty (as set forth by Dr. Yang Chuan). The eight-C properties should also be used in promoting public discourse on the bioethics of manipulating and cultivating human and other bios in medical research.

A global 'summit' of regulators and experts in gene editing took place in Washington, D.C., in December 2015, hosted by the U.S. National Academy of Sciences. Particularly controversial was the use of CRISPR technology in the human sperm line to eradicate hereditary diseases[38] and the genetic engineering of zygotes carrying material from three different origins.[39] Questions posed included (1) whether one should generate many embryos and then select the one free of the mutation responsible for a mutation and throw the others away and (2) whether for late-onset disorders such as inherited genetic heritage for developing kidney cysts one should do nothing in the hope that further medical breakthroughs will heal or control ensuing genetic disorders. And, of course, issues were brought up of 'enhancement' of individuals or as many future people as possible for better social or intellectual properties (or for Tour de France cyclists to improve their 'natural' erythropoietin production[40] without actually

---

[36] Sass HM 1998 Genotyping in Clinical Trials. Towards a Principle of Informed Contract, in: J Medicine and Philosophy 23(3)288-296.

[37] Sass HM 2006 Let probands and patients decide about moral risk in stem cell research and medical treatment, in: Cross-cultural Issues in Bioethics; the Example of Human Cloning. Roetz H ed., Amsterdam: Rodopi, 425-444; Sass HM 1996 Moral risk assessment in biotechnology, in: Changing Nature's Course; the Ethical Challenge of Biotechnology. Becker GK, Buchanan JP, Hongkong U Press, 127-144

[38] http://news.mit.edu/2015/overcome-crispr-cas9-genome-editing-hurdle-1201; http://motherboard.vice.com/read/this-week-top-genericists-want-todecide-if-gmo-humans-areok; http://www.kurzweilai.net/transhumansit-position-on-human-germline-genetic-modofication.

[39] Liang P et al., 2015 CRISPR/Cas9 mediated gene editing in human tripronuclear zygotes, in: Protein Cell 6:363-372.

[40] http://www.ncbi.nlm.nih.gov/pmc/articles/PMC2657498.

injecting themselves with additional erythropoietin, as Louis Armstrong did). But even less sensational breakthroughs than CRISPR provide great healing options, such as stem-cell therapy[41]. The remarkable progress in manipulating bios of these and other new technologies will soon be widely accessible and may encourage positive and negative deeds by good and bad people to cultivate or to destroy individual bios and biotopes, both human and non-human. In following Fritz Jahr's Bioethical Imperative, we should hold to the following premise: wherever intensified public discourses, human and civil right initiatives, and national laws and regulations lead us, the conscience of the individual closest to the decision should be respected and, if possible, treated accordingly.

EMBRYO TALKS ON EMBRYOID CONSTRUCTS
This is disgusting, said the 80 day old twin embryo to herself.
What do you mean?, asked her sister.
Embryo: The people construct artificial cells by transferring a somatic cell nucleus into an denucleid egg and call it 'embryo'.
Sister: This is an insult to us; these constructs have no father and no mother. Apples are not oranges, and we embryos are not embryoids as those products are.
Embryo: We are loved by our mother, we are in her womb. I love her. These cells are in an artificial solution in a dish, not loved and just manufactured for growing so called stem cells and derive specialized cell lines and tissue for medical help and cure of sick people.
Sister: Helping sick and poor people is very good; but they should not call these cells embryo. I love my mom, too, also my dad; I love you; you are so close to me.
Embryo: I feel our dad loves us, too; he is not quite healthy and our parents had to get medical help to transport his gametes into our mom's fallopian tube; they call this GIFT. Anyway, our genetic composition is different from either parent; we might also have a different individual composition in as far as our cytoplasm might have interacted differently with our nucleus after separation, and we definitely will become different as our genetic heredity will be influenced by different exposure to enzymatic, nutritional, physical, and social environments.
Sister: Medical help is good; doctors helped our parents; we would not be without those doctors.
Embryo: It would not be us two, it would be someone else or nobody, if the fertilized egg had not been split into the two of us or if the egg had not been merged with our daddy's sperm or if it had died shortly thereafter.

---

[41] Stem cells from embryos might be usable for creating dopamine-producing neurons in Parkinson's disease; bone marrow stem cells infused into coronary arteries may repair heart attack damage; reprogrammed adult skin stem cells become active beta cells and immune cells for diabetes patients; websites: International Society for Stem Cell Research; Parkinson Disease Foundation, last visited 08-20-16

Sister: So is life. But why do these people call those man-made artificial cells embryos?
Embryo: They do not think clearly, therefore they mix things up.
Sister: What do they mix up?
Embryo: Humans sometimes don't think clearly; sometimes they want to exercise power over others. Some even want to put these good doctors and scientists into prison.
Sister: Why would they do such a horrible thing?
Embryo: They say, they want to protect human beings, even unborn humans such as you and me; and they don't understand that embryoids are not embryos.
Sister: This is really stupid; it is irresponsible; they does not show respect for people or for us. I don't want to live in a world governed by those evil people.
Embryo: How can we jump ship? We cannot abort ourselves. We are loved by our parents, we are and will be a very happy family and happy people.
About 20 years later, the girls developed a severe form of diabetes. Treatment was easy and successful using remedies made by CRISPR technology and derived from embryonic constructs produced from their oocytes and somatic cells. They live happily ever after.

III. CARING FOR HUMAN BIOS

7. BEGINNINGS AND ENDS OF INDIVIDUAL HUMAN LIFE

STAGES IN HUMAN BIOS?

Everyone's life and its dwelling place are threefold: the womb of the mother, the earth, the heaven. In the first we get life only, with movement and the beginnings of conscience, in the second life, movement and the beginnings of knowledge, in the third the fullness of all. The firs life is a preparation for the second, the second for the third, the third goes off in itself without end ... The first and the second homes are like factories for developing the body to be used in the following life; the third home will bring the true completion and the enjoyment of both ... The passage from the first life to the second and from the second into the third is tight and painful, but in both passages only the closing and wraps are left (first only a secondary one, but then the prison of the body), such as from a broken eggshell comes the young.

J.A. Comenius[1]

7.1. Interpreting and Protecting Individual Human Life

Biologically, individual human life comes from other individual human lives interacting sexually with each other, with each of us having a mother and father. So have most other forms of so-called higher life. We individual humans also have our own personal microbial, geographical, and social biotopes. Aristotle recognized an individual drive and an innate 'knowledge' and competence of individual bios 'to create another being similar to them, animal to create animal and plant to create plant, in order to participate as much as they can to the eternal and divine; for all desire this and do for its sake whatever they do according to nature ... As living beings cannot participate to the eternal and divine by their permanent individual existence, for none of the perishable may remain the same, inalterable and numerically one, each participates to the divine in the way it can, other more other less. It does not remain the same but similar to it, not numerically one, but one in species'.[2]

We humans share individual finality with other individuals; we are born as individuals and die as individuals. But as humans we are gifted and challenged to develop our own concepts about the wheel of rotating bios, about life and non-life, about birth and death, about our bodies, souls, and feelings, our calls and duties, our angst and hopes. Other species might have more and better senses, but we humans seem to be superior in processing the input from our senses. Religious and philosophical debates past and present demonstrate a wide variety of positions and visions in regard to human life and our own individual lives in particular. As far as the evaluation of the individual human body and the begin-

---

[1] Amos Comenius: Didactica Magna, 1633ff, quoted in: Fritz Jahr 1933 Life after Death, in: Jahr l.c. 73f; cf. Jahr: Three stages in Life, (1938), l.c.:107-114.

[2] Aristotle De Anima, II, 415a28-415b8.

nings and ends of individual human life are concerned, the history of humankind presents a variety of concepts that have been pondered by our forefathers and foremothers for millennia. Countless individual and collective interpretations of biological facts have led to legal disputes and condemnations, to accusations, suicides, and murder. Various interpretations have been rejected by some but recognized by others as unique expressions of human dignity, setting us apart from other creatures.

7.2. Bioethical Interpretations of Biological Facts

This chapter focuses on the various interpretations of biological facts in discussing medical, religious, and philosophical understandings of the beginnings and ends of the human bios as individual life. Given the wide variety of concepts, values, and virtues involved in assessing the dignity of the steps of early human life and the dignity of the processes of dying and the lack of a global moral and cultural consensus, it should be ethical, prudent, and dignifying to *respect different positions*. These controversies might be unsolvable, as they go far beyond our individual bios. Therefore, we need to look for a formula that would recognize our perplexity with our own death and dying (and our being alive at all), rather than looking into a one-size-fits-all recipe for valuing and protecting the dignity of human life and of human beliefs and visions concerning it. A Uniform Life Protection Act based on medical facts needs to respect our different moral and cultural traditions, and it must include a Conscience Clause for individuals who hold different convictions, as informed by their conscience and beliefs.

Birth and death are biological facts, but they have been interpreted in various ways over the millennia by religious and cultural traditions. They have also been regulated differently by legal and regulatory authorities. A basic description of the individual human body and person is to define it from the time after birth and the beginning of breathing up to the end of breathing and heartbeat. Before birth it is *viscerum matris,* a part of the female body; after death, it is a decaying corpse. However, the human body is formed before birth, and some believe that human bios, even individual bios, will continue after death. Some positions hold that life itself is in permanent development and change: growing, modifying, transforming, decaying, and even interchanging from one species to the other or from physical to spiritual bios. Indeed, all forms of bios are interconnected – depending on each other, eating and being eaten. Many also believe in invisible forms of life such as spirits, angels, and devils. Contemporary quantum mechanics supports these old religious concepts to the extent that it might be scientifically more reasonable to assume that there is a multiverse rather than one single visible universe.

Buddhist and other concepts of metamorphosis envision a transmigration of spiritual life and souls from one species to another at birth and death. Hindu reasoning argues that everything was a dream of Vishnu before he brought it into existence, protecting it from danger and decay in various forms of his own avatars.[3] Similarly, monotheistic religions see God as the creator of all life, specifically individual human life. Some positions hold that God in person or an impersonal PrimeOne, Dao or a Big Bang started the process of life once and that from there on life continued to expand and develop on its own by trial and error, natural selection, and struggle and survival as described by Darwin and modern biology. Others hold that humans at least are individually animated by God to make them in his image: 'God formed man of dust from the ground, and breathed into his nostrils the breath of life; and man became a living being.'[4] The visionary and teacher Johan Amos Comenius presents a similarly wide picture, as the introductory quote shows.

Thomas More, Lord Chancellor of Great Britain, Christian martyr, and a Saint of the Roman Catholic Church, argued strongly for priest-suggested suicide. Documenting the Christian belief in resurrection, he suggested to a suffering patient: 'Let's face it, you will never be able to live a normal life. You are just a nuisance to other people and a burden to yourself – in fact, you are really living a sort of posthumous existence. So why go on feeding germs? Since your life is a misery to you, why do you hesitate to die? You are imprisoned in a torture-chamber – why don't you break out and escape to a better world? Or say the word, and we'll arrange for release. It's only common sense to cut your losses. It's also an act of piety to take the advice of a priest, because a priest speaks for God.'[5]. In Hinduism, death is not the end of life; life is a continuous stream of energy. Only individual life ends, re-incarnating into another human or non-human life. The teaching of the Bhagavad Gita comes close to Comenius' and Jahr's vision: 'Just like the body passes through childhood, youth, and old-age, it attains another body. Death therefore does not affect the wise ones … Just like a person discards old clothes and put on new ones, the Soul leaves the old body

---

[3] Sass HM, 2012 'Earth, Universe, and Multiverse are Living Beings.' Fritz Jahr and the Foundations of Global Bioethics, Muenster: Lit, 345-358.

[4] Genesis 2:7; the Muslim tradition is even more precise in regard to God's creation and animation of the individual human person: 'Truly, the creation of each of you begins in his mother's womb within 40 days (as a drop of sperm, *nutfa*); then he is for the same time a lump of blood (*alaqa*); thereafter for the same period of time a small lump of flesh (*mudga*); then He breathes the soul into him', hadith tradition, quoted in Ilkilic I, 2004 Der moralische Status des Embryos im Islam, in: Weltanschauliche Offenheit in der Bioethik, Berlin: Duncker & Humblot, p. 165; Larsen WJ 2001 Human Embryology. Amsterdam: Elsevier. The God of Abraham not only approved but requested surrogate motherhood and extramarital sex, directing Abraham to have a son with his Egyptian female slave Hagar; God promised Hagar to make her son Ish'mael 'a great nation.' Abraham's God also blessed the marriage with his half-sister Sarah and gave them their son Isaac; the Qu'ran comments about Isaac and Ish'mael: 'Among their offspring were some, who did good works and others who clearly sinned against their souls,' Qu'ran 17:120.

[5] Morus T (1516) 1965 Utopia, Turner P transl., Penguin Books, p. 102; cf Sass HM 1999 Significance of religious beliefs in end-of-life medical Decision-Making, in: Mulla Sadra Logic and Ethics, vol. 8, Chomenei SM ed., Tehran, p. 203-218.

and enters into a new one.'[6] Not too different is the Muslim faith expressed in the Qu'ran: 'the Lord of Creation, who made me, who gives me guidance, food and drink, who when I am sick, restores me, who will cause me to die, and then to live, and who, I pray, will forgive me my sins on the Day of Judgment.'[7]

Biology tells us how individual human life develops after sperm and oocyte merge and form a zygote, which about a week later nidates into the mother's uterus and grows until birth. But it is not a biological issue to answer the question about the moral status of an embryo conceived after in-vitro fertilization or various medical technologies such as GIFT (gamete into fallopian tube). Neither will biology tell us when morally recognizable human life begins or when it ends. Biomedical '*facts*' have been manipulated for the sake of a moral good, such as when medieval medical textbooks described rare 11-month pregnancies to make the biological stricture of 9-month pregnancy less stringent in calculating the time of cohabitation between husband and wife, thus 'liberating' the woman from a strict biological timeframe and defending her against husband, priests, lawyers, and the general public. The 11-month pregnancy medical 'law' became even more essential for European noblewomen, who kept their social and financial standing when bearing male offspring after 11 months.[8] Would such a professionally deceitful lying by doctors about a definite biological law be evidence that those physicians of bygone days manipulated (cultivated) biological laws based on wider bioethical principles in favour of '*women's liberation*'? The pseudo-scientific narrative of 11-month pregnancy, which according to Rabelais resulted in the giant Gargantua, was generated originally to circumvent the insight *mater semper certa, pater semper incertus* (the mother is always certain, the father uncertain). Nowadays we have surrogate mothers who carry the foetus of the biological mother, or mothers who carry a donated foetus from someone else with or without her husband or lover's oocyte. For these situations, the individuals to be born and the various mothers and fathers will have to develop their own narrative identity in regard to the family tree, family ethics, and self-identity – as we humans do in many other situations.[9]

We had and will have different sources for our beliefs and for the moral and cultural interpretations of biological and physical facts. Different understandings of the beginnings and ends of human life between religious and cultural positions and even within cultures are normal and should not be dealt

[6] Gita 2:3 and 22; see also Kishore KK 2003 End of life issues and moral certainty, in: Eubios J Asian and International Bioethics 13:210-213.

[7] Qu'ran 26: 78-82.

[8] Carranza AA 1630 De patu naturalii et legitimo. Geneva, Switzerland; Screech MA 1969 Eleven Month Pregnancies, in: Etudes Rabelaisiensis 7:94-106; Sass HM, 1992 Diagnosing the 11-month Pregnancy: Some Aspects of Moral and Cultural Foundations in Medical Judgment, in: The Ethics of Diagnosis, Dordrecht: Kluwer, 153-162.

[9] Ricoeur P 1991 Narrative Identity, in: Philosophy Today 35(1): 73-81, 263-275.

with by intimidation, indoctrination, incarceration, or murder.[10] Public and theological policy should respect the dignity of each citizen's conscience and his or her 'inalienable right to follow one's own conscience and to profess and practice one's own faith.' 'People must not attempt to impose their own "truth" on others', as Pope John Paul II underlined. When religious law becomes synonymous with civil law, it 'can stifle religious freedom, even going so far as to restrict or deny other inalienable human rights.... Intolerance can also result from the recurring temptation to fundamentalism, which easily leads to serious abuses, such as the radical suppression of all public manifestations of diversity.'[11]

It is precisely this dignity of human moral choice and challenge that we find in the controversies about the 'right' and 'wrong' interpretation of the 'will of God' or of the 'natural law' versus the perverse, the unnatural, the inhuman. Thus, the controversies, fights, indoctrinations, and even killings over the interpretation of moral traditions tell us that not facts but their interpretations are indicative of the validity and dignity of the human conscience.[12]

A Human Dignity Imperative therefore could read as follows: *Whenever theologians, politicians, teachers or groups disagree about the interpretation of facts and the right course of action, then human dignity must be protected primarily in the dignity of the individual conscience, which must be allowed and encouraged to make decisions for itself, its loved ones and its community based on personal responsibility and liability.*

7.3. Animation: Brain Life and Brain Death

Monotheistic religions and Western cultures believing that God personally animates each individual can distinguish between animate and non-animate human life, but Asian cultures of understanding bios have problems differentiating be-

---

[10] Andre Hellegers, the founder of the Kennedy Institute of Ethics at Georgetown University, once stressed, that 'it is not a function of science to prove, or disprove, where in this process (foetal development) human life begins, in the sense that those discussing the abortion issue so frequently use the word "life," i. e. human dignity, human personhood, or human inviolability. Such entities do not pertain to the science or art of medicine, but are rather of societal judgement'; cf. Hellegers A 1970 Foetal Development, in: Theological Studies 31, 3-9.

[11] John Paul II 1990 If You Want Peace, Respect the Conscience of Every Person. Vatican City (December 1990). The Pope could also have quoted Abu Hanifa, the 8th-century founder of the orthodox Sunni Islamic law school of Hanafi, who said: 'Differences of opinion in the congregation can be read as a special grace of God.' I quoted earlier a similar argument by Moses Mendelsohn: 'Diversity seems to have been the plan and goal of providence. None of us reasons and feels totally like his fellow humans. Why do we hide from each other in the most important issues of our lives by masquerade, as God purposely has given each of us one's own face?'

[12] Sass HM 1995 'Bioethical Issues in the Abortion Debate.' The Abortion Debate in Transatlantic Perspective [AICGS Seminar Papers, No 10, March 1995] 17-32; Sass HM 2016 Cultural Dimensions of Bios and Bioethics J Health and Culture 1(1)26-37.

tween the human body and the human soul.[13] A functioning brain is necessary for a functioning body, and also for understanding oneself, the world, and God. Thus, the absence of brain functioning has led to a medical designation of death, or 'brain death' as the 1980 USA Uniform Determination of Death Act (paragraph 1) defines it: 'An individual who has sustained either (1) irreversible cessation of circulatory or respiratory functions, or (2) irreversible cessation of all functions of the entire brain, including the brain stem, is dead. A determination of death has to be made in accordance with accepted medical standards.'[14] Bioethical issues remain with such a strictly clinical definition of this very personal, existential phenomenon: the formula does not discuss issues of dignity and care for patients in persistent vegetative states, for anencephalics, or for persons who want to be judged by less stringent terms.[15] Asian cultures in bioethics do not support organ-based criteria such as those for the brain. They base respect and responsibility for the dignity of human beings on interpersonal ethics, in particular on the virtue of filial piety. This attitude creates a strong, reliable impetus to not expose their loved ones to artificial life in intensive care units. Michael Tai argues that the principle of 'filial piety' should recognize artificiality as being unnatural: 'Artificial life relying on external means is not harmonious with nature. Keeping a PVS (persistent vegetative state) person on a respirator is unnatural. If medical procedures fail to revert a deteriorating health of a person and the treatments received prove to be futile, forgoing treatments is the way of the Tao and is just ethically justifiable.'[16]

Different from the brain-death concept, that of brain life faces higher hurdles, because the maturation of the foetal body and its brain is a continuous process with less visible sections in development and because life, not death, will be the outcome. This is one of the reasons that abortion causes great personal and societal uncertainties and conflicts in most cultures. But a bioethical evaluation of the moral significance of neuronal maturation at the beginning of life, similar to the cessation of neuronal functions at the end of life, might open a

---

[13] Tai MC 2004 The Asian Way of Bioethics. Taipei: Princeton Intern. Publ., p. 62f.

[14] USA National Conference of Commissioners on State Laws 1980 Uniform Determination of Death Act, paragraph 1; cf. Beecher KH, 1968 'A definition of irreversible coma: report of the Harvard Medical School to examine the definition of brain death'. JAMA 205,337-340.

[15] Hellegers A 1974 Allowing Anencephalics to Die, in: Obstetrics and Gynaecology News 9: 48; Zaner RM ed. 1988 Death; Beyond Whole-Brain Death Criteria. Dordrecht: Reidel; Veatch RM 1988 Whole Brain and Neocortical Definitions of Death, in: Bioethics, Adwards RB, Graber GC eds., New York: Harcourt Brace, 414-424.

[16] Tai MC 2004 The Way of Asian Bioethics. Taipei; Princeton Intern. Publ., p. 65; Tai suggest to remove life support from a PVS patient who cannot longer breath on his/her own: 'The removal of the system is to let Tao be Tao. Taoism however would oppose active euthanasia as it is an artificial way of end life. Palliative care will be the Taoist option to let nature take its course. Thus a Taoist will be in support of Hospice movement and in opposition to the Right to Die movement,' l.c., p. 63.

path to a consensus in recognizing the dignity of early human life, together with the dignity of the human conscience in interpreting the laws of God and nature and in making responsible choices. Bioethical criteria establishing a consensus on brain life similar to the understanding of brain death have to meet similar requirements: (a) compatibility with most of the major cultural traditions in existing pluralistic societies, (b) compatibility with the medical understanding and explanation of the process of human embryonic development and gestation, (c) simplicity of definition and diagnosis, and (d) a conscience clause for those who believe in stricter criteria than those of the uniform standard. In reviewing the consensus formation process that led to the widely accepted brain death criteria, we must discuss whether we can find a similar one for the beginning of human life. More precisely, we have to look into the process of neuromaturation and its biological and bioethical interpretations. Analogous to the definition of human death as brain death, all of these criteria are best met by relating the moral recognition of human life to the existence of brain life. The absence of brain-specific cells in early embryonic development has to be understood as the absence of brain life.[17]

Ontologically, the earliest possible manifestation of biomedical neurological facts, the beginning of synapse formation between postmitotic stationary neurons in the subplate zone, can be interpreted as a biological correlate to the beginning of brain life.[18] But no functional neurological brain tissue can be recognized at this time, even though spinal reflexes and brainstem activities have been documented around day 54 pc (post conceptionem). Only thereafter will cortical neuroblasts lose their ability to divide and soon start to interconnect by forming neurites, dendrites, and synapses during a process called synaptogenesis (i.e., the formation of brain tissue out of formerly isolated cells). Those neuro-neuronal interconnecting structures are the precondition of communication between individual neurons, neuron conglomerates, higher brain hemispheres, the parts of the brain, and the brain and the other parts of the body. The first appearances of synapse formation in the cortical plate and subplate zones occur in

---

[17] Biomedical facts in neuroscience provide information for bioethical interpretation; cf. Goldenring J 1985 The brain life theory: towards a consistent biological definition of humanness, in: Journal of Medical Ethics 11:198-204; Jones DG 1989 Brain birth and personal identity, in: Journal of Medical Ethics 15:173-178; Sass HM 1989 Brain life and brain death. a proposal for a normative agreement, in: Journal of Philosophy and Medicine 14:45-59.

[18] The Carnegie stages of neuromaturation identify in stage 7 (18th day pc) the first appearance of the neural plate, in stage 15 (33th day p. c.) the development of cerebral vesicles, in stage 22 (54th day p. c.) the appearance of the cortical plate formed by a single layer of postmitotic cortical neurons; cf. O'Rahilly R, Mueller F 1987 Developmental stages in human embryos. Meriden Press: Carnegie Inst. of Washington Publ. No. 637.

isolated areas around the 70th day pc[19] but may be transient. The stabilization of interneuronal synapses around and after the 151th day pc is the prerequisite for interneuronal information processing, which is required for learning, memory, awareness, and other complex mental processes.[20] The first stages in the structural ontogenesis of the cerebral cortex, the formation of synapses, are preconditions for all further intercommunication between neuroblasts and for the development of higher brain functioning. Synapse formation can be interpreted as the beginning of animating life. Prior to the 70th day pc, we have only biological, inanimate life. During the early stages of animating life, there definitely can be no functional higher brain life (i.e., no reasoning or controlling of bodily functions, no feeling of pain, no conscience or self-awareness). The isolated networks have to grow and to grow together, to interconnect, and to connect with other parts of the brain and the organs. This will take a long time and will continue postnatally, but it will happen in an evolutionary way without precisely identifiable steps of essential developmental or moral relevance. At this stage, the foetus cannot have a sentient, personal 'interest view' on life and survival.[21] A conservative moral assessment of neuromaturation therefore suggests that inanimate embryonic life prior to the 70th day pc (i.e., life absent higher brain function) would be the symmetrical correlate to brain death at the end of human life. Consequently, animating life as synapse formation after the 70th day pc, and animate life of early functioning synapse formation should be morally recognized and legally protected. Only from these stages on can we identify neurons, which start interconnecting and will finally represent what the tradition calls *Imago Dei, animal rationale*: ensouled body/human person.

7.4. Consensus on Symmetry between Brain Life and Brain Death?

A consensus on a symmetry of brain life and brain death, understood as the beginning and the end of animating and animate life and the end of dignified personal human life, can serve in moral recognition and legal protection of individual fellow humans. Such an understanding also provides moral advantages over disadvantages, preserves essential moral and cultural values, and reduces the moral risks associated with the extreme positions of dogmatic pro-life and pro-choice combatants. Synapse formation between post-mitotic stationary neocortical neurons can be evaluated as the physiological correlate and substratum

---

[19] Hinrichsen KV, 1990 Realisationsstufen in der vorgeburtlichen Entwicklunq des Menschen. Bochum: ZME; Kostovic I 1991 Entwicklung des Zentralnervensystems, in: Humanembryologie. Hinrichsen KV ed., Heidelberg: Springer.

[20] Sass HM 1994 The moral significance of brain-life criteria, in: The Beginnings of Human Life, Beller FK, Weir RF eds., Dordrecht: Kluwer, 57-70; Mahowald M 1996 The brain and the I. Neurodevelopment and personal identity, in: Journal of Social Philosophy 27(3): 49-60.

[21] Steinbock B, 2011, Life before birth. The moral and legal status of embryos and fetuses. Oxford: Oxford U Press, 2nd ed.

for animating human life. It is the biomedical, bioethical precondition for animate human life, enabling the significant functioning of control, command, communication, conscience and self-consciousness, and pain and pleasure in the person to be. Following the Judeo-Christian and Greco-Roman tradition of the theory of animation, I will call biological human life between conception and synapse formation '*inanimate*'; from the beginning of synapsis formation up to sometime after birth '*animating*'; and from then on '*animate*.' At the end of life, the pre-mortem status of brain death can be called '*post-animate*' life.

The shift from circulatory and respiratory to brain-related indicators of death can serve as a case study in successful consensus formation in applying differential ethics and value assessment to the bioethical challenges posed by new biomedical technologies. Traditionally, the death of a person was identical with the death of his or her organs. It was not necessary to differentiate between the cessation of particular organs' functioning and the death of the person, as long as cessation of breathing and heartbeat caused a chain of reactions, at the end of which all other organs ceased working. Intensive care technology supporting pulmonary and cardiovascular functions and the technical availability of heart transplantation and the artificial heart made it necessary to define the end of personal life morally and culturally in correlation to the functioning of particular organs. In 1968, after bioethical evaluation of biomedical facts concerning the processes of dying, an ad hoc commission of the Harvard Medical School came forward with a more precise biomedical criterion for a bioethical description of the death of a person: brain death. Their Uniform Determination of Death Act defined it as follows: 'An individual who has sustained either (1) irreversible cessation of circulatory and respiratory functions, or (2) irreversible cessation of at functions of the entire brain, including brain stem, is dead. A determination of death must be made in accordance with accepted medical standards.'[22] These criteria have since been accepted, with technical refinements, in most cultures having an underlying concept of a difference between body and soul.

The relatively smooth and widely accepted bioethical shift from cardiopulmonary death to whole-brain death was made possible by dormant values and principles in Western tradition, supported by the humanist Greco-Roman and the religious Judeo-Christian traditions. Such a shift to a brain-oriented definition of life and death has the following five medical, moral, legal, and cultural advantages: (a) Human life that meets the strict, well-defined biomedical criteria of whole-brain death does not deserve the same moral recognition and legal protection as other humans, while other forms of comatose or vegetative human life,

[22] Sass, 1992 l.c.; Sass 2015 l.c.; For early brain life and brain death discussion in the media cf. Steinfels P 1990 Scholar proposes brain birth law, in:, New York Times, Nov 8; Brain Waves: the beginning and the end in: The Plain Dealer Dec. 2, 1990; Wann beginnt das Leben?, in: Die Zeit, Nov 30, 1990; Darf man in Keimzellen eingreifen?, in: Die Zeit, June 1994, Nr 23/24:35.

including that involving cessation of neocortical functions, are not covered under this formula. (b) Moral, emotional, cultural, social, and economic costs that would have been associated with the artificial extension of brain-dead life can be saved. (c) Organs become available for patients who otherwise would die or face severe suffering, hardship, or inconvenience. (d) One single biomedical criterion serves as a correlate for a bioethical consensus on one specific scenario at the end of human life using the traditional difference between animate and inanimate life: 'cessation of all functions of the entire brain.' (e) People whose belief system does not support whole brain–related criteria of death will not be required to change their belief and conduct and can choose death to be diagnosed by traditional circulatory and respiratory criteria.

But three issues remain unaddressed by the Harvard formula: patients in persistent vegetative states, anencephalics, and specific values in different cultures.[23] Consensus-based public policy as well as patient-oriented medical ethics require either the introduction of a conscience clause into existing statutes or a global model statute reconfirming existing whole-brain death criteria as a uniform default position for determining human death (while respecting and encouraging self-determination by allowing competent individuals to opt for other criteria consistent with their system of belief). The U.S. President's Commission in 1981 based its moral assessment of a whole brain-oriented definition on two arguments: (1) that 'it is not known which portions of the brain are responsible for cognition and consciousness'[24] and (2) that those who still believe in the criteria of spontaneous breathing and heartbeat could live with the new definition. Such an overprotection for moral reasons is quite normal in assessing the use of a new technology for the first time. But patients, family, and the medical community are facing medical and moral conflicts associated with such a uniform, categorical statute.[25] A more flexible formula should allow for self-

---

[23] Hellegers A 1974 Allowing anencephalics to die, in: Obstetrics and Gynaecology News 9: 48; Veatch RM, 1988 'Whole Brain and Neocortical Definitions of Death', in: Bioethics. Adwards RB and Graber GC ed. New York: Harcourt Brace, 414-424; Sass HM 1992 l.c.; Zaner RM ed 1988 Death: Beyond Whole-Brain Criteria. Dordrecht; Tai MC 2004, The Way of Asian Bioethics. Taipei: Princeton Intern. Publ, 48: 62f., stressing the wholeness of body and mind, will not easily accept brain based criteria developed in Western culture.

[24] U.S., President's Commission, 1981, 40.

[25] Veatch, l.c., 422, underlines the importance to at least allow competent adults to choose higher brain death criteria, when and if they disagree with the whole brain death formula. Fletcher and Truog reformulate the Uniform Determination of Death Act by emphasizing the importance of the integrative function of the brain: 'People are dead if they have a distinct and precisely definable condition characterized by the absence of integrated brain function, such that somatic death is uniformly immanent' (Truog, Fletcher l.c., 208); such a reformulation of the original whole-brain death definition of the Harvard formula allows for covering anencephalic as well as the traditional brain death definition. Some Non-Western traditions, such as Parsi and Hindu religions, have no problem in understanding that at one time the body is ensouled and that at another time the soul will leave the body.

determination regarding medical interventions at the end of life according to individual quality-of-life assessments or cultural differences and preferences. Such a formula could read as follows: *In the absence of advanced directives, the irreversible cessation of all functions of the entire brain, including brain stem, will define death. Given global cultural diversity and different legal and religious traditions, states in promoting their interest in protecting life and dignity of their citizens in accordance with widely held values within their constituency may as a matter of public policy define different death criteria, such as those based on cessation of functions of the entire body or the heart, but should provide a conscience clause for individual choice. A determination of death must be made in accordance with accepted medical standards.*

Such a combination of uniform standard and conscience clause would allow for individual choice, cultural identity, patient-oriented clinical treatment, and a reduction of societal conflict. It would also include many advantages. Given wide differences in worldview and moral priorities in multicultural societies and in a world of diverse cultural traditions, only a conscience clause respects and supports individual self-determination and religious/cultural tolerance[26]. Legislation and regulation provide safe ethical and legal parameters for the full protection of life for those who do not wish to make their own choices regarding death and dying. Competent adults will not be sentenced by legalistic statutes to a slow dying process through various stages of vegetative life. Health care professionals will not be called upon to prolong vegetative human life against their own systems of belief, but they will not be allowed to take the life of a PVS patient without specific patient directives. Whole-brain death criteria might find even stronger support when they comprise a uniform default position. The fact that some intelligent people choose less strict criteria for the determination of their death signals that the default position might be too strict, but it is definitely not too loose or too liberal.

In strong contrast to the consensus regarding the end of life, our societies have no consensus regarding moral recognition and legal protection of its beginning. We have not even found a consensus on the methods and arguments necessary to start the consensus formation procedure. I propose using methods similar to those that led to the widely accepted consensus on brain-based criteria for the ethical evaluation of the end of human life. I also propose allowing for a conscience clause, particularity for pregnant women. If the difference of humans in regard to other living beings is our rational capacity for examination of conscience, for communication and tradition, and for debating right and wrong, then criteria related to the functioning of the brain will provide a moral and cultural

---

Hindu teaching of re-incarnation in fact denies individual death as compared to the death of the individual biological body.

[26] Schoene-Seifert B 2014 Hirntod, Ja Aber. Paderborn: Mentis.

basis for a societal consensus in regard to the beginning of morally significant human life.

Uniform brain life criteria for moral recognition of unborn human life have often been suggested by physicians,[27] theologians,[28] and philosophers.[29] We

---

[27] Goldenring J 1985 The brain life theory: towards a consistent biological definition of humanness, in: Journal of Medical Ethics11:198-204; Jones DG 1989 Brain birth and personal identity, in: Journal of Medical Ethics 15:173-178; 185. Jones argues that the first synapses 'are very few and far between and they are unlikely to be functional' and suggests that stages after the 151th day pc, from the 23th week of gestation up to 18 months after birth, develop a more distinctive characteristic of the networks in the human brain. EEG activity has been demonstrated as early as the 14th week, with more generalized activity during the 22th week, but this activity is 'discontinued with long periods of electrocerebral silence' up to the 32th week: 'If the EEG is to be taken as a guide to brain birth it is a highly conservative tool, placing the emergence of the semblance of an adult pattern at 32-36 weeks' gestation,' p. 176f. Goldenring concludes that functioning cortical brain, which according to our terminology would be the first manifestation of animating life, does not occur prior to the 22th to 28th week of gestation, while Jones, anatomist and neuroscientist, interprets the period between the 24th and 28th week of gestation, 'when most developmental sequences' of the brain have started, as the period of 'brain birth,' which 'demarcates the transition from non-personhood to personhood' following the maxim 'Whenever a functioning human brain is present, a human being is alive.' This proposal is more conservative and stops short of venturing into the moral evaluation of the stages of the evolutionary processes of the development of neuro-neuronal interconnecting and of forming the structures of the higher brain. It recognizes only the ontological differences that become manifest in the first transition from isolated to interconnected neurons in the cortical plate zone. Searching for the widest possible societal consensus regarding the protection of animate life, it is a morally safe and conservative judgment to refer only to the first biological evidence of synapse formation among postmitotic cerebral neurons as the prerequisite for cortical differentiation, which is the necessary physiological substratum and correlate to personal life.

[28] Haering B 1973 Medical Ethics. Notre Dame: Fides; Overhage P, Rahner K, 1961 Das Problem der Homisation, in: Questiones Disputatae 12(3). Freiburg: Herder. Rahner and Haering recognize that hominisation and personal life cannot be demonstrated theologically without the development of the biological conditions and presuppositions of personal life; both identify the cerebral cortex as the biological correlate to the Christian concept of personhood and 'imago Dei.'

[29] Brody 1982 l.c.; Kannegiesser H, 1988 Conception in the Test Tube. Melbourne: Macmillan. Kannegiesser, who is closest to our own moral assessment of neuromaturation, concludes that 'from about 10 weeks after conception until death, most human beings have sufficient moral value to warrant both care and protection.... The beginning of brain activity heralds the beginning of moral value while the cessation of brain activity (brain death) signals the end of the individual as a morally relevant entity.' He proposes ~~to~~ replacing criteria related to personhood by those related to brain functioning because of culturally different concepts of personhood. Using an ontological theory of essentialism, Brody argues that foetal humanity can only be based on brain functioning because 'a functioning brain (or at least, a brain that, if not functioning, is susceptible of function) is a property that every human being must have because it is essential for humans,' as evidenced by a

might even find a greater consensus for a definition of cortical life than we have been able to find for a definition of cortical death. Among the arguments favouring cortical brain life statutes are the following. (a) Other parts of the brain are still in development and maturation, so even though the brainstem shows earlier functions, these are transient and will be taken over by higher brain structures in adulthood. (b) There is no significant interrelation between developing and differentiating parts of the brain, so that the criteria proposed by Truog and Fletcher would not apply. (c) Other organs are not yet connected to the brain or functioning in a meaningful manner. (d) Aristotelian-Thomist ontology and anthropology, differentiating between an inanimate and an animate unborn, suggest cortex-related rather than whole-brain related criteria for recognizing personhood.

A universal Uniform Life Protection Act based on strong cultural traditions and on differentiating moral arguments would need to include a Conscience Clause and to consider integrated brain functioning, beginning with the presence of neuro-neuronal synapses in the subcortical plate and ending with the absence of brain functioning (cessation of higher or entire brain functioning). It would provide the following moral, cultural, legal, and political benefits. (1) One single statute protects the moral value of human life from beginning to end. (2) The symmetry between brain life and brain death criteria is conceptually clear. (3) Brain life and brain death criteria translate the ethos of strong ontological and moral traditions into the scenarios of modem biomedicine and its bioethical challenges. (4) Abortive, contraceptive, and contra-implantative interventions have to be assessed morally on grounds other than those of 'killing a person.' (5) Inanimate and postanimate forms of human life do not deserve the same moral recognition and legal protection as animating and animate life, thus reducing moral uncertainty and emotional stress in dealings with the beginnings and ends of human life. (6) A Conscience Clause protects decisions made by those who favour the full moral recognition of earlier stages of developing human life for religious or philosophical reasons. The diagnosis of animating life can be made in accordance with accepted standards of determining the age of the foetus by ultrasound and measuring its size by calculating post-ovulation days using human chorionic gonadotropin (HCG) testing. Given the accuracy of correlating the size of the embryo to its gestational and neuronal development, ultrasound diagnosis seems to be a sufficient indicator for determining the stage marking the earliest possible biological correlate to animate life.

7.6. Shortcomings of the Potentiality Argument

A special but deficient argument to protect human life from the moment of conception on has been prominently voiced by the Vatican and echoed by others as

wide consensus on brain death criteria, and that 'one ought to conclude that the foetus becomes a human being at some time between the 6. and the 12. week after its conception.'

well. It is the argument of *potentialitas*, that the *nasciturus* ('one who is to be born') has the potential to become a person in the future. This position suggests that rights can be claimed on the principle of potentiality,[30] and it has contributed significantly to the confrontational public debate and moral confusion over abortion. The argument inherits at least the following four logical as well as moral deficiencies: (a) We do not normally or regularity conclude that every potential requires moral actions for transformation into reality. (b) The argument is not supported by the moral tradition. (c) It is arbitrarily chosen to support one ontological stage in an evolutionary process over other potentialities. (d) The high natural abortion rate of around 50% suggests that abortion is as normal as implantation, or as much as the natural potentiality for nidation. In the Abraham story, both Hagar and Sarah had the potential to not become children, and Ismael and Isaac had the potential to be sacrificed by their father.

Potentiality is not reality, and the interrelatedness between both can have different forms, only some of which requiring an 'ought.' Potentiality in itself cannot establish rights – not the right to become President of the United States, to become the Pope in Rome, or to gain a certain position in society, even though the capabilities and potential might be there. In the worlds of bios, innumerable potentialities are not satisfied, and such a loss of realization has consequences beyond the potential of individual bios.[31] Honouring all potentials of all human persons by giving them rights would be moral malpractice because the claims cannot be realized. In fact, we habitually violate the potentiality principle. In fertility ethics, every lost opportunity for cohabitation violates it and so do all forms of contraception, whether they use hormonal or intrauterine devices or the so-called 'natural methods.' Chastity of priest and nuns, sexual acts not leading to fertilization, and abortions do not recognize 'potentiality' as a leading principle for making moral choices. Some moral choices disregarding or openly violating the potentiality principle have won cultural acceptance, while others have not. It is logically impossible to argue that rights can be derived from potentialities.[32]

Given the high natural abortion rate of around 50%, one can argue that it is the 'normal' potentiality of a zygote to not to reach the 16-cell stage.[33] Not only

[30] Congregation for the Doctrine of the Faith, 1987, Instruction on Respect for Human Life and its Origins and the Dignity of Procreation. Vatican.

[31] Crops for foodstuff and most trees and plants need fertilization by honeybees or other insects to fulfill their potential, but a pandemic among honeybees, sickness caused by Varroa mite parasites or neonicotinoid insecticides, or widespread total colony collapse disorder will have enormous consequences in these and other interconnected biotopes, including the human food chain and human culture.

[32] Sass, 1989. Schoene-Seifert B, 1990 Überlegungen zum moralischen Status des Embryos, Möglichkeiten und Grenzen der Forschung an Embryonen. Fuchs C ed., Stuttgart: Fischer, 99-111.

[33] Akerma, Karim: Lebensende und Lebensbeginn, Münster 2006:358.

is the potentiality argument morally unenforceable and logically weak; it does not represent the mainstream of theological teaching and philosophical tradition. Based on the theory of Divine animation, Mosaic Law did not recognize the nasciturus as a person with full rights: 'When men strive together, and hurt a woman with a child, so that there is a miscarriage, and yet no harm follows, the one who hurts her shall be fined. If any harm [to the woman] follows, then you shall give life for life, eye for eye.'[34] Roman Catholic theology has always argued ontologically, not teleologically, based on Aristotle and St. Thomas's concept of ensoulment.[35] Haering and Rahner presented ontological arguments favouring the understanding of neocortical reality rather than the potential of fertilized eggs as a necessary biological substratum for morally recognized life. Rahner asks whether the Church is really ready to teach and 'to accept that fifty per cent of all "human beings" – real human beings with 'immortal' souls and an eternal destiny – will never go beyond this first stage of human existence.'[36] In contrast to the recent teaching of the Vatican, Roman Catholic tradition is based on the centuries-old Aristotelian/Thomist theory of animation. St. Augustine, St. Thomas, and other fathers of the Church taught that early abortion prior to the 80th day did not require the same stiff canonical penalties as aborting animated or ensouled life, because it was not considered homicide. The change in Roman Catholic teaching regarding the moral recognition of unborn human life came in 1854 as a side effect of changes in the dogma of the Immaculate Conception. Pope Pius IX determined that in the first instant of her conception, the Virgin Mary was preserved and untouched by any taint of original sin,[37] as she was animated from the moment of conception. In 1869, another papal encyclical, following new Mariological teaching, extended the notion of ensoulment from the moment of conception to all human life. It thus abandoned the traditional approach of differentiating between inanimate or 'non-ensouled' and animate or 'ensouled' foetuses.[38] Thus, a change in dogmatic theory subsequently had severe side effects in moral theory and consensus formation. However, as late as 1896, Ligori's influential compendium on moral theology[39] used animation theory to discuss the difference between active and passive acts of sin as related to the difference between late and early abortion. Ligori suggests that in cases of aborted male foetuses after 40 but prior to 80 days pc, the abortion should be understood as terminating inanimate life, because it was not possible to know

---

[34] Exodus 21:22.

[35] Aristotle, De generatione animalium II, 736a32-b29; Thomas Aquinus, S.Th.l, q.118,a.2ad2; according to Augustinus, 'there cannot be said to be a live soul in a body which lacks sensation, when it is not formed into flesh and so not yet endowed with sense.'

[36] Overhage and Rahner, 1961.

[37] Bettenson H, 1963 Documents of the Christian Church. Oxford U. Press, Oxford, p. 381.

[38] General Synod Board for Social Responsibility, 1985, Personal Origins. London: Church Information Office Publ. 25.

[39] Ligori SA, 1898: Kb.lll, tractV, cap. IV, art.ll.

the sex of the foetus. The moral change accompanying the dogmatic rearrangement did not find full support among church members.[40]

The manner in which the potentiality principle is exclusively applied to the moment of conception makes it a hidden ontological argument favouring one of the developmental stages over the other and violating earlier potentialities at the cost of this one.[41] Also, if the potentially/'right to Be' principle were taken seriously, those holding these views would have to give research on the extremely high natural abortion rate of fertilized human eggs highest priority for moral reasons. Zygotes dying before they reach the 64-cell stage is as 'normal' or 'natural' as going beyond that stage and being born. No pro-life position so far has called for allocating funds to medical research to save approximately 50% of 'us' from 'premature death' (a much higher return in life years from invested funds than any other improvement in the existing health care systems). Finally, consider those holding the view that from the moment the sperm penetrates the *zona pellucida* of the egg an individual person exists that must be protected.

---

[40] An option open to the Roman Catholic moral teaching and supported by canonical reasoning would be the same the Church took in regard to the end of human life, when in 1957 Pope Pius XII declared that in cases of 'prolonged coma' the soul might already have left the body and no 'extraordinary means' would be required but that the determination of death should be left to the physicians. Not only might this option reconcile Church teaching and the conscience of the believers, it will contribute to the formation of societal consensus regarding the moral recognition of the beginning of human life as it contributed to the consensus regarding its end. In the light of biomedical understanding of the process of neuromaturation, Abrahamic traditions have great incentives to re-evaluate and reconfirm the traditional concept of individual 'ensoulment,' i.e., recognizing a biomedical correlate to the bioethical principle of moral recognition and legal protection of the *nasciturus*, as soon as the neuronal preconditions for the 'soul' become present.

[41] Applying the principle of potentiality to the moment of conception is arbitrary and should not be taken for granted without further argumentation and substantiation. The potential of 'new life' versus 'old life,' as expressed by haploid sets of chromosomes in each generated sperm and ovulated egg, would be the first prime candidate for the implementation of the principle of potentiality. The moral 'ought' would require seeing that as many potential oocytes would be transformed into reality. This has never been seriously considered, however, and would lead to multiple moral dilemmas. On the other hand, the potentiality of the fertilized egg immediately after conception does not yet express the individual new human genome; only later stages express the individual genetic code of the person to be. If genetic individuality is the substratum for potential persons, then the four-cell stage should be the first one to be protected; if it is not, then the potential of the oocytes has to be given strong moral standing and should not be disregarded. But when potential individuals ought to be protected by the potentiality principle, who or what deserves moral recognition: the four-cell conglomerate or each of the four totipotent cells, all of which have the potential to develop into a person. Protecting the potentiality of the conglomerate refuses to recognize the potential of the four individual cells, and protecting the potentiality of each of the four cells disregards the potential of the cell conglomerate. In general, the introduction of the potentiality principle into the debate of when to morally recognize and legally protect early human life results only in logical and moral confusion and causes logical and moral dilemmas and malpractice.

They have not elaborated on the potentiality of gametes representing earlier forms of 'new life' eager for support of their potential, or on the expression of the individual genome in the 4- to 8-cell stage. If those taking religious or philosophical positions really want to protect early human life based on the principle of potentiality, then they have to explain why they refrain from protecting oocytes as the earliest form of 'new' human life and why they have not yet suggested using cryo conservation of frozen sperm and zygotes to protect at least 50% of them from death. Since cryo storage is a proven method to preserve early human life, it seems to have the same moral and religious validity as surrogate motherhood or marriage among close relatives, as was the case with Abraham, Hagar, Sarah, Ishmael, and Isaac. Zygotes are early human bodies in development. In religious terms, we can say they are not yet animate and can compare them to brain-dead people who are no longer animated.

Damad summarizes the contemporary debate in a recent article about the tension between traditional Western attitudes and *figh* tradition (an Arabic term meaning "deep understanding" or "full comprehension") versus scientific possibilities in finding the most appropriate moral answer regarding the use of modern technology. 'Cloning new human life by inserting a somatic cell nucleus into a denucleid omnipotent or multipotent cell and transplanting the zygote into a uterus is genetic manipulation for the purpose to have an offspring. Many religions, philosophers and UNESCO see risks to individual human dignity, lineage, and culture in the use of cloning.'[42] Also, different from in-vitro fertilization or the use of other techniques to improve conception, in cloning the nucleus is either maternally or paternally imprinted (gynogenote or androgenote). In cases of nuclear transfer or newly developing methods of genetic editing by use of CRISPR/Cas9, mitochondrial and nucleus DNA can come from three contributing people. A multiplicity of moral, cultural, and familial issues arise.[43] How will we be able to solve them in solidarity with and in respect for individual and community bios?

7.7. Subsidiarity: Dignity of the Individual Conscience

Subsidiarity as a principle in social ethics was developed by Roman Catholics to support 'lower levels' of moral decision making (such as individuals, families, neighbourhoods, or small groups) against legal or ethical 'domination' by higher authorities (such as states or organizations).[44] Any global consensus statute on

[42] Damad M SM, 2012, Human cloning from the viewpoint of Islamic figh and ethics, in: Asian Bioethics Review 3(4)342-350.

[43] Park E 2016 Life, the Remix. A new technique that lets scientists edit DNA with ease is transforming science – and raises difficult questions, in: Time 188(1)42-48; see also chapter 3.

[44] The principle of subsidiarity was reformulated for the purpose of social policy in the Roman Catholic Church's confrontation with Fascist social policy, but can as such protect

such important, sensitive issues as the moral and legal recognition of a human life's beginning and end has to include conscience clauses for those who hold different views. In regard to its beginning, stricter views have to be legally protected and morally accepted. In regard to its end, individual concepts of life and death must be allowed to function as the prime criterion for defining one's own end of life within the parameters of a universal statute.[45] Therefore, individuals or groups holding stricter philosophical or religious views regarding the moral recognition of inanimate or vegetative life must have every right to hold on to them and act accordingly. Convictions applying more liberal concepts of animate versus post-animate life should be tolerated if the acts based on these beliefs will affect only the people who hold them. Their wishes could be conveyed in the form of advanced directives or living wills requesting higher brain

---

moral decisions and actions based on other individual and collective choices as well; cf. Papal encyclical 'Quadrogesimo Anno,' Rome 1934.

[45] Cf. Bagheri A, Afshar L 2011 Abortion in different Islamic jurisprudence. Case Studies, in: Asian Bioethics Review 3(4)351-365; this case study on Islamic abortion law shines a light on the reality of the subsidiarity principle. The case: Fatemeh, 15 weeks pregnant and a practicing Muslim with her husband Mohsin, is diagnosed as a carrier of beta thalassemia. They discuss abortion with their Muslim doctors and feel they have an argument in favor of terminating the pregnancy, even though rare and controversial: death or harm to the mother or the future child. Their option would be different depending on different religious and legal rules in various Muslim countries since the early Islamic law schools of Abu Hanifa, Ibn Malik, Ash-Shafi, and Ibn Hanabal in the 8th century, confirming Abu Hanifa's insight: 'Differences of opinion in the congregation can be read as a special grace of God' in different forms of execution. Saudi Arabian law: if life or health of the mother or serious anomaly of the fetus is of concern, abortion up to the 120th day pc is permitted, in some fatwas still only up to the 40th day pc; conservative Maliki and Gazali law schools allow abortion only when the life of the mother is threatened. Turkey (Presidency of Religious Affairs): abortion is *makruh* (disliked) at any time, but tolerated up to the 120th day upon the decision of a specialized physician and consent of the couple; often Imans are consulted as well. Egypt: Abortion is criminal; some schools allow it up to the 120th day pc if life of mother is endangered; fatwa number 336 of Mofti Al Deyar Al-Massriyyah, 2004: 'Any deformation that may be detected in the fetus are not considered a legal excuse for abortion, except they pose a risk to the mother's life. Allah Almighty knows best.' Iranian Parliament 2005 'Therapeutic Abortion Law': 'Therapeutic Abortion is permissible with definite diagnosis of three specialist physicians and approval of the Legal Medical Organization for cases in which fetus suffers from anomalies or (mental) retardations that causes hardship to mother and also for cases in which mother suffers from life threatening disease, before ensoulment (four month of pregnancy) with consent of mother and there is no penalty for consulting physicians. Violators of this act would be punished based on Islamic Punishment Act.' Malaysia (officially a multi-cultural state): Abortion is a crime; exception if a registered medical practitioner in good faith diagnoses risk to the mother's life or mental or physical wellbeing; National Fatwa Committee 2002 found that up to the 40th day abortion is disliked (*makruh*) and that husband and wife have to consent; tolerated after 120th day, only if harm to the mother is expected; after 120 days if harm to the mother due to severe deformity of the fetus.

death criteria for themselves in decisions of termination of medical intervention or organ transplantation.

A Uniform Life Protection Act would make abortion of inanimate life legal, as well as the use of contraceptives or devices that prevent nidation and the termination of clinical treatment after all brain functions have ceased, including those of the brain stem. The Bioethical Imperative, of course, calls for respecting inanimate, unborn life and post-animate human corpses as well, as we owe respect to all forms of bios. The specifics of this respect will be expressed in different ways, given the diverse cultural ceremonies and traditions involved amidst the goal of honouring the dignity of the individual conscience. No woman should be forced to accept abortion or contraception, as the moral assessment of these interventions depends on her own values and beliefs. Legislative or regulatory bodies might require mandatory consultation for pregnant juveniles prior to abortion. On the other hand, no individual or group should be allowed to dominate public policy, regulation, and legislation by imposing their views on the beginning and end of human life, life after life, or the moral status of the fertilized or unfertilized egg. Research on inanimate human life will require the involvement of bioethical experts or committees in preparing bioethical guidelines. Research on inanimate life or its use for diagnostic or therapeutic purposes will require the consent of those providing sperm, egg, or zygotes, the same way organ transplants cannot be done without the consent of the donor.

In contrast to Roe vs. Wade, I suggest the following formulation: 'For the stage prior to approximately the end of the 10th week of gestation, the abortion decision must be left to the pregnant woman, following medical consultation and spousal discussion where necessary. For stages subsequent to the 10th week, the state, in promoting its interest in the protection of unborn human life, may if it chooses, regulate, and even proscribe, abortion except where it is necessary, in appropriate medical judgment, for the preservation of the life or health of the mother.' I see two ways to start the process of consensus formation on protecting early human life. (a) A national consensus formation body, similar to the ad hoc Harvard committee on *'brain death'* in 1968, could set up the argumentative framework for establishing the biomedical criteria of *'brain life,'* allowing for bioethical evaluation and legal protection at the beginning of personal human life. A uniform statute should address the protection of human life from its beginning to its end. (b) A public debate could be initiated that would include information about the facts of embryonic and neuronal development and about the traditions of moral teaching and cultural history, both secular and religious. Such a debate among professionals and laypersons would represent a reflective moral equilibrium based on judgments, intuitions, and attitudes similar to those Fan finds in the Confucian traditions and Tai has outlined as the five virtues of compassion, righteousness, respect, responsibility, and 'no harm' (which in integrated form guide the way of Asian bioethics).[46]

How can we best protect the dignity of early human life and of dying fellow humans in harmony with the rich variety of ontological, moral, cultural, and religious visions and intuitions?[47] A combination of uniform standards and conscience clauses will guarantee individual choice, cultural identity, patient-oriented clinical treatment, and a reduction of societal conflict and confrontation. Conscience clauses regarding the beginning of life, when proxy decisions are made for unborn human life, should only allow for standards stricter than those covered by the uniform statute. Conscience clauses regarding the end of life, when competent adults make decisions for themselves, should allow for a variety of choices based on individual religious or philosophical understanding, some of which might be less strict than the default position backed by the national legal system.

We may, as a special application of the Bioethics Imperative to individual human life and dignity, thus formulate a Universal Life Protection Act:

A UNIVERSAL LIFE PROTECTION ACT

(1) *An individual developing or having integrated brain functions deserves moral recognition and legal protection. Biomedical facts suggest the protection of human life from early synapse formation in the cortical plate zone, when personal life becomes imminent, up to the absence of integrated brain functions, when somatic death is imminent.*

(2) *Given global cultural diversity and different moral and religious traditions, states in promoting their interest in protecting the life and dignity of their citizens in accordance with widely held values within their constituency may as a matter of public policy define brain life and brain death criteria based on accepted medical standards.*

(3) *States and laws must provide a Conscience Clause for individual choice in the moral recognition of earlier stages of unborn human life and in defining individual criteria for their death based on cessation of functions of the heart or higher brain.*

---

[46] Fan R 2009 Reconstructurist Confucianism. Rethinking Morality after the West. Heidelberg: Springer; Fan R, 2012, 'Confucian reflective equilibrium: why principlism is misleading for Chinese bioethics decision making,' Asian Review of Bioethics 4(1):8; Tai MC 2008 l.c.

[47] Rodriges S 2014 A Woman's 'Right to Know', in: Intern J Feminist Approaches to Bioethics 7(1)51-73; Kukla R et al. 2005 Finding Autonomy in Birth, in: Bioethics 23(1): 1-8; Brauer S 2016 Moral Implications of obstetric Technologies for Pregnancy and Motherhood, in: Med Health Care and Philosophy 19:45-54

(4) States with strict uniform laws should allow 'ethical tourism' without penalty when citizens disagree with those uniform laws based on their religious or moral conviction.

8. COMPETENT CARE FOR PERSONAL HEALTH

WE PEOPLE ARE DIFFERENT

'Non homo universalis curatur, set unus quique nostrum - It is not the universal person, we are to treat; he/she is an individual, unique, our patient.'

Galen, physician of Roman Emperor Augustus, 2nd century

8.1. Individual Health Profiles and Global Health Governance

We humans are of different individual bios, but we are also social bios and are integrated in the many habitats of persons within microbiome, with family and society, and in environmental harmony or disharmony. None of us can live alone, and we all need our co-bios. In interpreting the Fifth Commandment, *You shall not kill,* Fritz Jahr described three positive stages of self-preservation:[1] (1) not harming one's own life (e.g., maintaining health by avoiding anger and excessive drinking and eating); (2) protecting one's life, which also serves one's neighbor, community, and country; (3) following the inclusive Bioethical Imperative (to which the other two lead) to respect and treat, if possible, all bios as an end in itself. Jahr's interpretation of scriptural and philosophical texts corresponds to most recent environmental, social, genetic, and epigenetic knowledge. We are individually formed not only by our own DNA and genetic heritage, but also by epigenetic interactions from the earliest stages of life through interactions with social and natural habitats.[2] Personal and communal health and harmony go hand in hand,[3] depending on and enriching each other as integrated bios in symbiosis, as we discuss in other chapters. But implementations and applications remain far away. Except for the growing fitness movement, they seem to not be supported yet by public awareness and fashionable trends. While the expert doctor Galen insisted on treating each patient as an individual, he and many other great doctors were certainly aware of the individual as being integrated in the wider bios of society and nature.

Progress in molecular genetics and epigenetics, as well as new insights into the interactions of microbial, environmental, social, and individual human bios, has improved clinical knowledge in pharmacogenetics and in predictive and

[1] Jahr 2013 l.c. 77-84 (1934, Three Studies on the Fifth Commandment).

[2] Glucksman P et al. 2008 Effect of In-Utero and Early-Life Conditions on Adult Health and Disease, in: New England J Medicine 359(1)61-73; Dupras C, Ravitzky V, Williams-Jones B 2014 Epigenetics and the Environment, in: Bioethics 28(7)327-334; Chadwick R, O'Connor A 2013 Epigenetics and Personalized Medicine. Prospects and Ethical Issues, in: Personalized Medicine 10(5)463-471; Dupras C, Ravitsky V 2016 Epigenetics in the Neoliberal 'Regime of Truth,' in: Hastings Center Report 40(1)26-35. As to our interdependence with the multiple vast and changing microbial interconnections in our guts, living spaces and agricultures, see Montgomery DR, Bikle A 2016 The Hidden Half of Nature. The Microbial Roots of Life and Health. NY: Norton.

[3] Gostin LO 2012 A Framework Convention on Global Health. Health for All. Justice for All, in: JAMA 307(19):2087-2092.

preventive medicine. Unfortunately, most of this knowledge has not yet been put to work in personalized drug prescriptions, nutrigenomics, physical exercise and sport advice, personal health risk education, prediction and prevention, and lay promotion of health literacy. Due to their self-centered internal metabolisms, regulatory and political powers have not translated the wealth of new health knowledge into frameworks of supporting happy, healthy communities and societies. The international literature discusses various conflicts between issues of privacy, information property rights, and medical benefits in prescribing individualized, efficacious drugs and of informing and advising individuals on prevention and health care based on individual genetic profiles. New models of communication and cooperation in trust between experts and laypeople need to be developed. 'Not a matter of biology alone,' health care is 'a never ending journey towards the highest perfection of human being.'[4] Some traditional wisdom pertaining to good care for individual health has been replaced by an unfortunate repair mentality in a health care system focusing on a disease management paradigm for financial reasons.

New diagnostic knowledge in human epigenetics and pharmacogenetics makes sharing information and agency with citizens as future or actual patients both possible and mandatory. Based on Western and Eastern traditions of responsibility and self-determination within the individual's cultural environment, the obligation to know about one's genetic heritage and its relative advantages and uncertainties is a precondition for living a self-determined, risk-competent, educated life. Imparting this information would require a duty on the part of health care experts to inform, educate, and counsel the public, and to support the right to be told. In cases in which others are not affected negatively by individual self-determination, clients must have the right to refuse to follow health care advice. There seems to be no obligation to convey genetic information if diagnostic findings cannot result in advice or prescription; but one could make the argument that even in cases of interventional futility, citizens have the right to request it if they want to know.[5] If health risks are present or predictable, a right to know and an obligation to tell exist. A moral not a legal obligation to follow health care advice applies, however; and it becomes more pressing if health care costs are shared in solidarity.

Genetic and epigenetic diagnosis provides potentially important information for family members in regard to health risk, health status, and preventive measures essential for self-determination and quality-of-life decisions. Each person diagnosed with specific genetic properties will need to consider her or his responsibilities towards family. Postmodern cultures emphasize individual privacy, while in cultures of transition the love for and responsibility towards

---

[4] Peimin N , l.c., 42.

[5] Kielstein R, Sass HM 2002 Genetics in kidney disease; how much do we want to know? in: American J Kidney Dialysis 39:637-659.

immediate family still plays a high role among stakeholders, even within the wider family. As with severe genetic disorders, a higher-than-average risk of hypertension, forms of cancer, and metabolic disorders may run in families. Consequently, information about these risk factors would be vital to carriers, so that they seek frequent checkups and advice or can use preventive strategies to postpone onset or reduce impact. *Interactive family health care ethics* for dealing adequately with issues of family ethics still await development. Also, families may be influenced by unfounded feelings of guilt and shame, as well as by denial, accusations, divorce, suicide, and the breakdown of familial relations. The Golden Rule must be to avoid hiding behind traditional habits of secrecy and privacy. Instead, it calls for openly and aggressively informing and educating families while supporting dialogue in them and between them and society. These efforts follow the grain of traditional familial forms of communication and cooperation while honoring the will of the diagnosed carrier and making the best use of sometimes dormant principles of family responsibility and solidarity. In traditional settings, individual autonomy is embedded in family and community: 'Although a family is composed of many members, community starts not with the individual but with the unity of the family, which becomes the base of a macro vision of Confucian tradition for a harmonious universe.'[6] New, rapidly developing knowledge in interactive and integrated genetics and epigenetics among all forms of bios suggests building on such a 'family conceptor' model, which is similar to the religious/philosophical unifying of the integrated fate of bios and bioethics in biopolitics. In this sense, biopolitics is not a national but a global goal, responsibility, and strategy. In the words of Larry Gostin: 'The global governance system must be capable of exerting influence in multiple regimes that affect health. Intellectual property affects access to essential medicines, trade in services affects health worker migration, and climate change affects food, disease vectors, and natural disasters. Human rights laws cover socioeconomic determinants of health, while humanitarian law protects civilians caught in armed conflicts.'[7]

8.2. Health Information and Carrier Ethics

The individual is nevertheless at the center of caring for individual and collective health. Various cultural and social trends have weakened traditional concepts of the individual as being a part of the family and not an end and purpose in herself or himself. This cultural trend seems to give the individual more

[6] Tai MC, Lin CS 2001 Developing a culturally relevant bioethics for Asian people, in: J Medical Ethics 7:53; new and rapidly developing knowledge in interactive and integrated epigenetics among all shapes and shades of bios suggests building on this or other religious or philosophical unifying models of understanding the common and integrated fate of bios and bioethics.

[7] Gostin 2012 l.c. 2091.

responsibility and weight in global development. Therefore, in complex issues of family ethics, privacy, disclosure, right not to know, and duty to know, diagnosed carriers would be the prime moral agents making educated and responsible choices (a) to disclose, (b) to refuse disclosure of all or some information, or (c) to postpone hard choices such as informing family members. There will be hard cases in which information might be lifesaving to family members who could be carriers. Some time ago, the proposed guidelines[8] by the World Health Organization (WHO) on ethical issues in medical genetics suggested violating the principle of confidentiality somewhat in favor of informing and consulting family members, but guidelines of national organizations differ from such a stern position. In the future, responsible parenthood might include decisions regarding whether or not to (a) have children at all, (b) have prenatal testing and eventually elect abortion following positive testing, or (c) do nothing and trust to future breakthroughs in medical treatment. Data availability is a core principle beyond modern medicine, and it must be balanced with privacy and protection of data. The principle of data availability favors individual health care cards.

Since the discovery of blood types, reliable diagnosis, typing, and screening have become an essential part of emergency medicine and surgery, directly or indirectly saving millions of lives.[9] It is well known that we not only differ in types of blood but in many other individual properties. One example are cytochrome P450 isoforms, which control drug metabolism and cause non-efficacy, side effects, and even death in some types of metabolizers.[10] The fears that genotyping for drug metabolism will lead to discrimination are not convincing. Blood typing did not lead to discrimination, even though some people have rarer types (at least in certain populations), and therefore might have less access to blood replacement. Blood and medication profiles do not describe disorders (i.e.,

---

[8] WHO Report 2006 Medical Genetic Services in Developing Countries; WHO Report 2002 Review of Ethical Issues in Medical Genetics (refers to WHO 1998 Proposed International Guidelines on ethical issues in medical genetics and medical services).

[9] Sass HM 2010 Genetic Knowledge Is a Civil Right. Towards a New Model of Health Contract as Social Contract, in: Eubios. J Asian Intern Bioethics 20:2-9; cf. Paul NW, Roses AD 2003 Pharmacogenetics and pharmacogenomics: recent developments, their clinical relevance and some ethical, social and legal implications, in: J Molecular Medicine 81: 135-140

[10] In hypertension treatment, calcium antagonists are metabolized by the 3A enzyme in the cytochrome P450 isoform system, while beta blockers are metabolized by 2D6, so a switch from one to the other without proper drug metabolizing tests would be clinical and ethical malpractice; P450-2D6 enzymes metabolizing codeine for palliative care is absent in 7% of Caucasians, resulting in total non-efficacy in those individuals; P450-2C19 metabolizing diazepam (Valium) and other neuropharmaca is absent in 15% to 30% of Asians in comparison to Caucasians [www.drug-interactions.com]. As individual pharmacogenetic profiles for medication typing can be established the same way, we can easily establish individual profiles in blood typing, so that personalized drug delivery is both possible and ethically required.

an individual aberration from a generic image). Rather, they constitute different types and variations, none of which is the 'normal' one. Even in our basic genetic setup we have a model of variation, not one of order and disorder, similar to the rich diversities of human visions and goals in our cultural bios. It would be a crime against humanity and an inexcusable wrong towards all fellow humans who would die if their lives could not be saved by blood transfusion based on proper blood typing beforehand. In drug metabolism, as in every metabolic property, the concept of normal is moot, because only differences in expression and action have meaning. Genotyping for drug compatibility causes no significant ethical concerns other than those associated with blood typing: clinical reliability of typing procedures, equal access to typing services, and no intervention (i.e., medication prescribing) prior to typing. The new scenario of metabolism typing has consequences for the accepted bioethical setup of vaccine development, clinical trials, prescription procedures, and nutrition advice. Therefore, it should be considered unethical to omit genotyping from drug development and to fail to establish efficacy, dosage, and side effects for major types of metabolizers based on cytochrome P450 isoform properties and composition. Individuals have a civil right to information about their individual proteonomic and enzymatic properties for metabolizing drugs and nutrition.

Other individual variances of genomic properties are based on individual epigenetic dynamics during pregnancy and early childhood, combined with interactions with the social and biological environment.[11] Individual health risks vary, depending on one's epigenetic experiences and changes in the genetic setup. Epigenetic variances in diseases have been reported for obesity, diabetes type B, asthma, and various allergies and behavioral disorders, as well as for leukemia, Parkinson's, and Crohn's disease.[12] This, of course, is another challenge to the traditional 'one size fits all' form of therapy and preventive medicine based on inflexible WHO classifications of disease and reimbursement schemes. It is also a test for equality in health care, as we differ not only in our blood types but also in our epigenetic setup (and we exist in different microbial, social, and climate habitats). Because we lack a single standard genome and have individual and intergenerational variances along with different blood types, not only clinical medicine issues but also public health issues need to be revisited. As Stapleton, Schroeder-Baeck, and Townsend argue: 'Discoveries of the heightened sensitivity of the epigenome to environmental conditions during ear-

---

[11] Wellenreuther M, Hansson B 2016 Detecting Polygenic Evolution. Problems, Pitfalls and Promises, in: Trends in Genetics 32(3):155-164; Lunshoff JE et al 2010 Personal Genomes in Progress. From the Human Genome Project to the Personal Genome Project, in: Dialogues in Clinical Neuroscience 12:47-60; Ober C, Vercelli D 2011 Gene-Environment Interactions in Human Disease: Nuisance or Opportunity, in: Trends in Genetics 27:107-115.

[12] Stapleton G, Schroeder-Baeck P, Townsend D 2013 Equity in Public Health. An Epigenetic Perspective, in: Public Health Genomics 16: 137.

ly development, and possibly through international communication of effects, further complicate matters when considered alongside the diversity of phenomena documented as influencing the epigenome. Such findings undermine perceptions of justice in health that question the suitability of actions taken to address health inequalities.'[13]

These and other informational civil rights, based on individual genomics and epigenetics, are best served by providing inexpensive personal Drug and Nutrition Cards and access to information and education. First-class expert/lay communication and cooperation thus become even more essential for success in caring for health and happiness.

8.2. Individual Choice and Informed Contract

New areas of research need new models of control and quality assurance. Reforms are urgently needed in clinical trials and human experimentation based on new challenges and opportunities, particularly in regard to genetic research, DNA sampling, and DNA storing. My thesis is that the traditional soft-paternalism principle of *informed consent* must be replaced by that of *informed contract*, detailing rights and obligations for researchers and probands or patients and liberating the latter from their passive role of merely consenting to a more adequate position of being treated as a person. In particular, DNA sampling and research into drug metabolism and specific diseases cannot be justified without taking into account the probable benefits to patients or families. Modern medical research will find extensive information about pedigree and family members that cannot be taken care of by the concept of individual consent obtained only from those who participate in the research.

For genotyping in highly defined populations of patients receiving specific medication for certain subgroups of cancer or other diseases, it has been debated whether traditional models of informed consent would be enough for multipurpose, long-term DNA banking. Dealing efficiently with such banking and the probable benefits to patients and their families means overburdening the informed consent principle. Giving informed consent to draw blood for unspecified research might not be in the best interest of the patient, even though such consent might benefit the research and other patients in the future. Informed consent forms rarely address issues of multipurpose screening and long-term storage. One should work with a *contract model* because the probability of

---

[13] Stapleton G et al, l.c.: 142; Schroeder P 2004 Gendiagnostische Gerechtigkeit. Muenster: Lit, recommends a new principle 'Gendiagnostische Gerechtigkeit - *gendiagnostic justice*,' while Marx-Stoelting L 2007 Pharmakogenetik und Pharmakogentests. Biologische, wisssenschaftstheoretische und ethische Aspekte des Umgangs mit genetischen Varianten. Muenster: Lit, 148f, suggests including into the Georgetown four-principle model a *social-ethical principle* recognizing genetic and epigenetic differences and the different social environments in which these differences occur.

benefits in cross-purpose genotyping (and of future unspecified re-testing and new testing) is of great moral importance for the individual patient, patient groups, and the progress of clinical research. The model below describes the researchers' obligation to inform the patient on all or some of their findings and to establish a contract spelling out the obligations towards patient and family: 'We ask you to sign a contract for genetic testing on information and properties that might or might not be associated with your disease and if so how they are associated with it. This process might take a long time, and we might look for information we don't know yet. We make it our legal obligation to inform you about any findings that might benefit your treatment or members of your family. You or your representative have the right to cancel this contract at any time and to request that your biological properties be destroyed. If you want to share in possible financial gain associated with this particular research, we will provide you with a separate contract'.[14] Within the contract, patients or their legal representatives must be informed on standard data protection. To address complex issues such as privacy and disclosure, the right not to know, and the duty to know, the contract must allow patients to make their own choices (a) for mandating disclosure of individual predictive, preventive, or therapeutic knowledge, (b) for refusal of all or some information, and (c) for postponing such a decision for later based on future individual circumstances or clinical results. The moral issues of similarly informing and protecting family members will have to be addressed within the contract by allowing the patient to choose among a number of procedures by which family members of various degrees may or may not be involved, informed, or invited. Only recently has a 'Global Alliance' taken up the concept of fair and enforceable contracting in this domain among national legal systems.[15]

It is time to replace an *outdated informed-consent model* totally or in part with a contract one in which stakeholders such as probands, researchers, and sponsors delineate moral and legal contractual rights and obligations. Some informed-consent forms now include such features as informed contracts, but WHO and the European Forum for Good Clinical Practice have not yet produced proposals for genuine reform. An excellent example of how the ethics of diagnostic research are moving towards a more appropriate appreciation of individual and family health care competence and decision making as partners in research is an old statement by the Human Genome Organisation's international ethics advisory group on choices in data availability within a firm model of data and privacy protection: 'The choices and privacy of individuals, families and communities should be respected: (a) choices may be with regard to: donation, storage and use of samples and the information derived therefrom (e.g. specific,

[14] Sass 2001 l.c., 131.

[15] Global Alliance for Genomics and Health. Framework for Responsible Sharing of Genomic and Health-Related Data, 2015; http://genomicsandhealth.org.

related or other uses subject to authorization by an ethics committee, etc.). Informed consent may include notification of uses (actual or future), or opting out, or, in some cases, blanket consent. (b) Mechanisms should be established to ensure respect for such choices. (c) Participants should be informed about the degree of identifiability of their data (e.g. coded, anonymized, aggregate, etc.) and the security mechanisms in place to ensure confidentiality. (d) Participants should be told that samples or the information derived therefrom may be shared with other researchers including those from other countries, with commercial entities and through publication and availability on the WEB.'[16]

Recognizing the principle of autonomy and self-determination as a basic human and civil right, modern medicine allows for clinical research and medical treatment only if the proband or patient has given free and informed consent based on individual concepts of risk, benefit, values, fear, and hope. Global recognition of the informed-consent principle correlates to the vision of universal human rights as expressed by the United Nations Declaration in 1948 and is a fruit of the processes of emancipation since the European Age of Reason. If immediate medical treatment is required to save life, the informed-consent principle cannot be used because patient survival is the higher principle. As good as it looks theoretically, a number of well-documented cases demonstrate that the informed-consent principle does not always work and can be used in an abusive and exploitative manner: (1) If people do not clearly understand the risks and benefits associated with research and treatment, oral or written consent is void. (2) If people feel an obligation to sign forms, their consent is not given freely. (3) If researchers cannot or do not inform probands or physicians fail to advise their patients adequately, signed forms are a smokescreen to hide the fact that true informed consent is not given, despite the legal requirements being satisfied.

In general, the informed-consent principle was developed at a certain historical time during the last century under specific cultural conditions. It was a useful tool to protect vulnerable persons from abuse, and properly used it is the best tool available for the protection of human dignity and civil rights. Even if no abuse is intended, however, cultural obstacles seem to be associated, regrettably, with rigid implementation of it under the maxim 'one size fits all.'[17] We have already seen the following standard deviations from, exemptions from, and modifications of the general rules: (1) Consent for minors is given by their ethical and/or legal representatives, mostly the parents. (2) Competent adults may designate another person to give consent on their behalf, either immediately or

[16] HUGO 2003 Statement on genetic screening (November 2002), in: Eubios 13(3); see also Check Hayden E 2012 As Researchers Find More Uses for Data, Informed Consent Has Become a Source of Confusion, Something Has to Change, in: Nature 486, 312-314

[17] Truog RD 1999 Is Informed Consent Always Necessary for Randomized Controlled Trials?, in: New England J Medicine 340:804-807; Faden RR, Beauchamp TL, Kass NE 2014 Informed Consent, Comparative Effectiveness, and Learning Health Care, in: New England J Medicine 370:766-768.

under certain conditions in the future. (3) The consent required from psychiatric patients is related to their particular disease and situation at a given time; however, there are well-developed treatment contracts signed by patients and their caretakers for possible future situations known to and experienced by the patient.[18]

Even though they might be in transition towards individualism, some traditional cultures still have a strong sense of family ethics and decision making for the good of the individual family member, thus giving group consent for his or her good. The individualistic European model is seen as an intrusion into a different trust-and-responsibility structure and, if used, applies only legalistically, with no cultural/ethical authority or validity. Family consent is not without risk. It might be the elder male or female head of a variously sized family accepting responsibility for his or her relatives and trusted to make decisions, even far-reaching ones regarding marriage, education, or job training. Some individuals or branches of the family might not trust the proxy decision maker or elders might violate their trust. These are the situations leading to the rise of emancipation and the concept of individual choice in the European Age of Reason. But families and communities still exist for whom the model of an individual making autonomous decisions by and for herself is considered unethical or even decadent and perverse. In order to implement some of the visions and goals of the 'informed consent' principle, it might be helpful to at least work with a formula of 'informed consent plus X,'[19] X being features relating to specific cultural attitudes and modes of decision making.

As we have discussed, some moral or social communities handle ethical and social issues using community consent, even though individuals are primarily subject to risk. In Western civilization, religious orders and closely controlled religious groups obey decisions made by their superiors. The fact that various cultural and moral communities have different values, wishes, hopes, and fears is used well when proxy medical decisions are made for incompetent persons. Schools of communitarian ethics place great emphasis on supporting and respecting communal values. Ethics committees in pluralistic societies include neighborhood representatives or envoys from religious, moral, or social communities to which the incompetent persons belong. If a village or province shares convictions widely, then most likely individual preferences for participation in medical research or medical treatment would be similar. Also, decisions would be made by wise elders, elected or otherwise accepted if such a paradigm is part of the specific culture. Researchers required to inform, educate, and gain consent would be well advised to use the existing trust-and-responsibility structure for information and education and for contracting with the community

---

[18] Sass 2001 l.c.

[19] Zhai XM 2011 Diversified and in Harmony, but not Identical, in: Asian Review Bioethics 3(1)31-35.

and/or families and individuals.[20] Benefits for all of the above should be spelled out in detail. In the case of DNA sampling, contracts should be signed some time beforehand. The larger and the more complex the community, the riskier a communitarian approach will be and the more features will have to be developed and supported to protect dissenting individuals and groups. In communities in cultural transition or under indoctrinating, exploiting elders or oligarchic groups, the communitarian approach to protect vulnerable individuals and families will not work and should not be applied.

It is only common sense to recognize that probands in all kinds of research expect something for their participation. It can be personal recognition or attention, individual or general health care advice, better hygiene, fresh water or nursing care, money, or other benefits for themselves or the community. The Council for International Organizations of Medical Sciences' guidelines for medical research in 'populations and communities with limited resources' state as follows: 'the sponsor and the investigator must make every effort to ensure that: the research is responsive to the health needs and the priorities of the population or community in which it is to be carried out; and any intervention or product developed, or knowledge generated, will be made reasonable available for the benefit of that population or community.'[21] The Nuffield Council on Bioethics[22] suggests 'that sponsors of research should require that the development of local expertise in healthcare is an integral component of research proposals. Consideration should be given to the extent to which any strengthening of local healthcare facilities can be done in such a way that the changes are sustainable in the local context once the research is over.' The World Health Organization discusses issues of patenting individual DNA;[23] which should not be done without addressing the genetic property interest of the individual or family in contractual form.

8.3. Personal Health Care Cards

Given the diversity of individual and collective cultures in decision making, one size of consent does not fit all. It seems clear that the classical model of informed consent has outlived its useful life as a general standard for every personal, familial, communitarian, cultural, or legal situation. Whenever prevailing cultural attitudes and legal preconditions are missing to make the classical form of informed consent the tool of choice, it cannot be made a requirement

---

[20] Tai MC 2008 The Way of Asian Bioethics. Taipei: Princeton Intern. Publ.; Zhai XM 2002 Informed consent in medical research; Proceedings of the 4th Asian conference on bioethics. Seoul: Seoul National University, p. 6;

[21] CIOMS 2002 International Ethical Guidelines for Biomedical Research involving Human Subjects. Geneva CIOMS, p. 51.

[22] Nuffield Council on Bioethics 2002 The Ethics of Research related to Healthcare in Developing Countries, London Nuffield Trust, p.116

[23] WHO Report 2005 Genetics, Genomics and the Patenting of DNA.

that medical experts first change cultures and attitudes and then proceed with their medical work. It is also not acceptable that medical experts turn a blind eye to missing essential prerequisites for informed consent/contract work. We all have to work toward implementing human rights and free decision making by competent, risk-literate adults: this task cannot be put on physicians alone. Also, ethical situations might arise in which coherent trust-and-responsibility structures within families or communities are well developed by cultural or religious tradition and are working well in a number of cases. In those situations, it would be insensitive, counterproductive, and unethical to destroy a working network of trust, hope, responsibility, and reliability only to replace it by a model developed under different cultural and historical conditions.

Models of contracts with families or individuals rather than the use of one-sided, paternalistic consent might work better in all situations. All culturally sensitive models would need 'escape' or 'conscience' clauses allowing individuals to determine for themselves their place in a moral community in regard to values and decision making. Great emphasis should be placed on developing culturally sensitive tools and procedures for those who want to make their own choices, even though attitudes in their community or family suggest otherwise. Traditional cultures seem to be in transition from community-oriented ethics towards a heavier emphasis on the individual's goals, visions, and lifestyle, which might not align as closely with those of the family as it once did. Because medical ethics are not the prime instrument for changing culture or preventing it from changing, health care ethics and individual health competence need to make the best use of accepted models of autonomy, solidarity, and reciprocity. But they can contribute towards biocultural changes as well, as we are witnessing in the open markets of fitness centers and fashions.

We all know how to live with blood typing. It is only 100 years ago that the different types were discovered, making reliable testing available and lifesaving blood transfusion possible.[24] We also know how to handle privacy issues when dealing with blood typing, and we give medical and moral preference to data availability over data protection. Genotyping provides an entire set of new tools for humankind to better understand the human condition, to better care for health, and to fight sickness and disease. But like all tools, genotyping can be used either virtuously or viciously. Public discourse and education and the appropriate protection of human and civil rights will be needed to steward and accompany the transition into a new millennium of health literacy and care. Our charter into the new territories of self-understanding and self-destination, of better health care and improved quality of life for all, will not be made easier if we hold on to old models of control by various bureaucracies intent on protecting people from the dangers of progress but preventing it instead. Concomitantly,

---

[24] Landsteiner K 1901 Über Agglutinationserscheinungen normalen menschlichen Blutbildes, in: Wiener Klinische Wochenschrift 46:1132-1134.

they would prevent people from finding their own way to use the new properties of genetic knowledge for healthier people and societies and more liberty, justice, and happiness. Because of stronger familial ties and other virtues, traditional cultures seem to be better prepared for solidarity in the ethics of data sharing and availability. Many people still share the view of Tai and Lin: 'each person exists for the greater common good, for the greater good of the community of many different individuals.'[25] In the coming age of carrier ethics, a new moral action guide is required for determining individual and family priorities. Prominent among them are health literacy, self-determination and -understanding, the right and duty to learn about one's own genetic properties and risk profiles, and genetic solidarity with other fellow humans.

Since we differ as individuals in more than enzymes and protein metabolism, it would be only consequent to provide citizens with individual health care cards containing specific information on genetic or acquired properties, abilities, disabilities, and disorders such as risk of hypertension or diabetes. Data availability is the precondition for good diagnosis and prognosis, and subsequently for prevention and treatment. Digital technology allows us to pack a great deal of personal data into cards, clothing, or apps. Health care cards might include dos and don'ts in nutrition, fitness, and social interactions, as well as proactive personal reminders and other content for the cardholder, not the health care expert. Personal data, including data on health and health care, are the property of the individual. In other areas of life, we share these informational properties for our own benefit and convenience with others, such as credit card providers, supermarkets, libraries, online merchants, and insurers. Of course, we worry about the protection of private data. We have pertinent laws and regulations that work most of the time, and we accept these risks as we balance risk with benefit. Rights to individual health information should not be treated differently than other informational property rights.

Citizens are property owners of data concerning individual health status and health care. It is in their best interest to have health care cards and to share information with professionals in a protected framework as data availability becomes as important as data protection. Health care professionals cannot provide quality service if denied access to information necessary for providing it safely and efficaciously, but some information can also be kept just for the cardholder. It would be difficult to counter the argument that those who do not share personal health status data with professionals cannot request those services or receive the best possible service. If data are not stored and made available, rather than being generated anew each time, then costs will skyrocket without additional benefit. Therefore, those who do not entrust personal data to individual health care cards must accept the higher costs of more expensive

[25] Tai MC, Lin CS l.c., 53.

procedures.[26] As far as the principle of solidarity is concerned, data availability is not only a prerequisite for good health care, it is also a potential factor to reduce costs. Here is an eight-point Action Guide for stakeholders addressing different obligations and rights of stakeholders in promoting, protecting, and improving personal health in harmony and happiness:

STAKEHOLDERS IN CARING FOR PERSONAL HEALTH

1. The care for health involves and requires more than medical repair intervention; medicine and medical ethics are broader than applied natural science; they require compassionate, competent partnerships and the promotion of individual health care cards.

2. Educated, responsible people and families have a moral duty to learn about their genetic and epigenetic properties and how to make the most of them for health and happiness; they also have a moral duty to help fellow humans take care of their individual genetic properties, in particular members of their wider family.

3. Health care professionals are obligated to not suppress or withhold genetic and other information from patients and healthy people; they have the duty to do their utmost to acquire those data, to educate those who seek their advice and service, and to guide and to accompany them in the care for their health.

4. Laypersons and health care professionals should feel bound by an invisible civil contract of communication and cooperation in trust, sharing responsibilities, rights, and obligations in reciprocity and solidarity and also in the care of people less fortunate, less healthy, and less competent.

5. Health care centers such as hospitals, nursing homes, fitness centers, and health care advisors must integrate ethics and expertise in order to be valuable and trusted corporate neighbors.

6. Research corporations and national and international regulatory agencies have a prime and urgent duty to develop and regulate medicines based on individualized properties of fellow humans and to not hide their competence and skills behind developing and legalizing mass market products only.

7. Governments and national and international institutions and organizations must provide legal, regulatory, and information networks to protect human and civil rights, develop and improve health literacy, and for protect against exploitation and discrimination; regulatory ethics in human genetics should be based on the ethics of information and education, promotion of predictive services, and protection of privacy.

---

[26] For the growing role and benefit of digital data in active and proactive patient interaction and clinical care, see also Imison C, Castle-Clarke S, Watson R, Edwards N 2016 Delivering the Benefits of Digital Health Care. Nuffield Trust.

8. Discourse and commitment in civil society, the media, and education must focus on promoting competent, responsible care for personal health by individuals, families, and communities.

9. CITIZEN–EXPERT PARTNERSHIP IN CARING FOR HEALTH AND HAPPINESS

THE LITTLE PRINCE AND HIS JEWEL

Once upon a time there was a little prince named Adam. At birth his parents gave him a wonderful, singularly radiating jewel. All the other princesses and princes had their own unique radiating stones of different colours and radiance, shape, size, and weight. Through bio-energy they bestowed physical, emotional, intellectual, and spiritual strength on their owners.

The princes and princesses had to take good care of their jewels, as each had only one. If these precious gems were lost, taken away, or destroyed by accident, negligence, miscalculation, or mistreatment, the princehood and life were loss as well. Careful procedures had to be learned to maintain and even to improve their stones. Some went to the Internet for advice on wellness and health. Jewellery doctors were involved in researching the jewels' radiating faculties, in predicting and diagnosing problems and perils, and in repairing certain capacities, slowing down the aging process while enhancing and extending a joyful life.

Prince Adam was enthralled with the radiating bio-powers of his gem, and he shared them intellectually, economically, socially, and sexually with playmates of both sexes. He tended to go to extremes in seeking pleasure, enjoying the gardens of sex, drugs, foods, and sports. Prince Adam was smart (or thought he was); he went to the jewel repair shop whenever a failure occurred. But he kept living his high-speed life, burning life's candles at both ends. He remembered his parents telling him that the repair powers of the jewel doctors were limited and often produced unwarranted or painful side effects without any qualitative benefits. But one day it was too late. Something was very wrong with the gem's recharging capacities. The breakdown was comparable to cirrhosis of the liver in ordinary humans, or to an untreatable cardiologic or immunologic disorder. Specialized jewel doctors got involved, but no one could change the course of the gem's permanently decreasing bio-capacities, and the once powerfully radiating miracle bios ended its life in weird convulsions. The Prince became desolate, filled with sorrow and discomfort. In dying, he blamed himself for this premature dysfunction of his most precious possession.

The unfortunate fate of Prince Adam's gem is shared by an unnecessarily high number of radiating bio-stones in that principality. Some bio-jewels lose their radiation bio-power from natural causes; the rest are broken by various forms of malpractice by jewel doctors, by their owners' mistakes, and by natural or social disasters beyond the powers of humans.

9.1. Partnerships in Caring for Health and Happiness

The care for individual and public health, harmony, and happiness is more than interventions by experts in disease repair. As in most other successful human activities, the care for health requires the resolve of an individual who wants to be healthy and happy and communication/cooperation in trust with an expert in medicine, nutrition, and lifestyle. In the wider sense, a consideration of bioethics is a good exercise in integrating expert knowledge and individual or collective goals, wishes, and needs into harmonious, successful partnerships that integrate facts and visions, compassion and expertise. Therefore, the health care field is an exemplary model scenario for developing good expert–citizen partnerships in risk management and service provision in a service-based, civil society.

As far as expert service in health care is concerned, 15th-century Confucian doctor Gong Tingxian defined 10 interactive partnership rules for the advisor or therapist.[1] The first four require the study of Confucian philosophy in matters such as reading the pulse, being able to talk about death and life, and understanding the influence of climate and seasons on human health and well-being.

---

[1] Gong Tingxian (Ming Dynasties). *Ten Maxims for Physicians:* In the first place they should adopt a disposition of humaneness: this is a justified demand. They should make a very special effort to assist the people and to perform far-reaching good deeds. Secondly they should master the Confucian teachings. Confucian medical doctors are a precious help at all times. Their principles are valuable and enlightening; all of literature is open to them for consultation. Thirdly they should be versed in the details of the pulse. It is necessary that they discern 'interior' *[li]* and 'exterior' *[biao]*. If they but lower their fingers [on the pulse], everything will be clear to them. Thus they will be able to cure those who are gravely ill. Fourthly they are to recognize the causes of diseases. They have to be ready to speak about life and death. Only physicians who attain this stage are experts in their field. Fifthly they should know the types of climate *[ch'i]* and the macrocosmic phases *[yün]*, so as to understand the succession of the seasons. Accordingly they have to perform operations of replenishing [deficiencies] and reducing [over-abundances in the organism] with drugs of warm or cool temperature radiation, and to differentiate the treatments suitable at the time. Sixthly they should be familiar with the different types of transportation channels; their understanding of them is not to give rise to any errors. If they are equally informed on the palaces *[fu]* and the granaries *[tsang]* of the body, they embody Pien Ch'io in the present. Seventhly they should know the peculiarities of drugs and compose their prescriptions corresponding to the individual diseases. If they do not distinguish between warm and cool [qualities of drugs] they may endanger life. Eighthly they should be informed on the preparation of drugs. They have to be familiar with the intensity of the fire [for the boiling of drugs] and the degree of fineness [for the drugs which have to be cut], in order to know what is too much and what is too little, what is dangerous and what is harmless. Ninthly they should not be jealous, neither should they let themselves be guided by other people's favor or disfavor. The principles of heaven are lucid, they make us quickly aware of our mistakes. Tenthly they should not esteem profits too highly, but instead cultivate humaneness and righteousness. Although we distinguish between the poor and the rich, there is but one type of drugs. (English translation by courtesy of Qiu Renzong; German translation by Unschuld PU 1999 Zehn Regeln für Mediziner und Patienten, in: Medizin und Ethik, Sass HM ed., Stuttgart: Reclam, 352-355).

Only thereafter comes the study of acupuncture and herbal medicines.[2] In medicine as part of applied natural sciences, we have nowadays replaced the *Philosophicum* with a *Physicum*.

For the layperson, health literacy and compliance with doctor's prescriptions are recommended and required. As far as financial compensation is concerned, the expert is reminded that service should come from a humanitarian perspective, and the patient is advised to spend money rather than lose health or even life.[3] Modern science-based medicine set other ground rules: medical students worldwide take classes in natural sciences before they are introduced to medical care and clinical medicine. Today, we have replaced the care for personal health with objective classifications of diseases and reimbursement schemes, defined by national and international bodies and insurance companies.

Ethics and expertise belong to each other in all professional services and in every citizen's personal life, particularly in caring competently for one's health. Not far away from Confucian doctor Gong's advice to laypeople in caring for their health is the *Lay Citizen Health Care Action Guide* of Friedrich Hoffmann[4],

---

[2] In his influential 'Great Physician's Manual of the 7th century, Sun Simiao requests: 'A great physician must be tranquil, free from desires and accountable of what he does. To be compassionate is the first requirement of physicians who must be devoted to treat the ill and helping whoever is in need'; cf. Su Chung-shu 1997 The Medical History of China. Taipei: Cheng-chung, 78; Tai 2008 The Ways of Asian Bioethics. Taipei: Princeton, 17.

[3] Gong Tingxian (Ming Dynasties). *Ten Maxims for Patients:* In the first place they are to choose 'enlightened physicians' *[ming-i]* and thereby receive help in their ailment. They have to be careful, because life and death follow each other closely. Secondly they should be willing to take remedies. With their help even a person who has already fallen ill can yet get rid of his ailment. There are many foolish people who hinder themselves [by not taking remedies] Thirdly they should have the treatment started at an early stage. At the beginning it is still simple. Whoever fails to be careful in hoarfrost will suddenly be surprised by solid ice. Fourthly they should not have sexual intercourse, then their sufferings will cease by themselves. If however they act contrary to this maxim, even a divine physician will be at his wits' end. Fifthly they should guard against any excitement and should be very careful in this respect. If a person is angry, the flames flare up in him. This creates great difficulties in bringing help and in checking [the disease]. Sixthly they should beware of wrong thoughts and take care of themselves in peace. If they avoid all troubles, the mind will find peace by itself. Seventhly they should eat and drink moderately. The preparation of food is to follow the rules. Too much is harmful to the mind; satiation is difficult to digest. Eighthly they should be concerned about their getting up and their getting rest. They have to reduce their social life; even slightly increased stress will drain the vitality. Ninthly they should not believe in the heterodoxical [in medicine]. Such a belief is harmful. Alien principles are misleading: they deceive the people and make them uncertain. Tenthly they should not fear expenses. What sense is there in economizing here! I ask you, what is more precious, life or material goods? (English translation by courtesy of Qiu Renzong; German translation by Unschuld PU 1999 Zehn Regeln für Mediziner und Patienten, in: Medizin und Ethik, Sass HM ed., Stuttgart: Reclam, 352-355).

[4] Tinctures based on Friedrich Hoffmanns formula (Hoffmann Tropfen) can still be bought in German apothecaries today.

an 18th-century pharmacist and physician in Halle an der Saale and the founder of its Medical Faculty: '1. Stay away from everything which is unnatural. 2. Be careful with changes, as routine becomes our second nature. 3. Be happy and balanced; that is the best remedy. Stay in clear air, well-tempered, as long as possible. 5. Buy the best nutrition which goes easily in and out of the body. 6. Choose foods according to your bodily activity and relaxation. 7. When you love to be healthy, run away from physicians and from all drugs.'[5] Interestingly, Hoffmann reflects on selfish and immoral business practices by physicians, quacks, and incompetent persons – advice we find in other cultures and that can be considered an essential part of lay responsibility in interacting with medical professionals. Doctor Gong expressed this requirement in more positive terms when advising his readers to carefully choose 'enlighted physicians' only.

Most professional clinical services by physicians (who comprise only one sector of health care specialists) require compassionate competence. Other professional services require less compassion and a high level of technical expertise, such as blood sampling, brain surgery, or car repair. But different from a mechanic repairing a car, a brain surgeon is involved in evaluating and discussing surgical goals. In other situations, physicians make primarily value decisions, either alone or in partnership with the client, such as whether to perform an abortion or to assist in artificial insemination or euthanasia. In a later chapter discussing corporate bios, we will try to translate the original two-partner interaction for a larger group of stakeholders involved in modern health care: regulators, hospitals, physicians, and patients. Other professionals are encouraged to draft similar guidelines for expert-lay communication and cooperation in their area of expertise, such as business or politics. Here we concentrate on experts helping the individual layperson in developing and supporting a personalized health care plan.

In general, we find transcultural agreement regarding respecting professional ethics and protecting professional profiles and procedures. A conceptual foundation of the European medical tradition, the Hippocratic Oath states: 'Into whatever houses I go, I will do so only for the benefit of the sick, avoiding all willful injustice and harm, in particular all forms of sexual relationship with women, also with men, free men and slaves.'[6] Hippocratic professional ethics finds a counterpart in Confucian thought as expressed in the influential book by Sun Simiao of the Tang Dynasty, 'On the Absolute Sincerity of Great Physicians.'[7] 'A Great Physician should not pay attention to status, wealth or age; neither should he question whether the particular person is attractive or unattractive, whether he is an enemy or fried, whether he is a Chinese or a foreigner, or

[5] Friedrich Hoffmann (1666-1742) in: Mueller I, Wilhelm I eds 1991 Iatromechanische Theorie und ärztliche Praxis im Vergleich zur galenischen Medizin. Stuttgart, 260.

[6] Hippocratic Oath, in: Sass HM ed, 1999 Medizin und Ethik, Stuttgart: Reclam, 352.

[7] Quoted in Qiu R 1988 Medicine, the Art of Humanness, in: J Medicine and Philosophy 13(3):288.

finally, whether he is uneducated or educated. He should meet everyone on equal grounds. He should always act as if he were thinking of his close relatives.'

Other issues remain controversial, as we discussed in regard to abortion and euthanasia. Asian professional cultures and expectations of patients/clients seem to have been much more open to medical services in enhancing health, happiness, and longevity than modern Western medicine, which could be compared to a repair shop for sick bodies or confused minds. Many differences arise between the two cultures in the details of medical intervention, in the treatment of patients, and in enhancing health. Some traditions favor protecting and enhancing health in lieu of curing diseases; others devote medical and ethical efforts to alleviating suffering and caring for the terminally ill, arguing that enhancement is against nature. Medical ethics is indeed a fascinating field for cross-cultural studies because the challenges are not that different among different cultures: to care for health, to heal or to manage sickness, to alleviate suffering and accompany those who are frail, confused, or dying. *No expertise without ethics; no ethics without expertise*. Expertise without ethics is blind, unguided, and uncontrolled; it is dangerous and should not be applied. Ethics without expertise is helpless, powerless, sentimental, dangerous, and inapplicable. According to Aristotle, the master of a craft must know how and why to do things. He or she also has to be able to teach the craft and to explain the purpose and proper use of the product. In Confucian teaching, physicians should combine expertise (*ji*) and humaneness (*ren*). The same must be required for professional scientific and administrative work in our complex, modern technological societies: ethics and expertise belong together, always and everywhere.

Requirements for ethics being integrated into professional activities, as well as the interaction between ethics and expertise in the expert-lay setting, were traditionally expressed in terms of virtues or maxims. To a lesser degree (and only recently) were they informed by ethical principles. Whenever prudent self-interest or professional rules of conduct can be expected, then the appeal to virtues is the most effective. But when virtues are not strongly supported by traditions and attitudes, as is often the case in modern pluralistic civil societies, then an appeal to principles seems to be a better choice. In good decision making, one principle alone rarely governs most moral and technological challenges. Of course, the relevance and combination of each of the eight-C principles/virtues we discussed in chapter 3 need balancing, depending on the challenges of specific moral, cultural, and technical aspects governing situations, stakeholders, processes, and applications. Therefore, training based on case studies will be important in health care ethics as well as in other fields of professional service.

9.2. Competence in Professional Ethics

Galen, the personal physician to Roman Emperor Augustus in the 2nd century, defined the mandate of professional medical expertise and ethics: '*non homo universalis curatur, set unus quique nostrum.* 'It is not the universal person we are to treat; it is an individual, unique, our patient.' In presenting a set of virtues in ethics and expertise, Confucian physician Yang Chuan stated 1,700 years ago that because of the primary role of professional responsibility, 'we only can trust or rely on such physicians who have the heart of humaneness and compassion, are clever and wise, sincere and honest,'[8] (i.e., having both interacting virtues, ethics and expertise). A description of the character traits, virtues, and professional expertise necessary for applying medical knowledge correctly displays the combined relevance of ethics and expertise. Based in Hippocratic tradition, Edmund Pellegrino developed maxims for the 'virtuous physician,' including the traditional virtue of striving for the highest medical and technical expertise possible.[9]

Victor von Weizsaecker criticized the simplistic application of natural science in medicine and referred to a 'bi-personal transaction' between doctor and patient, based on solidarity and reciprocity. He named three fundamentals: knowledge of nature (*Naturerkenntnis*), knowledge of man (*Menschenkenntnis*), and craftsmanship (*Kunstfertigkeit*).[10] Transactions in medicine such as treatment, healing, and consulting are based on biological 'vital attachments' (*Vitalverbindungen*) among humans. Fernando Lolas-Stepke called them 'those biological relationships which tie together the members of a family or a group. For the word to be a socially effective tool in the moral sense, attachments are a precondition. They do not possess in and by themselves a moral character, but constitute the foundation for its development provided they are adequately transformed during lifetime. To be effective, moral norms have to be grounded in attraction but at the same time are related to hostility and repulsion. Other derived *Vitalverbindungen*, like those represented by fear, shame or custom, may help to establish obligations in a moral sense'.[11] Spanish physician and medical ethicist Lain Entralgo uses the term *transjective knowledge* to underline the non-subjective knowledge of doctor and patient in their successful implementation of reciprocity and solidarity[12]. Transjective knowledge gained by the physician depends essentially on the input of the patient in a true reciprocal partnership. Fritz

[8] Mencius, in: The Chinese Classics, Legge J ed., vol. 2, Oxford: Clarendon 1895:285f.

[9] Pellegrino ED, Thomasma DC 1988 For the Patient's Good, New York: Oxford, 205.

[10] Weizsaecker V v 1944 Die Grundlagen der Medizin, in: Gesammelte Schriften, Frankfurt: Suhrkamp 1987ff, vol. 7:7; cf. Lolas Stepke F 2015 The medizinische Anthropologie oft he Heidelberg School; Implikacations for Bioethics, in: Jahr 2015, 6(1):9-28.

[11] Lolas Stepke F 2015 The medizinische Anthropologie of the Heidelberg School; Implications for Bioethics, in: Jahr 2015, 6(1):19.

[12] Entralgo L 1950 Heilkunde in geschichtlicher Entscheidung, Salzburg: Muller, 20; also Lolas-Stepke l.c. 20.

Hartmann has pointed out that the patient has to 'help' the doctor to become a good healer and advisor.[13]

Other recommendations for physicians' professional ethics refer only to general rules of conduct in personal and professional life. Kishore applies the Indian Buddhist perspective and names the virtues of 'dharma: love, trust, righteousness, compassion, tolerance, fairness, forgiveness, beneficence, sacrifice, and concern for the weak.' From these character traits of a truly educated, cultured person also derive the moral values of 'justice, equality, autonomy, benignancy, altruism, human solidarity, respect for the dead, respect for other forms of life, and preservation if life'[14] for the physician and other experts. Michael Tai focuses on a set of five principles 'rooted in Asian culture': '*ahimsa* (nonmaleficence), compassion, respect, righteousness, *dharma* (responsibility).[15] *Dharma*, a Sanskrit word meaning the pattern and destiny of 'living right,' is not only a Buddhist maxim. It is also known in Confucian traditions of self-responsibility, including situations both private and professional. Mencius said that: 'Between father and son, there should be affection, between ruler and minister, there should be righteousness, between husband and wife there should be attention in their separate functions, between old and young, there should be a proper order, and between friends there should be faithfulness.'[16] Can today's expert or layperson embrace the wisdom of Mencius and say that between them 'there should be competent and compassionate cooperation'? Such a trust-based partnership between the professional on one side and the client on the other would be successful not only in the care for health and happiness: it would definitely be a broader interaction in the care for health than much clinical or primary medical care.

9.3. Principles and Guides in Health Care Ethics

Professional principles in modern health care differ from those of Hippocrates and Yang Chuan. Health care is seen primarily as an application of knowledge in the natural sciences, biology, and medicine. The most widely used guides are the three principles of 'autonomy, beneficence, justice,'[17] that led to a new mod-

---

[13] Hartmann F 2003 Kranke als Gehilfen ihrer Ärzte. Bochum: ZME 2. Ed; Hartmann F 2003 Der Beitrag erfahrungsgesättigter Therapie (EBM) zu einer ärztlichen Indikationen-Lehre. Bochum: ZME.

[14] Kishore RR 2003 End of life issues and moral certainty; a discovery through Hinduism, in: Eubios Asian and Intern J 13:210-2103.

[15] Tai MC 1999 The principles of medical ethics of Asians and for Asians. Proceedings of the 2nd Asian Bioethics Seminar, Tokyo, University Research Center Nihan University, 42-51; Tai MC 2008 The Asian Way of Bioethics. Taiwan: Princeton Intern Publ, 187-193.

[16] Mencius, l.c., 3.

[17] US Department of Health and Human Services 1979 The Belmont Report. Ethical Principles and Guidelines for the Protection of Human Subjects in Research [45 CFR 46].

el of respecting 'the patient as a person.'[18] Originally developed as common ethical denominators in a multicultural society, these principles were intended to guarantee a wide spectrum of public support for human experimentation and clinical research. They emphasized informed consent of the research subject (replacing the benevolence or humaneness of the physician), the traditional principle of no harm, and the principle of justice (e.g., that no vulnerable populations such as prisoners or those who could not give consent were used in potentially risky experiments). These three principles were originally devised to guide human experimentation within a civil society grounded in basic constitutional laws and rights as opposed to specific religious traditions. Beauchamp and Childress later included the concept 'nonmaleficence,' and because of the enormous influence of their publication the four principles of autonomy, nonmalefi-nonmaleficence, beneficence, and justice were called the 'Georgetown Mantra.' They now make up the most commonly used framework for clinical ethics and medical ethics teaching, both in the United States and abroad. [19] Also referred to as a model of common morality, they are used in most medical guidelines. It has been said that these principles represent an individualist approach to ethics while neglecting traditional models of family and community responsibility in making decisions. But if the principles of personal autonomy and self-determination are not respected by the community or family, then these communities have a moral problem. Some bioethicists such as Tai, take issue with the individualistic Kantian/European view of autonomy: 'In a society where family is the center of all attention, autonomy becomes collective rather than individualistic. The center of each person's life is not himself or herself but the family. Thus autonomy can only be spoken of as a collective right rather than an individual privilege. Although family is composed of many members, community starts not with individual but the unit of the family which becomes the base of a macro-vision of Confucian tradition for a harmonious universe. Each person exists for a greater common good or for a greater collective individual.'[20]

All four principles must be implemented professionally by individuals or committees to fulfill the requirement of treating probands or patients ethically. A module developed next to the original process of research or treatment serves as a quality-control feature for the process itself. The four principles are used routinely for quality control, for reviewing cases, and for education. When used as ethics principles separately, they are not integrated with requirements for the highest professional expertise in technical matters (as in Yang Chuan's model), nor do they make explicit requirements for experts to cultivate character traits. In Europe, another set of bioethics principles discusses 'autonomy, dignity, in-

[18] Ramsey P 1970 The Patient as Person. Exploration in Medical Ethics. New Haven: Yale U Press.

[19] Beauchamp TL, Childress J 2013 Principles of Biomedical Ethics. New York: Oxford, 7th ed.

[20] Tai M 2008 The Way of Asian Bioethics, Taiwan: Princeton Intern. Publ., 50f.

tegrity, and vulnerability' as more responsive to the European tradition.[21] The sets of virtues discussed by Tai and Kishore, on the other hand, emphasize self-cultivation within the process of personal and professional moral duty. But all of these sets focus on one side of an interaction: the provider group that calls the shots from the viewpoint of paternalistic morality. 'Patient knows best' instead of 'doctor knows best' replaces the principal active player with another one within the educational framework for doctors.

Virtues and principles in the ethics of health care and in the interactions among its stakeholders today should cover more than caring for the sick and frail. Predictive, preventive medicine allows for measure to protect and improve health before it deteriorates. This paradigm gives educated laypersons more power and responsibility in protecting and enhancing their health. Peimin Ni quotes the Western Han Dynasty health care expert Huang Di Nei Jing as saying: 'the sages do not wait until the sickness is there to cure the sickness, they cure it before it takes place.... If one only waits until the sickness is there and then uses medicine to cure it, that is no different from waiting until one is thirsty and then starting to dig a well.' He also quotes Sun Simiao on public health, health education and preventive medicine: 'a superior doctor takes care of the state, an average doctor takes care of the person, an inferior doctor takes care of the disease.'[22] The Hippocratic dietetic rules of respect for the *res non naturales* refer to a similar model of empowering the layperson to take health care into her/his own hands, with or without expert help. Health enhancement and anti-aging, those millennia-old dreams of humankind, can be achieved to a certain degree today, taking into account various costs and risks. Together lay health care ethics, those enhancement issues have not yet become a prime focus in contemporary bioethics. Dormant cultural traditions have not yet been re-activated in lay health education and competence and in physicians' obligations to advise and assist in health care protection (and, if possible, enhancement). Limits to anti-aging and health enhancement will need to be discussed using classical models of the Golden Rule of avoiding extremes (and following the Doctrine of the Mean, dormant in Western and Asian cultures as well).

Individuals will react differently to the challenge of health protection, health enhancement, and anti-aging. As far as the healing arts and medical professions are concerned, one finds in general two contrasting models. One is a fiduciary culture built around a partnership or stakeholder relationship of physicians, nurses, patients, healthy and sick clients, and their families. The other is a partnership/stakeholder relationship retreating in extreme cases to more parental models of care for the suffering and helpless, as called for by the virtue of com-

[21] Rendtorff JD 2002 Basic ethical principles in European bioethics and biolaw: autonomy, dignity, integrity and vulnerability – towards a foundation of bioethics and biolaw. in: Medical Health Care Philosophy 5 (2002) 235-244,

[22] Ni Peimin 1999 Confucian virtues and personal health, in: Confucian Bioethics, Fan R ed., London: Kluwer, 31.

passion. Because individuals have different visions and wishes for their lives, physicians need to use the partnership model to treat their patients humanely and respectfully. In summary, different cultures have come to use different terms, virtues, principles, or modes of interaction in integrating ethics with expertise in communication and cooperation with stakeholders. These include humaneness, compassion, cleverness, wisdom, sincerity, and honesty (Yang Chuan); nonmaleficence, compassion, respect, righteousness, and responsibility (Tai); autonomy, nonmaleficence, beneficence, and justice (Beauchamp and Childress); autonomy, dignity, integrity, and vulnerability (Rentdorff); and balancing self-determination with compliance, quality of life with length of life, nonmaleficence with beneficence, and self-determination with respect for others (Sass).[23]

9.4. Partnership Covenants

Close to the interactive partnership model of Gong Tingxian, Robert Veatch has proposed a 'Covenant between Physicians and Citizens' that accepts beneficence, nonmaleficence, autonomy, and justice in balance but adds *fidelity to promises, veracity, and avoidance of killing* to guide those four mid-level principles.[24] For Veatch, a covenant includes more than legal, technical, or ethical principles: it is 'a kind of contractual relationship with special emphasis on the morally binding communal qualities of mutual loyalty and reciprocity that are essential to all contractual relationships.'[25] Successful professional–lay interactions thus occur within the wider social, economic, and political biotope, supported by a triple contract theory: 'The first contract specifies the basic content of an ethical system. It is what contractors taking the moral point of view (the outlook that other people's welfare is considered on the same scale as one's own) would invent or discover or have revealed to them as the basic ethical principles for society. Real human beings, being finite, can only approximate this hypothetical condition, but it is the best system we have for knowing the basic content of an ethical system. It is a system usable by those who are convinced that morality is objective and absolute (whether they derive their ethical theory from a theological system, attempt to determine the ethical principles by use of reason, or believe they can use the moral sentiments to discover them). It

[23] Just to prove a different methodological scheme in applying a not yet used combination of six different aspects to review the controversial issue of human cloning and stem-cell research in medical ethics, I have used the set of 'risk-reward, precision, solidarity, traditional basket, minimax of risk-reward, dignity'; see Sass HM 2006 Bioethics Principles in Medical Research, in: Sass HM 2006 Bioethics and Biopolitics. Xian: Press fmmu.sn.cn, 302-338.

[24] Veatch RM 1981 A Theory of Medical Ethics. New York: Basic Books, 'A Draft Medical Ethical Covenant': 327-330; cf. Veatch RM Ethical Dimensions of Advance Directives and Surrogate Decision Making, in: Advance Directives and Surrogate Decision Making in Health Care, Sass HM, Veatch RM, Kimura eds. Baltimore: Johns Hopkins U Press, 81f.

[25] Veatch l.c., 125f.

is also usable by those who are convinced that morality is subjective. (They would see real people coming together assuming the moral point of view for more practical purposes of trying to reach an agreement on a system that would lead to joint harmonious survival) … Once the basic social contract articulates these fundamental principles, a second contract, one between the society and a profession, can then spell out (again from the moral point of view) the special role-specific duties regarding interactions between lay people and professionals. The only limit of that second contract will be that as a whole it cannot contravene the morality of the prior, more basic, contract social contract. – Finally, within the content of these two contracts, individual professionals and lay persons (or the groups that function as individual units) have the opportunity to spell out further the terms, moral and otherwise, of their relationship.'[26]

Veatch's triple-contract model builds on broad traditions in the social contract theory present in many cultures, whether in a religious, conservative, or individualistic philosophy based on human rights. It can and should be used for other fields of expert–citizen interaction in modern societies defined by divisions of labor, expertise, expectation, and vision. However, systems of value are part of the complex and highly adaptable bios of human life and will change over time.[27] The scope of change will have to be debated in each new situation and historical period by focusing on basic human and civil rights.[28]

After 2,400 years, it is time to say goodbye to the paternalistic beneficence of physicians and to some of the principles of Hippocratic ethics. New prominence should be given to the public's literacy and responsibility in regard to the *res non-naturales* (i.e., the things we as individuals have to recognize in our biotope and then prudently act on). The principles expressed in the prevailing Hippocratic tradition are not optimal for supporting citizens' health competence or patient–physician interaction in determining health care goals or in recognizing a patient's self-determination as an integral part of her or his individual human and civil rights. The traditional paternalism of elitist professionals fails to address the quest for developing patients' ethics and individual health responsibility in the realms of predictive and preventive medicine. Neither does it recognize the plurality of values and wishes patients might have in regard to health care and quality/length of life.

At least four factors call for a major shift in future health care ethics. Progress is necessary (a) in predictive and preventive medicine, (b) in intensive care and in methods of prolonging life and mitigating suffering, (c) in growing opportunities and visions in enhancement of health and happiness, and (d) in

[26] Veatch l.c. 137f

[27] Sakamoto H 1999 Global Bioethics as Inter-cultural Tuning Technology, in: Proceedings of the Second Asian Bioethics Seminar, Nihon University. Tokyo, 5.

[28] Ten Have H 2016 Global Bioethics. An Introduction. London: Routledge calls for 'global health governance' (138ff) and 'bioethics governance' (157ff) to steward those changing values and virtues within the process of culture.

ascertaining emotional, ethical, and economic limits in providing every medical intervention possible. Together these considerations comprise the following prime challenge in global health care cultures: developing and supporting an ethos of individualized health care that places the health-competent, health-responsible citizen in the driver's seat. Lay competence in evaluating risk and in mastering principles for taking care of one's own health should be given priority over secondary issues in physicians' ethics. The latter must change from paternalism to partnership. The global richness in individual, familial, and communal cultures calls for health care services geared to the values and wishes of the client or patient, not those of the doctor or system providing care. While contemporary European and Asian bioethics still concentrate on teaching and refining physicians' ethics in a paternalistic way, Anglo-American bioethics emphasizes the values of interactive lay-expert exchange in determining individual health care parameters, establishing self-determination and self-responsibility in predictive and preventive health care, and identifying goals and limits for acute and intensive care intervention. The teaching, theory, and practice of health care ethics will have to focus on interactive virtues in caring for healthy people and communities. Public health systems must also accommodate and support individual health priorities, as discussed in the next chapter. Caring for individual health in the 21th century is not possible without caring for diversity in visions, values and wishes. Engelhardt puts the issue uncompromising this way: 'A secular bioethics that is to transcend the battles of the culture wars and offer a means for morally authoritative collaboration in the face of intractable moral diversity will need to take seriously the role of agreements, contracts, the market, and limited constitutional polities ... At the very least, we can by default find procedures, strategies to live together as moral strangers in the face of irresolvable moral diversity'.[29]

In conclusion, I follow the interactive models of Gong Tingxian and Robert Veatch a broad, covenant-type model of interactive contractual relations and responsibilities among citizens, experts, service providers, and regulators[30] can also be used for devising similar guidelines *in other fields of modern civil societies* supported and enriched by contracts, limited regulations, diversity structures

[29] Engelhardt HT 2006 Global Bioethics. An Introduction to the Collapse of Consensus. New York: Scrivener, 17.

[30] For earlier versions on interactive rules for physicians and laypeople, see: Sass HM 1994 Formulating Global Post-Hippocratic Health Care Virtues. European Philosophy of Medicine and Health Care, 2(1), 1994, 6-10 [also in: Eubios Ethics Institute. Newsletter, 4 (1+2); Japan. Transl, in: Journal of Health Care, Medicine and Community, 5, 1994, 3-6; Cantonese transl, in: Newsletter. Centre for Applied Ethics, Hong Kong Baptist College, 2(1), 1994, 8-15; Italian transl. in: Kos, 118, 1995: 46-51; French transl., in: Journal International de Bioethique / International Journal of Bioethics, 1995, 6(1), 5-7. Interactive Virtue Catalogues for Health Politicians and Regulators, Corporate Service Providers, Citizens and Physicians, in: Sass HM 2006 Differentialethik. Anwendungen in Medizin, Wirtschaft und Politik, Baumann E, Brink A, May AT eds, 175f.

of solidarity and subsidiarity, respect for individual conscience and choice and the opportunities of market forces.

A COVENANT FOR INTERACTIVE VIRTUES IN THE CARE FOR HEALTH

For the Citizen

1. *Find truly educated, trustworthy health experts.*
2. *Develop competence and responsibility in health risk management.*
3. *Make extended use of predictive and preventive medicine.*
4. *Expect healing or relief from acute medicine, but be aware of the limits and risks of any medical intervention.*
5. *Be a responsible partner with experts in medicine and care.*
6. *Expect good communication and cooperation from experts and discuss relevant issues with them.*
7. *Recognize weakness and disease as a challenge in developing your personal quality of life.*
8. *Define and implement your sense of qualities of life, from childhood to old age, in sickness and in health.*
9. *Prepare advance directives and name proxy decision makers for situations of emergency or incompetence and discuss those with them.*
10. *Act responsibly in using communal health care funds.*

For the Professional

1. *Treat your patient as a person, not just his or her symptoms.*
2. *Assist your patient in developing health risk competence and health responsibility.*
3. *Integrate the 'clinical' and 'value' status of your patient into differential ethics, diagnosis, and prognosis.*
4. *Be aware of the benefits, limits, and risks of acute intervention and discuss them with your patient.*
5. *Be an expert partner in decision making with your client or patient and respect, if possible, her or his wishes and values.*
6. *Integrate ethics and expertise into intervention and advice.*
7. *Continuously educate yourself to provide the best possible clinical and personal service.*
8. *Select probands for health care research based on their medical status but also on their value status.*
9. *Assist your clients and patients in preparing value profiles and advance directives and work with proxies for the benefit of your patient.*
10. *Support personal responsibility and act responsibly in the use of communal health care funds.*

IV. COMPETENCE IN BIOETHICS

10. Cultivating Cyberspace Territories

'This is no game, it is the real world!' [1]

'Cyberspace is not like any other landscape, because it is formed solely by the desires, values, attitudes, beliefs, and perceptions of its creators. Therefore it is a totally cultural landscape because it is an expression of human thought and creativity. People have long dreamed of the creation of a perfect world, and there are many now who hold a utopian view of cyberspace. For the most part, however, people realize that cyberspace will not bring about either perfection or total chaos. It is also obvious, however, that cyberspace is already bringing about significant impacts on cultures around the world. Moreover, the cultural changes are not random incidents. Instead, they are products of human choices'[2].

10.1. Populating new Territories in Cyberspace

We humans live in real geographic biotopes, but also in non-geographical biotopes created in dreams and narratives; communications with gods, goddesses, angels, and devils; books, songs, theater, and art; and more recently in the so-called virtual world of the Internet. But the Internet is not less real in individual and collective human bios than eating, drinking, fighting, loving, reading, or praying. Since its debut in 2004, the online *World of Warcraft* game had over 100 million accounts.[3] More than 12 million players are routinely (and mostly daily) in active interaction with its natural and imaginary interactive environments, which are called *virtual reality* (VR). *Second Life*, a VR platform founded in 1999, calls itself a '*global community*', where I can be seen and act 'as a real person'; the new 'Project Sansar' promises to even more 'democratize virtual reality as a creative medium; it will empower people to easily create, share, and ultimately monetize their own interactive social experiences'[4]. In VR, 'real people' fight and cooperate with other real (not virtual) players, enjoying social recognition and friendship, taking part in (virtual) commercial transactions involving auctions of gold and other valuables. Millions of people around the globe from different cultures and traditions populate social website meeting places for love, sex, special interests, and hobbies.[5] Big-city citizens raise fish or crops and flowers daily in real (virtual) biotopes of *Happy Aquarium* or *Farmville*, where over 30 million 'farmers' tend daily to their vegetables, fruit trees,

---

[1] Promotional slogan for 'World of Warcraft' website, visited 2016-08-20.

[2] GEOG-597i: Critical Geospatial Thinking and Application. https://www.e-educarion.psu.edu/geog597i_02/node/880.

[3] www.battle.net; Wikipedia: World of Warcraft.

[4] Website Second Life, press release 2016-04-26, visited 2016-08-20.

[5] Rosen C 2007 Virtual Friendship and the New Narcissism, in: The New Atlantis 14: 124-126; Gorry G 2010 Avatars in the Workplace, in: The New Atlantis 127: 126-129.

cows, etc., exchange flowers or fruits with real (virtual) friends in those territories. The terms 'real' and 'virtual' still needs to be defined, but no one seems to care about academic definitions as long as VR (virtual reality) is RR (real reality) for those involved.[6] While these newly created and populated environments enlarge traditional, non-geographic biotopes of human culture, they have also been criticized as unhealthy in that they replace real 'I-Thou' communication and cooperation with new forms of escapism; in fact, Internet abuse has been diagnosed as a new and very difficult to treat form of addiction.[7]

After being challenged by the devil to use his spiritual powers to create bread, Jesus reasoned that 'man shall not live by bread alone, but by every word that proceeds from the mouth of God,' and he refused to use his powers to gain richness and power.[8] We have always dreamed and told stories that became essential to our individual and collective bios, and those non-geographical segments of our human bios were instrumental in determining our actions, our identity, our success, and our happiness. I have witnessed my cat and my dog having dreams, but I don't know their content. It might be that my goldfish, living room plant, or apple tree has something like dreams or contemplations or something non-geographical in its bios that will favor its specific natural selection in struggling for its own form of life. Hegel praised the birth of Greek philosophy, saying 'not before have people started walking on their heads'[9], but he was wrong. Narratives, visions, contemplations, and calculations have always been a part of human bios as we know it; this can be documented in all cultural traditions and histories. Human individual and communal bios has always transcended geographical spaces via dreams, telling narratives from generation to generation, communicating with gods and goddesses, with good and evil spirits, angels and devils, making up stories, inventing heroes, reading books, watching theater and movies, enjoying radio and television. The recent fashion trend of hunting for virtual monsters in real environments (such as *Pokemon Go*)

---

[6] Cf Mizrach S ,Lost in Cyberspace. Cultural Geography of Cyberspace, last visited 2016-08-20: 'The laws of physics do not apply to in cyberspace, and thus neither do standard limitations on human modes of locomotion, self-representation, or capabilities … What patterns of social relations play out in the kinds of virtual places that exist in cyberspace? Are we erecting virtual *agoras* or simply electronic *disneylands*? How does power shape the nature and experience we have in cyberspace? .. To the pioneers of virtuality, there is a sense that this all could be a whole new phase in human evolution. All this talk about "downloading" personalities into digital form represents, in a new form, the human ambition for transcending the body and cheating death … So in the future, any geographer who ignores cyberspace and its impact on the human ordering of space may be doing so at their own peril'.

[7] Sass HM 2012 Ludwig Feuerbach über virtuelle Realität im Internet, in: Aufklärung und Kritik 2/2012:29-37; oral information by Volker Kielstein MD, Magdeburg, a therapist expert in treating addiction.

[8] Matth 4:4.

[9] Hegel GWF (1833) Geschichte der Philosophie, Michelet KL ed 1833, vol. 13.

can easily change 'our connected-in-real-life, location-based, augmented-reality future in a way that is bigger than a game.'[10] In similar augmented-reality bios, I can replace the funny Pokemon with my friend or lover, with my most hated foe, or an unpleasant head of state; I can also replace hunting with hugging or beating or any other interaction with my real-virtual partner/friend/foe.

The invention, discovery, and colonization of new territories via digital equipment have definitely broadened our outreach into human territories and cultures within the last generation beyond anything we could have imagined. The Internet has broadened our natural and cultivated geographical ecosystems into new cyberspace territories and ecosystems. We humans always had supportive and encouraging interactions with non-geographical religious and spiritual powers, some or all of them shaped by human contemplation, calculation, and interpretation. But never before had we built fully interactive worlds of non-geographical territory as we did during the current era. We fellow humans joined religious communities believing in the same God, but now we communicate and cooperate in social websites of love, friendship and special interests, as well as in adaptive digital systems of mail, trade, health care, and business advice. Brick-and-mortar centers of learning and education have already been supplemented by cyberspace programs of all sorts; in fact, some of the best universities are expanding into cyberspace, making courses available everywhere. Clinics and other local health care centers are complemented by cyberspace-situated medical advice and guidance sites and e-health care communities. When I go for free to my favorite online Tai Chi video on the internet, I meet my good friend and adored teacher and enjoy her private, 50-minute class; also, I can stop or start anytime or just do a selection of movements whenever I choose.[11]

New business and trade alliances and totally new marketplaces are developing in cyberspace. When I look for a flight connection on a travel site, I get additional, unsolicited offers to include a hotel or rental car. Like walking in an Oriental marketplace, other merchants selling similar goods follow me. As America Online co-founder Steve Case predicts,[12] a third wave will form new ecosystems as a natural extension of cultivated cyberspace. In this iteration, alliances between regulators, businesses, entrepreneurs, and citizens in different fields must experiment with new dynamic interactions and adaptations that blend cooperation and competition.

Of course, new Internet territories include factors similar to those in geographical ones: love and hate, mutual aid and extortion, power and dependency, corruption and gratitude, self-identity, self-destruction, self-cultivation. In the

[10] Mims C 2016 'Pokemon Go' Surged by Building Community, in: Wall Street J 07-25-2016: B4.

[11] You Tube: Tai Chi Chih by Carmen Brocklehurst for New Mexico PBS; cf. www.taichichih.org.

[12] Case S 2016 The Third Wave. An Entrepreneur's Vision of the Future. New York: Simon & Schuster.

old days, some religious people have responded to the loss of social integration and obligations in RR (real reality) by fleeing into eremite-like lifestyles in VR (virtual reality), which may or may not have made them happier and more in harmony with themselves and their vision. In cyberspace territories such as the virtual world Second Life, I may become a symphony conductor, an admired doctor, an eminent lawyer, a great hero saving the world from destruction, or a distinguished scientist, - all by working hard and being accepted by others, while still being an underachiever among my geographical neighbors in RR.

I discuss below new avenues of communication in the care for health and the democratization of traditionally privileged professional knowledge in medicine as just one of many possible illustrations for the new powers, benefits, and hazards of venturing into these new territories for personal or professional reasons.[13]

10.2. Instant Equal Access to Previously Privileged Knowledge

The internet opens new landscapes and geographies previously closed for many people. The availability of information, advice, hand-holding, camaraderie and many integrated forms of cooperation in many fields of life is one of the most fascinating scientific and interdisciplinary breakthroughs of our times. As far as the care for health is concerned, this may well lead to vast cultural changes such as new individual and collective attitudes or abilities, cooperation in fighting or preventing disease, and alliances in protecting and enhancing health. The Internet provides a wealth of information and advice, establishes new cyberspace communities concerned with health and health care, and makes previously privileged medical knowledge available globally 24 hours a day, 7 days a week.[14]

New information networks have changed medicine and health care in the following three areas. (1) 'E-health' sites communicate information and advice to laypeople in accessible language. Among their goals are to promote individual health care competence by de-professionalizing vast areas of previously privileged knowledge and to create new global rooms for interactive cyberspace communities, thus changing individual and cultural attitudes towards health and disease and towards traditional systems of providing and financing the treatment of sickness. E-health addresses issues of individual wellness and well-being, not just medical issues in health care. (2) 'E-medicine' uses the Internet to improve and to modify traditional forms of diagnosis, therapy, quality control, and biomedical research via competence networks in medicine. (3) Public-health

[13] Schroeder P 2002 Vom Sprechzimmer zum Internetcafé. Medizinische Information und ärztliche Beratung im 21. Jahrhundert. Bochum: ZME.

[14] Fox S, Duggan M 2013 Information Triage: Health Online. Washington DC: PEW Research Center, 55 p, report that 72% of internet users in 2012 visited health information sites; van Mielo 2014 The 1% Rule in Four Digital Health Social Networtks, in: Intern J Medical Informatics 16(2):133

Internet networks provide training, coordinate preparedness, and promote timely interaction among partners in community and public health in emergency situations.

E-health is 'an emerging field in the intersection of medical informatics, public health and business, referring to health services and information delivered or enhanced through the Internet, and related technologies. In a broader sense, the term characterizes not only a technical development, but also a state-of-mind, a way of thinking, an attitude, and a commitment for networked, global thinking, to improve health locally, regionally, and worldwide by using information and communication technology.'[15] In 2001, Eysenbach proposed the following '*10 E's in E-Health*': '1. Efficiency – one of the promises of e-health is to increase efficiency in health care, thereby decreasing costs. One possible way of decreasing costs would be by avoiding duplicative or unnecessary diagnostic or therapeutic interventions, through enhanced communication possibilities between health care establishments, and through patient involvement. 2. Enhancing quality of care – increasing efficiency involves not only reducing costs, but at the same time improving quality. E-health may enhance the quality of health care for example by allowing comparisons between different providers, involving consumers as additional power for quality assurance, and directing patient streams to the best quality providers. 3. Evidence based – e-health interventions should be evidence-based in a sense that their effectiveness and efficiency should not be assumed but proven by rigorous scientific evaluation. Much work still has to be done in this area. 4. Empowerment of consumers and patients – by making the knowledge bases of medicine and personal electronic records accessible to consumers over the Internet, e-health opens new avenues for patient-centered medicine, and enables evidence-based patient choice. 5. Encouragement of a new relationship between the patient and health professional, towards a true partnership, where decisions are made in a shared manner. 6. Education of physicians through online sources (continuing medical education) and consumers (health education, tailored preventive information for consumers). 7. Enabling information exchange and communication in a standardized way between health care establishments. 8. Extending the scope of health care beyond its conventional boundaries. This is meant in both a geographical sense as well as in a conceptual sense, e-health enables consumers to easily obtain health services online from global providers. These services can range from simple advice to more complex interventions or products such a pharmaceuticals. 9. Ethics – e-health involves new forms of patient-physician interaction and poses new challenges and threats to ethical issues such as online professional practice, informed consent, privacy and equity issues. 10. Equity – to make health care more equitable is one of the promises of e-health, but at the same time there is a

[15] Eysenbach G 2001 What Is E-Health?, in: J Med Internet Res 3(2):e20 (www.jmir.org); accessed 07-24-2016.

considerable threat that e-health may deepen the gap between the "haves" and "have-nots." People who do not have the money, skills, and access to computers and networks, cannot use computers effectively. As a result, these patient populations (which would actually benefit the most from health information) are those who are the least likely to benefit from advances in information technology, unless political measures ensure equitable access for all. The digital divide currently runs between rural vs. urban populations, rich vs. poor, young vs. old, male vs. female people, and between neglected/rare vs. common diseases.' - Eysenbach suggests three additional criteria for good e-health platforms: '*easy to use, entertaining (no one will use something that is boring), and exciting.*' Thus, medical information on e-health sites will have to differ essentially from content in medical textbooks and professional journals, especially in regard to avoiding jargon. While established health care systems have increasingly become disease-treatment systems for a variety of reasons, their success has also 'medicalized' multiple issues of health and well-being related to lifestyle and stress.

10.3. Promoting New Cultures in the Care for Health

Addressing more than specific medical issues, e-health sites also discuss the wider framework of health protection and enhancement of health and well-being, emphasizing health and lifestyle attitudes over medical treatment. Driven by the consumers, the rise of e-health sites has occurred outside of the established health care system. The central and yet-to-be-evaluated role of e-health seems to in empowering the layperson to take control of her or his own health risk and health care. If knowledge begets self-determination, independence, and contribution to family, community, and society, then literacy – including health literacy – allows individuals to make their own choices, including ones in regard to lifestyle, quality of life, and wellness while contributing to family, community, and society. Literacy programs supported by UNESCO and other agencies have indirectly improved living and health conditions of millions of people. The promotion of health literacy by e-health sites and other means is the logical next step to empower people to take better care of their health and that of their loved ones. Health literacy is 'the degree to which individuals have the capacity to obtain, process, and understand basic health information and services needed to make appropriate health decisions.'[16]

Modern medicine knows a lot about predictable risk to health, prevention of disease, management of chronic disease, and individual proteonomics vis à vis drug metabolism. We have the communication and education tools to provide individuals with information on risk prevention, health care management, and disease management.[17] But traditional health care systems have so far failed to

[16] http://www.healthypeople.gov.

[17] Schroeder P 2003 Patientenaufklaerung und Gesundheitskommunikation im Internet, in: Sass HM ed, Patientenaufklaerung bei genetischem Risiko. Münster: Lit, 57-78.

translate the new wealth of information into knowledge tools for the individual citizen or for promoting individual health care competence and new models of lay–expert partnerships. Information and advice provided by e-health seems to be absorbed more successfully than educational public health initiatives.

We seem to value more what we actively search for through our own initiative than what comes to us from authorities.[18] The U.S. Department of Health website *medlineplus.gov* provides a helpful guide for reviewing the reliability of e-health websites.[19] More and more health information has become available outside of the traditional sickness care system of hospitals or physicians' offices. Health food stores, health clubs, and 'new age' stores offer more health care information than can be found in the traditional sickness treatment system. Sites that are easy to understand and use (such as *www.webmd.com*, with more than 20 million visitors per week) represent an information revolution on health care matters, venturing far beyond simple information and advice for treating diseases.[20] When a German medical journal presented a study reviewing German citizens' desire for medical information beyond that provided by the existing health care system, results showed that 59% of those interviewed wanted the most recent information on their particular disease or disorder, 53% a 'second opinion,' 42% information on alternative medicine, 41% information about specialized local physicians, and 39% advice on how to deal with health insurance.[21] According to a poll by the Kaiser Family Foundation, 75% of young adults in the United States aged 15–24 have searched the Internet for health-related issues. Health information was more often sought than music for copying (72%) or sports information (46%). Of these online health seekers, 15% look into health-related sites once a week and 24% once a month. Cancer, diabetes, and health care related to sexual activity were the subjects of the most searches.[22]

E-health sites are perused by all types of citizens, both well and sick. Some visit for advice on how to stay healthy or to get information or second opinions on the disorders of loved ones. Predictive, preventive, and lifestyle-enhancing health information that is reliable and easy to understand either supplements or replaces advice from a personal physician. A number of health care insurers now

---

[18] Dutta-Bergmann MJ 2004 Health attitudes, health cognitions, and health behaviors among Internet health information seekers, in: J Medical Internet Res 6(2):e20 (jmir.org).

[19] https://medlineplus.gov/evaluatinghealthinformation.html; accessed 07-24-2016.

[20] Collste G 2002 The Internet Doctor and Medical Ethics, in: Medicine, Health Care and Philosophy 5: 121-125; Winkler MA et al 2000 Guidelines for Medical Health Information Sites in the Internet, in: JAMA 283:1600-1606.

[21] Noiting HD, Wasem J 2002 Was mündige Patienten erwarten, in: Deutsche Ärztezeitung, May 15, 2002.

[22] Kaiser Family Foundation 2001 How Young People Use the Internet for Health Information, 46 pages, https://kaiserfamilyfoundation.files.wordpress.com/2001/11/3202-genrx-report.pdf.

cooperate with Internet health information providers or Internet physicians advising patients on attitudes, medication, and treatment. Patients and insurers are willing to pay for those services, sometimes saving money and getting better results (or at least a second opinion) from another physician. E-health empowers people to understand the importance of staying healthy and to find advice and support in reducing health risks. As far as the right to literacy is a human and civil right, the promotion of health literacy is one of the most basic ways to support citizens' well-being and autonomy. Health education by e-health vehicles 'challenges individuals, communities, and professionals – indeed all of us – to take specific steps to ensure good health, as well as long life, are enjoyed by all.'[23] A survey documented that customers seeking medical news on the Internet were 'more health conscious and health information oriented, held stronger health beliefs, and were more likely to engage in healthy activities.'[24]

Because of their anonymity, e-health sites allow for personal questions and advice relating to health care and lifestyle that are rarely asked in the doctor's office. Ilkilic[25] found such a Turkish site, which discussed issues of very personal concern and counted the visits of customers to each of the issues. These were the most-visited pages in August 2003 on the site www.kekimce.com: premature ejaculation (883); worries about impotence (857); how to lose 3 kg weight in 7 days (777); diseases of the prostate (763); losing weight without fasting (677); skin care (671); and hepatitis (668). Because drug addiction, smoking, drinking, and sexual activities that might result in infections are often of a shameful, secret nature, e-health sites are of particular importance. They are a powerful tool for educating and supporting people struggling with obesity, smoking, drinking, drugs, and other issues, as well as people with lifestyle problems they don't want to talk about in public or to their doctor with lifestyle problems they don't want to talk about in public or to their doctor directly.

10.4. Meeting Places for Health Communities

The Internet provides new avenues for information, education, communication, discussions, and advice on topics such as medical news and services, drugs and medications, specific diseases, and healthy lifestyles.[26] Called 'portals,' different

---

23 www.healthypeople.gov.

24 Dutta-Bergmann l.c., 8.

25 Ilkilic I, Ince I, Pourgholam-Ernst A 2004 E-Health im muslemischen Kulturen. Bochum: ZME, 13; www.kekimce.com, accessed August 2003; the site has since changed its format, last accessed 07-25-2016.

26 The Internet is full of health information websites in many languages and with different quality of authorship, information, and reliability; e.g. in 2006 Chinese sites included www.dzwww.com/jk/ by the Da-zhong Daily group and www.jkb.cn/ by the Health Newspaper; the site www.jkzw.com.cn by Shenzhen Quanwangxun Development Co. and the www.39.net site are subdivided into different rooms and lay emphasis on prevention of

sites offer different services to different communities, including the following eight: (1) Internet-based or -supported medical education, medical–ethical education, and continuing education for health care professionals; (2) medical expert competence networks and cyberspace rounds for individual patient management of a complex nature; (3) general health information and health care sites for laypeople to educate themselves on basic or specific matters of health care, exercise, lifestyle and nutrition, basic health risks, and common afflictions such as colds, stomach pain, etc.; (4) specialized interactive sites for individual medical checkups with or without a personal advisor or physician involved; (5) cyberspace visits to a doctor for a brief diagnosis or a 'second opinion' referring to existing personal clinical or laboratory data; (6) sites provided by insur-insurers, drug companies, or other stakeholders in health care management for information or advice to their constituency; (7) sites to order or review prescriptions and medicinal drugs; (8) sites for cyberspace-based health-care communities of self-selected communication seekers such as patients suffering from diabetes, obesity, hypertension, drug abuse, or genetic disorders.

Some sites provide more than one service, and others serve only paying subscribers or licensed personnel. Many e-health portals, particularly ones specializing in specific disciplines such as oncology or diabetes, also provide 'self-test' questionnaires for lay visitors. Some are integrated with 'private consultation' links and professional 'competence-nets' with two levels. (Private consultation requires registration and fees for service.) Self-diagnosis test sites such as *www.real-age.com* do not charge; they combine advice on lifestyle modification, nutrition, and physical exercise with medical information and encouragement, including tips on how to deal with specific issues or where to turn for more personal advice. They finance themselves by advertising wellness products, physical exercise equipment, vitamins, etc.

Health-literate citizens visiting sites such as www.realage.com receive a free diagnosis, specific individual prognosis, and advice on how to lower their real age. Although initial diagnosis and counseling is free, they also offer additional paid checkups and education on nutrition, exercise, and lifestyle. Reliability of information, potential fraud, and exploitation are issues in these new rooms, just as they are in traditional ones providing health information and services. The Internet is particularly vulnerable to fraud and exploitation. Drugs sold there might not be efficacious and are often harmful or dangerous. As laypeople look for alternative means of healing, sites offering an array of supposedly efficacious products become popular, but efficacy is difficult to establish. More studies need to be done, and bioethicists should be involved in governance and quality control. Drug company Pfizer uses the Internet to promote and provide information about its lifestyle drug Viagra, but it also warns

disease and lifestyle advice; cf. Sass HM 2006 Bioethics and Biopolitics. Xian:press.fmmu.sn.en, 256-276.

consumers about bogus Viagra. Many other websites and emailers offer sexual stimulants and health remedies with questionable efficacy.

An earlier report by the European Commission stressed both the economic and health benefits of e-health: 'When combined with organizational changes and the development of new skills, e-health can help to deliver better care for less money within citizen-centered health delivery systems ... There are many examples of successful e-health developments including health information networks, electronic health records, telemedicine services, wearable and portable monitoring systems, and health portals. Today, at least four out of five European doctors have an Internet connection, and a quarter of Europeans use the Internet for health information.'[27] E-medicine sites for professionals often include or are interlinked to e-health sites for laypeople. A service of the U.S. National Institute of Health, *www.clinicaltrials.gov*,[28] lists more than 220,000 trials and explains in plain language the goals and risks of trials and their potential outcomes. The success and reliability of these and other different locales of e-health depends on two requirements: technical skills and moral authority. Confucian physician Gong Tingxian's advice to laypeople quoted earlier remains relevant: 'choose enlightened physicians [*ming-i*] and thereby receive help in their ailment; they have to be careful, because life and death follow each other closely.' Like conventional health care partnerships or any other field of technology and service, e-health must integrate ethics and expertise, humaneness and skill.

Of particular cultural and ethical importance are new forms of communities in cyberspace, dwelling beyond the limits of time and geography. Developed outside of the established medical system, these health-oriented communities have a global reach. Establishing a global community for patients and families of a rare genetic disorder of the kidney called von Hippel-Lindau syndrome (VHL) was the vision of Joyce Graff. She is the widow of a victim of this genetic disorder, which is inherited by 3 in 100,000 people. The site *www.vhl.org* not only provides information on recent research and advice on treatment, nutrition, and lifestyle, it is also a global friendship network, with friends sending birthday greetings and recipes for cakes and cookies. Carriers and their families become friends and virtual neighbors, supporting each other and sharing sentiments, good and bad news, and visions and fears. Most of them know each other better than their neighbors next door, who may have no idea what VHL disorder means. Similar but much larger sites exist for the community of carriers of polycystic kidney diseases.[29] Closeness and friendship on the Internet is not just

---

[27] Eysenbach 2001 l.c.

[28] Accessed 07-25-2016.

[29] Supported by a grant from the DFG foundation, the Bochum Zentrum fuer Medizinische Ethik built a German language site named www.zystennieren.de for information and interactive communication. To our surprise and without much fanfare, we had over 18,000 hits within the first 18 months, mostly from young carriers who have no symptoms yet and do not see a doctor, but surfed for and found a place to get information and to communicate

virtual. It is real, but in a different way than neighborly or friendly relations in geography.[30]. *WebMD* provides health information, drug information, weight loss, foods and recipies, fitness and exercise, sex and relationships, balanced lifestyle and a special for 50+ netizens called 'living better, longer'. *RealAge,* founded by Michael Roizen in 1999 and now a part of *Sharecare*, offers an easy-to-understand online physical check-up, called 'RealAge', checking your real biological age and potential against your actual diagnostic and lifestyle information; your real-age might be lower or higher than your birthday age, the difference between those two will give you incentives to change your lifestyle.[31]

10.5. Should Cyber Territories Be Regulated?

In all areas of human activity, new techniques and instruments can be used to promote or to hurt human cultures and fellow humans. Why should it be different with such powerful new tools as the combination of research and results in biomedicine and information technology? The wealth of information and communication developing around the Internet is naturally seen as a competitive force by existing players in the fields of disease management. Without much integration with the existing health care system so far, e-health is growing parallel to the existing sickness care system. It often lacks quality control and can be primarily profit-oriented, but these temptations are well known to the traditional existing sickness care system as well. Some voices have called for Internet rules of good behavior and have proposed a set of ethics rules for professional conduct of stakeholders in e-health information and communication. The Commission of the European Communities[32] has published preliminary guidelines for quality-control criteria related to websites. Certification is probably

---

with others on issues such as getting married, having children, etc. We had an extensive, sometimes emotional and controversial debate among young carriers about telling the truth to one's fiancé prior to or after engagement or not telling at all. A separate room, monitored by a physician who was himself a carrier, discussed a dozen of the most common issues for ADPKD carriers; the webmaster of this room also followed up in private emails once in a while. The site is closed now because of loss of funding; cf. Sass HM 2007 Gesundheit und Wellness durch E-Health? Die vier K von E-Health: Kultur, Kommunikation, Kooperation, Kompetenz, in: Gross D, Jakobs EM eds, E-Health und technisierte Medizin. Neue Herausforderungen im Gesundheitswesen. Münster: Lit 29-49, includes action guides for e-health surfers and providers.

[30] Boyd B 2006 The Dotcomrade. The Many Faces of Online Friendship, in: the New Atlantis 14:124-126.

[31] The questionnaire can be completed in 20 minutes and includes questions regarding eating, drinking, social habits, hobbies, fitness and exercise, also 'how many friends to you have?'; returning visitors are complimented, if their exercise has continued and if they had increased the number of friends and leisure activities, in case those had been too few.

[32] Commission of the European Communities (2004) E-health — making healthcare better for European citizens: An action plan for a European e-Health Area. COM (2004)356, 2004-04-30.

preferable to regulation, but even that may not be strong enough to promote and protect professional and ethical quality standards in websites for both laypeople and experts. Codes of conduct have been proposed by nongovernmental organizations such as Health on the Net Foundation[33] and Health Internet Ethics.[34] But e-health cultures and customs have yet to develop. In 2002, UNESCO bioethics unit director Ten Have argued that 'the only feasible approach, precisely because of the nature of the Internet, is self-regulation and self-binding of providers and consumers.'[35] Of course, nation states and international bodies, concerned about the content provided internet territories should use all opportunities to educate citizens about the risks, benefits, and evil powers in cyberspace; they may issue rules and regulations as they do in geography, and they might compete with market forces in providing cyberspace territories for information, meeting, communication and cooperation, camaraderie and care.

E-Health communication and cooperation may be vital for quick emergency health communication during a mega crisis or terrorist attack.[36] E-health has been suggested as a useful tool for improving medical and health information in developing countries[37] and for the elderly.[38] Even in countries with low levels of Internet access, it can be used to communicate with 'health ambassadors,' health care providers, and social service agencies in remote rural areas.[39] The Internet's increasing power of promulgating health information, communication, and advice could become a great means to promote health literacy and competence. Independent certification boards or agencies need to support quality control and issue quality certificates without hampering competition and the Internet's diversity of information, support, and communication. The *eEurope 2002* report by the Commission of the European Communities writes: 'it is critical that e-health content and services are developed efficiently, are available for all, and health related web sites comply with established quality criteria.' It will depend on good cooperation between the experts and sources of medicine, informatics, and education to serve the people in protecting and enhancing health, in avoiding, managing and healing diseases, and in supporting those who are sick, frail, old, or confused.

---

[33] www.hon.ch/honcode/conduct.html, accessed 07-25-2016.

[34] www.hiethics.org, accessed 07-25-2016.

[35] Ten Have H 2002 Cybermedicine and E-Ethics, in: Medicine, Health Care and Philosophy 5:119.

[36] Kittler AF, Hobbs J, Volk LA, Kreps GL, Bates DM 2004 The Internet as a vehicle to communicate health information during a public health emergency, in: J Med Internet Med 6(1):e8; see also chapter 15 in this book.

[37] Drury P 2005 eHealth. A Model for Developing Countries, in: eHealth International 2:19-26

[38] Bashur R 2007 Global Telemedicine and the Elderly, in: eHealth International 3:1-6.

[39] Sass HM 2006 l.c. 256-276.

While e-health has all the properties to emancipate laypeople from the unnecessary paternalism of experts and from the dominance of protected and privileged knowledge, only honest and virtuous physicians can take the lead to develop the new cyberspace rooms and communities for health care information seekers. These and other new web-based places of communication and cooperation certainly need to be open to competitive market forces, but certain levels of quality assurance and quality control are crucial for protecting people from fraud and disinformation and for making communication in trust possible. As integrated in e-health, the merging of medical knowledge, common-sense lifestyle advice, and information technology certainly becomes a new tool for information, advice, compassion, and solidarity in the concern and care for individual and public health. Yet as with all tools, it can be used for unhealthy, immoral, and inhumane purposes. Following the interactive 15th-century rules of doctor Gong Tingxian for patients and physicians, Xiaomei Zhai and I have developed action guides for today's health care surfers and providers of cyberspace health information and advice.[40]

ACTION GUIDE FOR E-HEALTH NETIZENS AND HEALTH CARE SURFERS

1. Wellness and well-being depend, among other causes, on good self-care information and both medical and non-medical advice. They also require a personal commitment to deal responsibly with medical and non-medical risks to health, quality of life, and length of life.

2. Be a critical consumer of cyberspace-based communication on the protection and promotion of health and on dealing with diseases and disorders. Be critical and verify information and advice by using more than one source. Do not trust those who promise everlasting health, wonder drugs, or sensational cures and remedies.

3. Be a courteous, civilized partner, helpful, understanding neighbor, and trustworthy friend in cyberspace health care communities; protect your privacy and meet close friends in private outside of community rooms.

4. E-health communication can never replace local health care. Use private consultation rooms in cyberspace but keep in personal contact with health care experts and local institutions you trust in your neighborhood.

ACTION GUIDE FOR E-HEALTH PROPERTY OWNERS

1. Provide clear, scientifically sound, evidence-based information on medical and non-medical strategies for a healthy and enjoyable life. Encourage health care surfers to deal responsibly with their health and wellness risks, and help them develop their own concept of quality of life and live accordingly.

[40] Zhai XM, Sass HM 2004 E-Health Ethics: A Yet to Be Recognized Issue in Medicine and Medical Ethics, in: Eubios J Asian Intern Bioethics 14:147-148.

2. Never promise what you cannot deliver responsibly, and respond to trusting clients honestly and fairly. Providing health care is not just a profit-oriented business, either in local or cyberspace communities. Seek certification and professional oversight of your services, and employ only persons of the highest per-personal and professional standing.
3. Provide and promote rooms for health care communities. Allow them to create their own culture in sharing information and emotion, in supporting each other, and in building networks and groups. Never allow uncivilized or offensive behavior in your rooms.
4. Advise health care surfers to seek medical diagnosis and personal advice from experts in their neighborhood outside of cyberspace and to keep in personal contact with a trusted health care expert. Provide rooms for private consultation and guarantee privacy and quality service in private as well as in public services.

11. Solidarity and Subsidiarity in Healthy Markets

SUBSIDIARITY AND SOLIDARITY BUILD STABLE COMMUNITIES

As history abundantly proves, it is true that on account of changed conditions many things which were done by small associations in former times cannot be done now save by large associations. Still, that most weighty principle, which cannot be set aside or changed, remains fixed and unshaken in social philosophy: Just as it is gravely wrong to take from individuals what they can accomplish by their own initiative and industry and give it to the community, so also it is an injustice and at the same time a grave evil and disturbance of right order to assign to a greater and higher association what lesser and subordinate organizations can do. For every social activity ought of its very nature to furnish help to the members of the body social, and never destroy and absorb them. The supreme authority of the State ought, therefore, to let subordinate groups handle matters and concerns of lesser importance, which would otherwise dissipate its efforts greatly. Thereby the State will more freely, powerfully, and effectively do all those things that belong to it alone because it alone can do them: directing, watching, urging, restraining, as occasion requires and necessity demands. Therefore, those in power should be sure that the more perfectly a graduated order is kept among the various associations, in observance of the principle of 'subsidiary function,' the stronger social authority and effectiveness will be the happier and more prosperous the condition of the State.

Pope Pius XI: *Quadrogesimo Anno*, 1931[1]

11.1. Vested Interests in Modern Health Repair Shops

Over the last decades, contemporary health care systems (HCS) in developed countries have built ever bigger and more costly inflexible supertankers carrying only one type of cargo: health repair technology and services. The medical services offered by hospitals and doctors in private practice are similar to the engineering and technical services offered by car repair shops for automobiles. It would be more accurate to call them health repair systems (HRS) The difference, however, between car and health repair is that we pay for the former directly out of pocket, whereas HRS services are paid for by complex and increasingly complicated models of statutory or private insurance schemes, or by socialized medicine's bureaucracies and state agencies.

Owners of these HRS supertankers and their cargo have a vested interest in neither modifying the load nor redirecting the course. Politicians, conditioning the

---

[1] Pius XI 1931 Quadrogesimo Anno. Encyclical of Pope Pius XI on Reconstruction of the Social Order to our Venerable Brethren, the Patriarchs, Primates, Archbishops, Bishops, and other Ordinaries in Peace and Communion with the Apostolic Sea, and likewise to all the Faithful of the Catholic World, paragraphs 79 and 80; cf. St. Thomas: Contra Gentiles, III, 71; Waschkuhn A 1995 Was ist Subsidiaritaet? Ein sozialphilosophisches Ordnungsprinzip. Von Thomas von Aquin bis zur 'Civil Society.' Opladen.

regulators, are thinking in the short term, from one election period to the next, and thus ignore both issues. Medical schools focus on researching and teaching ever more specialized repair competencies. Regulatory authorities prevent market forces from focusing on people's health rather than on medical repairs. They do not primarily support morally and economically sound health initiatives, including making the citizen the most important stakeholder in the care, support, and improvement of health. Consequently, health insurers and hospital operators and owners reduce their responsibilities to micromanagement within the given regulatory and financial parameters. Statistical evidence from many national health care systems documents that the percentage of health care expenditures within the Gross National Product (GNP) does not correlate at all positively to life expectancy and health status in those countries, with the United States and Greece having the most negative connection. All stakeholders (except citizens as clients, i.e., patients and potential patients) have little incentive[2] to change the course of the ship and the content of the cargo (i.e., to include services of prevention and prediction, to include teaching and training in health literacy, and make health the responsibility of the citizen as the central stakeholder interested in a healthy and enjoyable life). A revolution of Copernican dimensions is necessary to change the course of these HRS supertankers. But no rebellion or major cultural attitude change on the part of clients is in sight that would be strong enough to force the cartels of vested interests to unbundle unfair restrictions in the care for health. For financial reasons, existing systems of repair will not be able to apply ever-expanding medical knowledge to everyone in the future; nor will every person in an aging society be treated by all available standardized medical procedures based on personal choice and lifestyle vision. The HRS, already not living up to its goals, is unavoidably doomed to collapse sooner or later. We therefore will need a conceptual and organizational transformation of Copernican dimensions away from the single, inflexible solidarity pillar towards flexible subsidiarity and a healthy, fair, and integrated HCS broadly based on the triad of *responsibility, solidarity, and subsidiarity* in the care for health in the 21st century.

Prioritizing of repair services occurs in most models under the term *rationalization,* which actually means rationing.[3] The cost side is where the discussions and fights occur right now and where various national models differ as they unsuc-

---

[2] The US Institute of Medicine in 2002 recognized that a broad collaborative stakeholder approach might be the most prudent way to care for the public's health; cf. IOM (US Institute of Medicine) Board on Health Promotion and Disease Prevention, 2002: The Future of the Public's Health in the 21st Century. The National Academies Press: 'There is a growing recognition that individuals, communities, and various social institutions can form powerful collaborative relationships to improve health that government cannot replicate… The determinants that interact to create good or ill health derive from various sources and sectors.'

[3] Huster S 2011 Soziale Gesundheitsgerechtigkeit. Berlin: Wagenbach, 34-54.

cessfully micromanage the repair system. Thus, the content of the cargo is unfortunately not under discussion; rather the focus is on implicit tactics to reduce the cost of the load. Various forms of saving money are visible, whether called rationalizing or rationing. These include sanctioning un-acceptably long waiting lines for essential services and lifesaving interventions; reducing service capacities or eliminating some non-profitable services; delayed, limited, or denied approval of new drugs and technologies; and so-called quality norms for medical interventions and associated generic reimbursement schemes for services based on individual requirements. Some regulatory and legal restrictions eliminate competition and market forces for better service, such as the requirement that stronger Sickness Funds in Germany support weaker ones financially. Other legal and regulatory features provide different schemes for different people, such as special first-class insurance benefits for members of the U.S. Congress and Senate, voted into existence by the same people who benefit from them. Preferential health care services for military veterans exist not only in the United States but in many other countries.

A more viable and just system of caring for each other in competent and compassionate community life would be a three-tiered, interactive bios of (1) health education and literacy, basic medical services, and full pain care paid for in different ways by competitive public–private markets; (2) supplementary medical and lifestyle-related services paid for by the beneficiaries; and (3) subsidiary services by existing and new charities for those who fall through the grids of medical and social networks and by 'moral friends' for culturally controversial interventions such as abortions, assistance in dying, cosmetic surgery, or lifestyle enhancement.[4] Of course, the health literacy and responsibility of citizens will be the basic platform of a reformed, just, and successful new culture of caring for health.

11.2. Replacing Health Repair with Health Care

The definition of 'health' by the World Health Organization reflects the narrow contemporary understanding of care for health as being reduced to medical repair intervention. It is wrongly suggested that health is an entitlement of citizens to be delivered and provided by health care authorities to achieve a state of 'complete physical, mental and social wellbeing and not merely the absence of disease and infirmity.'[5] But health is a much more complex phenomenon; rather

---

[4] Cf. Sass HM 1990 Zielkonflikte im Wohlfahrtsstaat, in: Grundfragen der Sozialpolitik, Sachsse C. ed., Frankfurt: Suhrkamp, 71-84; ibid. 1993 Gesundheitsvorsorge durch Gesundheitsverantwortung. Plädoyer für eine radikale Reform der gesetzlichen Krankenversicherung, in: Liberal 993; 35(1):8-23; ibid. 1995 The new Triad: Responsibility, Solidarity and Subsidiarity, in: J Medicine and Philosophy 20(6):587-594; ibid. 2008 Public Health Ethik ist Partnerschaftsethik, in: Bundesgesundheitsblatt 51:164-174.

[5] Preamble to the Constitution of the World Health Organization as adopted by the International Health Conference, New York, 19-22 June, 1946; signed on 22 July 1946 by the

than a state, it is a process of challenge and response, of understanding, balancing, protecting, and managing well-being. As I wrote in 2006, 'Health is a process and a balanced result of health-literate and health-competent care of one's own physical, emotional, and social wellbeing, achieved by competent understanding, modification and enhancement of individual genetic, social, and environmental risk factors and challenges, with the support of health care professionals and through equal and fair access to health care service, including health education and preventive services.'[6]

Self-interest as well as prudence and responsibility should tell individuals that caring for their health is of prime importance for long life, quality of life, fulfilment in life, and for reaching goals. Health-literate citizens can make educated choices for care, but health-illiterate people cannot. Health-literate people make better patients because educated consumers in general are better customers.[7] But citizens as current or prospective patients are held hostage in bureaucratic and paternalistic HRS systems of disease management that deal with one aspect of health care only: managing acute and chronic disease. Of course, to remain healthy despite genetic disparities or social disadvantages is an issue of social justice, and special considerations apply in regard to genetic and epigenetic heritage and social disadvantages and harm.[8] But services in repair and redistribution will never achieve what services in education and empowerment can do for the life-competent, health-competent citizen.[9] What is needed is a transition from existing disease management cultures towards attitudes and cultures in HCS systems that reflect true concern for health. Thus, health care is primarily an issue for individual self-determination and responsibility; only secondarily is it an obligation of the community or government. Individual citizens are the prime beneficiaries, customers, and consumers of health care services. Assisting people in caring for their health and reducing health and health care risks could and should be a successful business, a good investment,

---

representatives of 61 States (Official Records of the World Health Organization, no. 2, p. 100) and entered into force on 7 April 1948.

[6] Sass HM 2006 Cultivating and Harmonizing Virtues and Principles, in: Asian Bioethics Review 3(1)38.

[7] Cf. Herder-Dorneich 1983; Herder-Dorneich P 1983 Ordnungstheorie des Sozialstaates. Tuebingen: Mohr; Goodman JC, Musgrave GL 1993 Patient Power. Solving America's Health Care Crisis. Washington: Cato Institute.

[8] Powers M, Faden R 2006 Social Justice: The Moral Foundations of Public Health and Health Policy. Oxford: Oxford U Press.

[9] 'Collective action' to care for children's health definitely is a priority in social justice, as Powers M and Faden R 2006 Social Justice: The Moral Foundations of Public Health. Oxford: Oxford U Press, 92-95, rightly point out; but without associated health education and care education and the empowerment for health literacy and health responsibility, the social goal of levelling disparities in genetic and social background will never be reached.

and the prime obligation of HCS public policy.[10] The prime moral agent for good personal and communal health has been lost and needs be found and empowered: the health-literate, health-competent, and health-responsible citizen.

Providing service for one of the most fundamental human needs holds great social, cultural, and ethical merit. Modern medicine has improved success rates in intervention, prediction, and prevention and provides extended opportunities for beneficiaries and those in the business of health care services, but systems of insurance and of providing health care have not been allowed to change accordingly. Healthy people make healthy communities, and healthy people and healthy communities can make healthy social and natural environments in a mingling of integrative and integrated health. Modern medicine is performed in regulatory, institutional, and financial settings that determine the maxims under which stakeholders interact successfully. Health care ethics thus become a firm foundation for a future system of care and insurance. Health care policy, health care insurance, health care providers, and above all health care regulators need to empower the citizen as a consumer of professional health care services[11]. A health-literate citizen makes a better customer and partner in health care and disease management, as well as a healthier, happier, and more independent health-literate and health-responsible person. Except for a few small steps, neither governments nor insurers nor hospitals have yet exploited the vast opportunities of the Internet for educating and advising citizens on caring for and improving health.[12]

As health is a basic human good, transition periods such as ours fare best when traditional medical and moral principles are reassessed in the light of new and expanded opportunities, not when new ones are invented. The cultural and medical overconcentration on medical repair services has brushed aside centuries of lay health literacy and responsibility, such as the prudent recognition of the six *res non naturals* as cultivated attitudes for harmonious, healthy, and hap-

---

[10] A study on 'Effects of lowering LDL cholesterol with statin therapy in people at low risk of vascular disease: meta-analysis of individual data from 27 randomized trials' by Cholesterol Treatment Trialists (CTT) Collaborators, in: The Lancet, Early Online Publication, 17 May 2012 (doi:10.1016/S0140-6736(12)60367-5) suggests that an upfront general prescription of statins to everyone over 50 would be cheaper for the NHS than coronary and stroke care in later years. In whose interest is it to use statins or similar remedies as universal elixirs for the reduction of national health care expenditures, rather than educating and encouraging people to take care of their health with or without statins?

[11] Using Veatch's three-level Covenant model, as discussed in chapter 9, will be helpful not only in reforming health care but also other parts of the political body.

[12] Cf. Sass, HM: Gesundheitskulturen im Internet. E-Health: Möglichkeiten, Leistungen und Risiken, Bochum: Zentrum für medizinische Ethik, 2006, Heft 166. Sass, HM: Wellness durch E-Health? Die vier K von E-Health: Kultur, Kommunikation, Kooperation, Kompetenz, E-Health und technisierte Medizin, hg D. Gross, EA Jakobs, Münster: Lit 2007, 29-49. Sass, HM: E-Health: Health Promotion and Wellness Communities Eubios J Asian and Intern Bioethics 2004, 14:170-174.

py lifestyles by Roman doctor Galen: light and air *(aer)*, eating and drinking *(cibus et potus)*, work and rest *(motus et quies)*, sleep and wake *(somnus et vigilia)*, secretion and excretion *(secreta et excreta)*, and stimulation of the mind *(affectus animi)*.

We already discussed health care action guides by Galen, Confucian doctor Gong, and German doctor and pharmacist Hoffmann. These and other traditional visions of health and good health care need to be adapted for the 21st century into the institutional settings of health information, education, and training in health literacy and individual health responsibility. They can support developing cultures of prevention by changing attitudes towards nutrition, physical exercise, mental activity, and many other easily available lifestyle modifications for people living in stressful urban environments.[13] Fashionable contemporary movements of translational medicine[14] have yet to explore these potentials of translating traditional health care knowledge into the modern world of repair medicine.

Tang Dynasty physician Sun Simiao once differentiated between mediocre, average, and superior doctors: 'a superior doctor takes care of the state, an average doctor takes care of the person, an inferior doctor takes care of the disease.'[15] In regard to modern health care systems, we could translate Dr. Sun this way: 'A superior health care system sets a framework for promoting and protecting health literacy and responsibility, healthy people and communities, healthy environments, and healthy forms of solidarity and subsidiarity; an average health care system focuses on patients as persons and not just on repairing their diseases; an inferior system of health care just repairs illnesses and diseases.' What would such a superior HCS look like, and who would be responsible for building, protecting, running, enjoying, and improving it? A Learning Health Care System (LHS) needs to 'preserve the value of personal care and even ...

---

[13] Fritz Jahr, the father of modern bioethics, had such an integrative and integrating understanding of caring for health. In an essay on the Fifth Commandment 'thou shall not kill', as already mentioned, he describes three integrated fields for translating the old rule into the modern world of health care: (a) 'duties towards one's own life ... by not taking one's own life, not shortening it, not harming or endangering it, not weakening one's health by unchastity, excesses in eating and drinking, heavy anger, frivolous foolhardiness and daredevilry, etc.; (b) public health 'whoever protects his own life in this regard, he fulfils one's duty also towards the community'; (c) the general Bioethical Imperative, 'respect every living being in principle as an end in itself and treat it, if possible, as such.' (Jahr (1934) in Muzur, Sass ed., 2012:34f).

[14] The new field of translational medicine has not yet recognized the vast potential of empowering citizens to become literate and responsible prime agents in the care, protection and improvement of their health and life; cf. also Kagarise MJ, Sheldon GF (2000) Translational Ethics. A Perspective for a New Millennium, in: Archives of Surgery, 135(1):39 and Cribbs A 2010 Translational Ethics. The Theory-Practice Gap, in: Medical Ethics. J Med Eth 36:207-210.

[15] Sass HM 2006 Bioethics and Biopolitics. Xian: press.ffmu.sn.cn 203.

enhance it by partnering with patients in achieving the goals of learning health care'[16].

11.3. Basic Health Care Is a Moral and Cultural Obligation

We all have to grow, learn, and work to find our place in society and to develop ourselves. Confucius once pointed out that people are like raw pearls, precious but in need of polishing. We learn by accepting and internalizing social norms, lifestyles, rules, and attitudes; therefore, family background and neighbourhood attitudes are important in the early formation of character. But we also learn math and history, reading and writing in school. Health literacy and health care knowledge are rarely included, neither in general education nor in special education and training. Printed, audio, and visual media selectively provide information and advice on health issues, as do special e-health sites (with realage.com or the now-defunct healthypeople.org being among the better ones). If there is a human and civil right to education, then health education is a prime candidate for such a right. Health education and health care competence can also level differences in family background and social opportunities. Thus, political and cultural support of e-health sites and other forms of providing access to information and advice would be the first step in allowing people to take charge of their lifestyle decisions and to de-professionalize vast areas of protected knowledge. Actually, the successes of modern repair medicine seem to have made preventive health care obsolete. Hospitals, as reliable and trustworthy corporate citizens, can play an important role in offering outreach programs for educating individuals and communities on the basics of lifestyle-related health knowledge, such as seasonal health risks. An additional effect of making such knowledge available to everyone will be the reduction of social inequalities and the development of more equal and harmonious communities.

Of course, basic medical intervention and protection of life is an obligation of solidarity and compassion as well. Routine diagnostic services belong to basic care for health, as do access to fitness outlets and lifestyle advice. Medical service to take out an inflamed appendix or tooth is a moral obligation; the replacement of teeth, however, is not a basic service, particularly not in the age of processed food. Aging is a normal process, and anti-aging remedies don't belong to basic medical care, for everyone must come to terms with aging one way or the other. Pain care, on the other hand, is an obligation we owe to all on the basis of solidarity and compassion. Care for the demented is a moral obligation as well, and the growing number of senile fellow humans can never be cared for in an inflexible system without the involvement of families, neighbourhoods, and charities. As some of us are born with genetic traits requiring special medi-

[16] Miller FG, Kim SYH 2015 Personal Care in Learning Health Care Systems, in: Kennedy Inst of Ethics J 25(4): 443

cal care, solidarity demands that we alleviate these special burdens also.[17] Therefore, genetic testing and consultation is one of the basic preconditions for making citizens health literate and competent. Predictive medical information services belong to the basic package, as they provide essential information for prevention and health improvement. But to pay in solidarity for health repair caused by unhealthy lifestyles is ethically controversial.

Basic health care can be financed in a competitive market by one or more payers. If someone cannot pay health insurance premiums, the community should pay. Market competition and transparency are essential for financial stability and success, which can be measured in better health and happiness amongst an ever-larger number of people. Basic health insurance should focus on making citizens health competent and on creating a culture of healthy, happy lifestyles. It must include reasonably fair[18] basic medical intervention and repair services in saving lives and alleviating pain.

11.4. Supplementary Care, Individual Preferences and Finances

Most highly successful but expensive services were not around two generations ago, so it is only a small comfort to exclude them from basic financial packages. A stronger argument for exclusion is that payment for each intervention has led to a repair mentality among citizens in HRS systems and to the reduction of self-care and health care competence. We have not been given a chance to live

[17] Genetic testing and detailed consultation for inherited genetic anomalies that can be influenced by lifestyle modification is a basic civil right that must become an ever-more important instrument in allowing people to take care of their health. A prime candidate for empowering carriers to exercise their health competence is ADPKD (polycystic kidney disease), as it allows for postponing the onset of acute symptoms by means of controlling hypertension, avoiding contact sports, and other practices. Other candidates for 'the right to know' are BRCA1 and BRCA2 (breast and ovarian cancer), MLH1 and MSH2 (Lynch syndrome), and FBN1 (Marfin syndrome); cf. Kielstein R and Sass HM 2001 Genetics: Ethical Issues in Kidney Disease, in: Ethics and the Kidney, Levinsky NG. Oxford U Press, 167-182; for a civil right of non-discrimination cf. Kious BM, 2010 Genetic Non-discrimination and Health Care as an Entitlement, in: Journal of Medicine and Philosophy 35(2)86-100.

[18] Of course, the discussion about a decent – better: a reasonably fair – basic minimum of emergency medicine and health repair services will depend on changing cultural priorities and, most of all, on political will and majority. In developing a fair basic package of services, it might be prudent to start with 35% of the funds spent yearly over the last 5 years and prioritize services according to urgency, basic necessity, efficacy, and price, then add 5% for predictive and preventive services and 10% for individual elected supplementary services. This would bring down costs immensely, if supported by the community and stakeholders, and it would leave financial room for supplementary insurance based on individual choice and funds. The government must contribute its share by introducing health education in all levels of public education and by competing in the health care information market with a first class e-health platform. Of course, service for severe individual genetic risk factors is part of the 35% basic care.

healthy lives based on our own health care competence and responsibility. But if we want to pay extra for additional services, we can use the model of special supplementary insurance for health risk such as taken out for skiing, racing, or hunting. We can also pay extra for automotive or occupational health risk insurance. As we are different in values and lifestyles, there will be different sets of supplementary services in medicine and health care. Not everyone will be able to pay for all possible or desired supplementary services, and not everyone will be able to buy an automobile of his or her choice. This is unfortunate but not unjust, and charities and friends might help out.

11.5. Charitable Care for Controversial Services and the Needy

All cultures over the centuries have supported impressive works and institutions of charitable service. In the age of full payment for all requested services, these charities still are there, but they have lost support and moral and cultural influence. Whatever a future model of caring for the sick, the frail, and the poor will be, there will always be a need for charity and supplementary services for those who fall through the grid of even the best possible social networks. So said Fra Gerard, 900 years ago. He was the founder of the Order of St John of the Hospital in Jerusalem, which serves pilgrims, Christians, Muslims, and Jews alike.[19] Buddhism, Christianity, Islam, and various secular movements have traditionally cared for the needy, desperate, hungry, and sick, and an integrated and interacting model of health care will give these and other traditions a new field of care and help. The fact that we believe in different gods and goddesses or in none is an additional reason to allow for diversity in service among providers and recipients of charitable work.

Some medical services are morally or culturally controversial, such as contraceptives or anti-nidativa, abortion, testosterone treatment, shortening the process of dying or euthanasia, hormonal and surgical modification and reparation treatment for transsexuals, and extremely expensive life-prolonging medications or interventions. There will always be people for and against these and other medications and procedures. It would contribute to peaceable, compassionate communication and cooperation if, instead of quarrelling about these services being in the basic package, politicians and supporting groups would allow and even encourage charities to collect tax-favoured donations and to take care of the additional requests not shared by all.

[19] The meditation 'Our brotherhood will not end because the soil, in which this plant grows, is the misery of the world, and because, God willing, there always will be fellow humans working to reduce suffering and to make misery more bearable' has been attributed to Fra Gerard (1090-1120), Head of the Hospital at Jerusalem of the Order of St. John the Baptist.

11.6. Competent Compassion in Solidarity and Subsidiarity

We witness today the painful financial and moral destruction of overblown social and medical repair systems in some parts of the world, and the absence of even the most basic communal and political support systems elsewhere. Benedikt Spinoza, in his *Tractato Theologico-Politicus* of 1670, argued that peace and the fabric of society would not fall apart when state-provided tutelage is abandoned and liberty and freedom are given, allowing individuals to make their own choices based on their personal visions and values. Rather, peace in the community and respect for persons would be threatened if people were not allowed to be prime moral agents in making life decisions. Even if a 'natural right to health care'[20] could be established by a *volonté général,* it must not be confused with medical repair rights. Social justice, as outlined by Powers and Faden, must contain a central civil right to education, empowerment, and the distribution (or quite often redistribution) of justice. Modern welfare systems unfortunately favour redistribution over empowerment; therefore, the misappropriation of funds and justice in HRS is only one sector of unhealthy social policy. Of course, 'the fact that we recognize health as a good, for which social inequalities should be without consequences,' is an 'achievement of civilization which we should not easily throw away,'[21] but good health can and must be achieved and improved though true and fair health care – not by repair services alone. Preferably, it should be embraced by educated, empowered citizens ready to take care of their health and lives. Engelhardt discussed a 'global collapse' in criticizing ill-conceived quests for consensus.[22] I would go one step further and call this form of so-called 'consensus' a quest for uniformity, which in health care would translate into uniform repair bureaucracies and their final collapse. We all have different visions and values for life, health, fun, success, and risk.

More than two millennia ago, Lao Tzu (who was definitely not akin to a freewheeling modern market ideologue) addressed the limited efficacy and potential dangers of anti-liberty rules and regulatory paternalism: 'the more taboos and inhabitations there are in the world, the poorer the people become, the more articulate the laws and ordinances, the more thieves and robbers arise.'[23] Can the Tao be used as a blueprint for a critical political, moral, financial, and organizational review of so-called health care systems, and can the forward-looking statement of Spinoza be used as a guide for replacing our unjust and uncivilized HRS with true and just health care cultures and institutions[24] for integrating the

[20] Eberl JT, Kinney ED, William MJ 2011 Foundation for a Natural Right to Health Care, in: J Medicine and Philosophy 36(6)537-557.

[21] Huster S 2011 l.c.

[22] Engelhardt HT 2006 The Search for Global Morality, in: Global Bioethics. The Collapse of Consensus, Engelhardt HT ed., Salem MA; Scrivener Press, 18-49.

[23] Tao Te Ching 57.

[24] Cf. Sass HM 2008 l.c. for the SEMPER model of public health strategy in developing and protecting individual and communal health in partnership with individuals, communities,

values and virtues of responsibility, solidarity, and subsidiarity in basic care, in personal and free choice for supplementary services, and in charity for many other needs and services? UNESCOs 2005 *Universal Declaration on Bioethics and Human Rights* emphasized that cultural diversity has to be taken into account in the assessment of ethical challenges. Ten Have and Gordin have pointed out that 'respect for cultural diversity depends also on the weight that we give to the role of the individual person (which is itself a point of view that is heavily determined by a specific liberal cultural stance).'[25]

At a time when the discussion and promotion of ever-more rights to full, free 'health care' are timely and fashionable (at least in the Western world), this critical review of health repair systems will most likely not find much support from academic colleagues, short-term-oriented politicians, regulators, or a public culture expecting full-and-free service and instant repair gratification.[26] The time of change and awakening will come when people are fed up with rationing and waiting in lines, when higher premiums are asked for others' lifestyle repair needs or for old-age issues being confused with disease. Alternative markets in promoting healthy lifestyles already find prosperous and rewarding niches for the rich outside of our HRS. When that time comes, the following action guides might be helpful for politicians and regulators, for citizens as prime beneficiaries and agents of good health, for health care experts as coaches, and for health care insurers as enablers and promoters of health and health care.

STAKEHOLDER ACTION GUIDES IN SUBSIDIARITY AND SOLIDARITY

Eight Health Care Rules for Politicians and Regulators

1. Base health care policy broadly on solidarity, free choice, and subsidiarity.
2. Make solidarity the principle for health education and for basic medical services and good pain care.
3. Cover individual risk profiles in basic insurance.
4. Support competition in health services and insurance markets.
5. Regulate quality in health services and insurance.
6. Make health care competence a prime political and educational goal.
7. Encourage protection for those who cannot care for themselves, for charities, and pro-bono services.
8. Promote a fair and competitive market for all stakeholders.

Eight Health Care Rules for the Layperson

1. Find truly educated and trustworthy health care experts.

---

and corporate neighbours and partners, SEMPER standing for the public health principles Safety, Education, Minimax, Efficacy, Partnership, Review.

[25] Ten Have H, Gordijn B, 2011 Diversity and Bioethics, in: Med Health Care and Philos 14:227f

[26] Sass HM 2006 Differentialethik. Münster: Lit, 153-162, 163-176.

2. Develop health care competence and responsibility.
3. Make extended use of predictive and preventive services.
4. Expect healing or relief from medical services, but be aware of limits and risks in medical interventions.
5. Request information and advice from medical experts and be a fair partner in communication and cooperation.
6. Define and implement your sense of qualities of life, from childhood to old age, in sickness and in health.
7. Help your neighbour in need; prepare your own Advance Directives for situations of compromised capacity to make prudent decisions.
8. Act responsibly in spending funds in the care for health and happiness.

Eight Health Care Rules for the Health Professional
1. Treat people as fellow humans, not just as carriers of symptoms.
2. Assist clients and patient to develop health risk competence.
3. Integrate the 'clinical status' and the 'value status' of your patient into differential ethics, diagnosis, and prognosis.
4. Be aware of benefits, limits, and risks of medical intervention and share them with your patient.
5. Be a fair expert partner in communication and cooperation to those who seek your services, while respecting their values and wishes.
6. Provide excellent professional and personal services; continue to educate yourself and to improve them.
7. Provide 'pro bono' services to the needy, and be a fair partner to proxy decision makers.
8. Act responsibly in the use of communal and private health care financing.

Eight Health Care Rules for the Insurance Professional
1. Offer insurance for people as stakeholder partners, not for profit alone.
2. Provide basic medical insurance for health care, nursing care, and good pain care.
3. Recognize individual differences in health risk profiles and include those in basic insurance based on the principle of solidarity.
4. Offer competitive insurance for supplementary health care services based on client preferences and risk profiles.
5. Use health information as a competitive edge in providing even better services in the promotion of health care.
6. Provide incentives or reduce premiums for partners with proven health care competence and action.

7. Cooperate with charities; respect your client's choices.
8. Protect the values and interests of all stakeholders in caring and paying for health.

12. Training and Learning in Biocultures

THE GREAT WAY OF LEARNING
'Non scholae sed vitae discimus' – We don't learn for school, but for life.
Seneca[1]

The Great Learning (Da Xue 大學): Investigate things, extend knowledge, make the will sincere, rectify the heart-mind, cultivate the person, regulate the family, govern the state well, bring peace to the world. – The Way of Great Learning lies in illuminating bright virtue, in holding dear the people, in stopping only at utmost goodness ... Wanting to illuminate bright virtue under heaven, the ancients first governed their states. Wanting to govern their states, they first put their families in order. Wanting to put their families in order, they first cultivated their body. Wanting to cultivate their body, they first rectified their heart. Wanting to rectify their heart, they first made their intentions sincere. Wanting to make their intentions sincere, they first extended their knowledge. The extension of knowledge lies in the investigation of things '.
Confucius[2]

12.1. We learn and train for Life, not for School

Learning is more than reading books or memorizing names and data; we learn in order to become successful, productive, respected, acknowledged, integrated, and happy people within our social, cultural, and political biotope. Educating and learning are tools of human bios 'for survival and the improvement of living conditions.'[3] We don't learn for our teachers; we learn for ourselves. Learning by doing and doing by learning are two of the most successful ways to gain knowledge and competence, to become successful and valued partners in a professional and social culture, and to contribute to the stability and cultivation of a social and political biotope. As already mentioned, Victor von Weizsaecker[4] required three things for the competent professional: knowledge of man, knowledge of facts, and craftsmanship in an integrated form, and Aristotle ar-

---

[1] Seneca A 65 Epistolae ad Lucilium

[2] Confucius, The Great Learning, in: The Chinese Classics, Legge J ed.London 1861: 355-381, digitalized version in the internet.

[3] Sass HM 1980 Education is one of man's indispensable tools, in: Impact of Science on Society 30(2)93; cf. 'Only if we actively assimilate past experience – distilled in history, literature and art – and keep it alive in our own culture and educational system, shall we preserve for ourselves the wisdom necessary to make positive and judicious use of the world of modern technology as a means for achieving a genuinely human civilization,' l.c., 99; ibid. 1999 Educating and Sensitizing Health Professionals on Human Rights and Ethical Considerations: The Interactive Role of Ethics and Expertise, in: Intern J Bioethics 10(1-2)69-81.

[4] See Chapter 3.

gued that the master in a craft must be able to know to produce a tool, to use a tool, and to know the function of the tool within society. For all biotopes of worthwhile and successful learning, we can refer to the models of partner/partner or master/disciple rather than that of teacher/student. A good master will have a good apprentice; apprenticeship traditionally is the most favored and successful way of learning in all crafts, whether in building, painting, healing, or leading. Close, valued interpersonal relations have been reported between master and disciple in all cultures and disciplines. Partners and stakeholders communicate with each other to find better situational solutions for cooperation and to stabilize and even improve competency. Confucius gives us the full scale of didactic goals in education and training: (a) recognize and learn the fact and thus improve and enlarge your scientific and technical knowledge and expertise; (b) recognize and learn about your own values and thus strengthen your resolve, thereafter re-integrating your intellectual and moral powers anew; (c) this will result developing in your personal culture well and in educating and influencing your immediate biotope, such as your family; (d) only thereafter will you be truly successful in leadership positions locally and internationally, as everyone is called to bring peace and to cultivate the worlds of bios. Learning and leadership are not just for a few selected by family origin or by successful network building; they are for all! There are many ways to learn and grow.[5] In his drama *Dr. Faustus*, Goethe described two ways to learn: the way of Dr. Faustus, by studying books and philosophizing, and Gretchen's way, by means of pain, suffering, and guilt after Dr. Faustus had made her pregnant. Not caring for his former girlfriend in need, Dr. Faustus of course was not a learned man in the Confucian sense; he is not a good role model for learning successfully. Learning changes the person, not just his or her skills. We humans don't have mostly hard-wired biological properties such as microbes and other species do; therefore we have to train, to educate, and to cultivate them. And we don't learn for our teachers, as Seneca reminds us, but for ourselves. Only lifelong learning brings and keeps us in sync with the complex worlds of bios, which are both adaptable and integrating.

Below, I present a few instruments for situation-and-case based learning in interdisciplinary and social settings, integrating facts, values, and people. (1) A *Checklist*, which I have used in occupational, professional, social, and political assessment and for preparation and review of successful decision making in business. (2) a Medical-Ethical *Questionnaire*[6], developed together with Herbert

---

[5] Sass HM 1980 Education as an Indispensable Tool, in: Impact of Science on Society 30(2):93-99; ibid. 1986 Technische Risiken im Aspekt der Sozialpolitik, in: Technische Risiken in der Industriegesellschaft. Compes PC ed., Bonn: Gesellschaft fuer Sicherheitswissenschaft, 425-449; ibid. 1997 Moral Aspects of Risk and Innovation, in: Artificial Organs 21(11)1217-1221.

[6] The Bochum Questionnaire has been translated into many languages, for an English translation see Advance Directives and Surrogate Decision Making in Health Care 1998. Kimura

Viefhues for single-case medical-technical and medical-ethical decision making, which can be modified for other occupational and professional situations (3) a *Case-based Training Course* in Medical Ethics[7], originally developed for participants of the World Congress of Bioethics in Rijeka, (4) a model to *prepare for yet unknown situations*, i.e. educate individuals in preparation for executing Personal Advanced Directives, originally developed together with Rita Kielstein, which can be used in preparing for other yet unknown personal or professional situations, (5) finally a list of *narratives for theoretically unsolvable challenges*, which cannot find theoretical or academic solutions because of a genuine character that only the person in a *real-life decision making* situation can make[8].

12.2. Integrated Training for successful Decision Making

I have used the following general checklist successfully in different preparatory and strategic situations for risk assessment in technology, business, and everyday personal challenges. Traditional classical religious or philosophical reasoning and in ethics and political science was integrated whenever it seemed relevant, but they did not play the leading role. The checklist does not represent a classical utilitarian model either, as it takes values supported by individuals and groups as serious as facts of biology, technology, or business. Rather it follows Thomas Aquinas' advice *actiones humanae secundum circumstantias sunt bone vel male* – human actions are good or bad depending on the circumstances[9]. In certain situations, the virtue of compassion is most prominent, in others technical competence might be the prime imperative. While differential diagnosis in medicine collects and evaluates facts by different means of diagnosis, *differential ethics* follows the same model in collecting and evaluating values, visions and taboos and integrates those with the findings in medical diagnosis for an integrated action-driven strategy of optimizing success and minimizing failure or catastrophe[10].

R, Sass HM, Veatch R eds, John's Hopkins U Press; cf. Kielstein R, Sass HM 1993 Using Stories to assess Values and establish Medical Directives, in: Kennedy Institute of Ethics J 3:303-325

[7] See Borovecki A, Sass HM 2008 Upotreba Postupnika u Klinickoj Etici. The Use of Checklists in Clinical Ethics. Special Edition for the 9th World Congress in Bioethics of the International Association of Bioethics. Zagreb [Croatian and English language]; the English language version also in www.practical-ethics.de, a Spanish version Directivas Anticipdas. La Historia Clinica oriente a Valores. Kielstein R, Mainetti JA, Manzini JL, Roubicek M, Sass HM, Viefhues H eds., Muenster: Lit 2002.

[8] Cf Sass HM 2006 Bioethics and Biopolitics. Xian, chapter 4, Chinese/English

[9] Summa Theologiae 81,II,qu18.3

[10] Sass HM 2006 Differentialethik. Anwendungen in Medizin, Wirtschaft und Politik. Baumann E, Brink A, May AT eds, Berlin: Lit; Sass HM 1992 Ethische Risiken m wirtschaftlichen Risiko, in: Ethik und Wirtschaft. Lenk H ed., Stuttgart: Reclam 214-234; Sass HM 1987 Philosophical and Moral Aspects of Manipulation and Risk, in: Swiss Biotech 5(22a)50-56

The checklist method is superior to religious or ideological moralism, which has proven often and often to be unhealthy for individuals and communities and unsuccessful in establishing and stabilizing harmonious cultures and societies. In integrating technical and ethical risk assessment, such a checklist allows for identifying major individual and collective players and the strength and significance of their involvement in integrating ethics and expertise. I have used this method in academic teaching as well as in consulting in real-life risk assessment in business, politics, and in interdisciplinary academic and applied research. Such an analytical and evaluative method of differential ethics can be used in all kinds of technology assessment and application assessment, definitely also in family medicine and primary health care, in developing policy options for public policy, in scenario evaluation schemes in situations of professional activity, and in anticipatory assessment of new technology and of introducing new technology into business, social and cultural contexts. Ethical assessment is intertwined with technology assessment and situational challenges are given priority over the application of theories. Principles and rules supported by one or the other theory are used to develop different courses of possible action and the most suited one for the specific general scenario or individual case is selected competitively. Only when principles or virtues will contradict each other due to different worldviews or theories, then theories have to become involved and have to undergo a critical checkup by stakeholders and among stakeholders. The Confucian 'Doctrine of the Mean', a very early stakeholders model, puts emphasis on the need of stakeholders to be open to criticism and self-criticism, resulting in the self-cultivation of stakeholders and in best possible harmonious solutions and procedures.

Using the checklist in interdisciplinary or intercultural settings first of all develops *a mutually shared vocabulary and language*, also personal experience in arguing and respecting each other's positions, which makes it easier for everyone to change or to modify a position. *Ethics is neither to be confused with emotion nor with etiquette.* When new groups come tighter for the first time, is might be helpful to prepare future decisions and evaluation by discussing 'other people's' cases or scenarios first in order to develop a familiarity with each other's style of argumentation, personality and priorities. Important is also to anticipate in step four real cases and scenarios which do not fit well to the selected course of action.

MEDICAL AND MORAL RISK ASSESSMENT SCHEME

1. IDENTIFY DATA AND ISSUES
- *a. Collect technical data*
- *b. Collect significant human data*
- *c. Identify value elements*
- *d. Discuss relations between technical and moral issues*

2. DEVELOP ALTERNATIVE SCENARIOS FOR ACTION
- *a. Establish reasonable possibilities for each scenario*
- *b. Identify stakeholders*
- *c. Identify principles uncertainties*
- *d. Discuss ethical and technical risk and uncertainty*

3. PRESENT A SET OF ALTERNATIVE SCENARIOS
- *a. Discuss uncertainty in each scenario prognosis*
- *b. Assess technical and moral benefits and risks*
- *c. Discuss assessments with stakeholders*
- *d. Evaluate differences in benefit-risk balances*

4. FORMULATE A JUSTIFICATION FOR YOUR SELECTION
- *a. Specify your reasons for selected course of action*
- *b. Include stakeholders in reviewing decisions*
- *c. Understand ethical shortcomings of justification*
- *d. Anticipate and discuss objections to your selection*

12.3. Integrating Technology Assessment and Value Assessment

This virtual training course in personalized medicine and clinical ethics builds on a checklist, originally was developed and widely tested in clinical and family practice 1987 at the Bochum Center for Medical Ethics. That checklist also is known as the *Bochum Questionnaire* and available in Brazilian, Chinese, Croatian, Dutch, English, German, Italian, Spanish, Swedish, and Turkish language, also on the internet[11]. Checklists are used routinely in many fields of life.

[11] Sass HM, Viefhues H 1987 Bochumer Arbeitsbogen zur medizinethischen Praxis. Bochum: ZME; subsequent translations into Chinese (Qiu Renzong), Croatian (Ana Borovecki) Dutch (Henk ten Have), English (Stuart Spicker), Italian (Antonio Autiero) , Japanese (A-kio Sakai), Portuguese (Juan Batistiole), Spanish (Jose Alberto Mainetti), Turkish (Ilhan Ilkilic), and other languages; see www.ethik-in-der-praxis.de for the questionnaire and additional lists of questions for specific situations. – This soft-paternalism approach earned us criticism from US colleagues; they argued that we were too timid to honor the self-determination of the patient as a person when asking 'to what degree should the physician permit this patient to determine the treatment plan?'; but we got a warmer response from Asian colleagues for respecting values and wishes of patients and their families in clinical and other decision making.

In medicine, checklists are in use by family practitioners to collect basic medical and laboratory data of patients and to note details of prognosis, treatment and prescriptions, therapeutic or chronic improvement, by hospitals at time of admission and later to document clinical patient data, in research to document patient/subject's reaction. Checklists are useful for documentation and review; they also guarantee that a wide range of issues are known and considered rather than only a few with most intriguing and acute details. Checklists must be short, must allow for precise documentation, and eventually need to be complemented by special additional checklists such as working with a special type of client/patient, different lists documenting laboratory tests or sonograms or special ethical issues in different fields of service. The flowing checklist has been used since 1987, but colleagues have modified it and students have been encouraged to critically review this and other checklist.

Traditionally, checklists for patient's values and wishes were not necessary, because the family doctor knew his/her patients and their families very well, medical knowledge was only basic and options for different treatments were not available, and because physicians could assume that patients were representatives of a consistent moral and cultural environment having quite similar moral, religious, and cultural views and expectations from medicine and their doctors. When used in the global settings of clinical treatment and care checklists have to be open and may not predetermine the outcome of deliberations and decisions. Open checklists such as this one are helpful, when patients of different personal and cultural background are treated in Bangkok, Berlin, Buenos Aires, Bagdad, Beijing and elsewhere, where no uniform and robust value system can be assumed equally for all, as it was in the old days. Teaching of medical ethics to students and training in clinical ethics to teams and individuals will use cases to be as close to reality as possible, so does this training course.

'A. The Medical Status. Medical-Scientific Diagnosis of the Medical Status
The evaluation of the medical-scientific diagnosis follows traditional patterns. *General considerations:* What is the patient's diagnosis and prognosis? – What type of treatment is recommended regarding the diagnosis and prognosis? What alternative treatments could be offered? What are the anticipated outcomes of these various treatment options? – If the recommended treatment is neither offered to, nor accepted by, the patient, what is the prognosis? – *Special considerations:* Will the preferred medical treatment be helpful to the patient? – Will the treatment selected lead to a positive prognosis in the particular case? If it does, to what degree? – Could the selected treatment harm or injure the patient? To what degree? – How can benefits, harms, and risks be evaluated? – *Medical practice:* Are any other medical treatments equally adequate? – What consideration should be given to (1) the most recent medical advances due to biomedical research as well as (2) the physician's extensive clinical experience? What relevant facts are unknown or unavailable? Are the terms employed cor-

rectly, are they precise? – *Summary:* What is the optimal treatment after considering all the available scientific-medical knowledge?

Case: Medical Status: Mrs. A., 38 years old, overweight, employed as an office clerk, complains to her doctor about dizziness during the day and some sleeplessness at night. He diagnoses high blood pressure and recommends that she lose weight and start physical exercise. He does not take a careful medical history, including family history; otherwise he would have found that all four of her grandparents died in their 40s and 50s, probably of high blood pressure or a stroke or heart attack related to genetically inherited high blood pressure. If he had known the family history, he might have prescribed medicine in addition to physical exercise and a change in eating habits. – Questions: Do you use checklist forms to document first visits and routine checkups? Are you happy with the anamnesis forms you use? Did you or your colleagues experience similar omissions, and/or too quick recommendations, as in the case of Mrs. A.? Provide a few cases which demonstrate that careful information on the patient's medical status and history is essential for good treatment! Review the first section of the Bochum Checklist based on your experience! Do you have recommendations for improvement or modification of this list; do you already have your own list?

B. The Value Status. Medical-Ethical Diagnosis of the Value-and-Wish Status

The diagnosis of the value-and wish status of the patient follows three principles: *Health and well-being of the patient:* What harm or injury may arise as a result of selecting a specific method of treatment? – How might the treatment compromise the patient's well-being, cause extensive pain, or even shorten his/her life? – Might it cause physical or mental deterioration? – Might it produce fear or grave anxiety in the patient? – *Self-determination and the patient's autonomy:* What is known about the patient's values, wishes, fears and expectations? – What is the patient's understanding of intensive or palliative treatment, as well as resuscitation criteria? – Is the patient well-informed about diagnosis, prognosis, and the various treatment options available for him/her? – How is it possible to satisfy the patient's preferences in formulating the treatment plan? – To what degree should the physician permit this patient to determine the treatment plan? – Who else, if anyone, could or should make decisions on behalf of a patient and his/her best interests? Must the patient agree with the chosen therapy? – *Medical responsibility:* Have any conflicts surfaced between the physician, the patient, the staff, or the patient's family? – Is it possible to eliminate or resolve such conflicts by selecting a particular treatment option or plan? – How can one work to assure that the following values will be re-affirmed? – (1) Establishing mutual trust between patient and physician; (2) Honouring the principle of truth-telling in all discussions; and (3) Respecting the patient's privacy and protecting his/her confidentiality? – What relevant facts are unknown

or unavailable? – Have the salient ethical issues been adequately formulated, clarified, and addressed within the physician-patient relationship?
Summary: What kind of treatment is optimal given thorough attention to the salient and relevant clinical [medical]-ethical issues?

Case in Hospital Care: Mrs. M, 38 years-old, had her left breast removed 5 years ago because she had breast cancer. Now she has increasing pain in her lower back, and her physicians have determined that the cancer has metastasized to her bones. They recommend chemotherapy to reduce pain and to prevent or slow down the spread of cancer. Mrs. M. undergoes chemotherapy with uncomfortable side effects. Her pain increases and is not treated adequately. The physicians do not tell the 'full truth', that chemotherapy will not kill the cancer but might prolong her life. Mrs. M. dies in the hospital 8 months later, not as she had wished, at home. Without chemotherapy she might have died a few months earlier. - Questions: What did the physicians know about Mrs. M.'s wishes and values when making treatment decisions? How would you have incorporated your medical-ethical diagnosis in treatment decisions? Does the doctor have to treat the disease or the patient as a person? Is full and professional palliative care a basic right of each and every patient? Would you follow patients' Advance Directives or wishes based on their value-and-wish profile, even when that differs from your own? - Describe and discuss some cases which demonstrate that careful information on the patient's medical status and history is essential for good treatment! Review the second section of the Bochum Checklist based on your experience! Do you have recommendations for improvement or modification to this list; do you have your own list already?

C. Integrating Medical Status and Value Status
Treating the Patient as a Person.
Which options (alternative possible solutions) are available in the face of potential conflict between the medical-scientific and the medical-ethical aspects? – Which of the aforementioned scientific and ethical criteria are most affected by these alternative options? – Which options are most appropriate given the particular value profile of this patient? – Who, if anyone, should be consulted to serve as an advisor to the physician? – Is referral of the patient necessary for either medical or ethical reasons? – What are the moral (in contrast to the legal) obligations of the physician with regard to the chosen treatment? – What are the moral obligations of the patient, staff, family, health care institution and system? – What, if any, are the arguments for rejecting the selected treatment? – How would or should the physician respond to these arguments? – Does the treatment decision require achieving an ethical consensus? - Consensus by whom and with whom, and to which degree? – Why? – Was/Is the treatment decision adequately discussed with the patient? – Did he/she agree? – Should the decision process be reassessed and the decision actually revised? – *Summary:* What decision was

made after assessing the scientific and ethical aspects of the case? – How can the physician most accurately represent the medical-ethical issues and the process of evaluating the medical and ethical benefits, risks, and harms?

Case for Interactive Communication and Cooperation: Mr. C., 79 years-old and dependent on others. He seems to have lost all interest in life. At times he is confused and does not recognize others, even close family members or nurses. He has pain in his legs and can only walk short distances because of poor blood supply to his legs, which is caused by previous smoking. Blood vessel surgery might improve his mobility and reduce pain, also make nursing care easier, thus improving his quality of life. Mr. C. does not understand the issue and cannot make his preferences clear; he had not executed an Advance Directive when he was better off in earlier days. One of his sons and a daughter and the nurses favor surgery while his daughter is opposed. – Questions: Which of the 8 C virtues/principles of communication and cooperation, competence and competition, contemplation and calculation, compassion and cultivation need to be applied in this case and in what mixture? Please, develop your own checklist for this and similar cases? How would you want to be treated in this case? Rewrite this narrative o that it would fit your personal wish-and-value profile.

A Case of a Patient Refusing Treatment: Mr. D., a 44 years-old diabetes patient, has been blind for 4 years now. Two years ago, he became a patient in the neighborhood dialysis center. After first refusing dialysis treatment, he finally accepted it. A year ago, his right leg had to be amputated; he consented because he wanted to live long enough to witness the wedding of his daughter and the birth and baptism of his first grandchild, both of which he enjoyed very much. Now, lifesaving amputation of his left arm is mandated. He refuses the surgery and also dialysis treatment, stays at home, glides into a coma and dies, as he had wished, 10 days after his last dialysis treatment. – Questions: What would you do as a physician having the final word in the case of a patient with compromised competence to understand and/or to make decisions or to consent to treatment? How would you react in a complex situation to a patient refusing life-saving treatment? On what arguments – medical and/or non-medical – would you base your decision? How far would you take arguments from family members and/or from the nurses caring for him/her into account? Would you recognize an Advance Directive as authoritative if there had been one? Would you recognize someone, having a durable Health Care Power of Attorney as a partner in decision making or as the prime decision maker? Would you include other advisors such as priests or pastors of his/her religious belief, or friends of the patient into final treatment decisions, and how far? Under which circumstances would you refuse to treat the patient and rather refer the patient to a colleague or another institution? – Describe and discuss your own cases in which complex medical and moral decision making and complex institutional settings made it difficult to find a good patient-oriented solution! Review the de-

cision-making section of the Bochum Checklist based on your experience! Do you have recommendations for improvement or modification of this list; do you have your own list already?

Questions regarding Informed Consent and Decision Making: 1. Does this patient want treatment based on paternalistic or autonomous decision-making, or on partnership? – 2. Does the patient want to include the spouse or family members or someone else in making decisions or consenting? – 3. What are the special challenges for physician's practice and ethics to include others in decision making? – 4. What can/should be done to guarantee that each and every patient is treated according to her/his system of belief, independently, whether Christian or secular humanist, Taoist, Hindu, Confucian, Jewish or Muslim, and according to her/his value-and-wish profile?'

12.4. An Alternative Checklist in Health Care Ethics

The Bochum Checklist was developed 1986 for 20th century European family medicine and hospital treatment and then has found a place in medical-ethical teaching and in clinical medicine review and consultation elsewhere around the globe. The basic principles of competent and compassionate care, of communication and cooperation, and of on-going efforts to cultivate professional and personal lives, are similar in all cultures independent of religious or philosophical traditions and customs. But different cultures have their own values and principles which are more easily referred to than to imported principles. Michael Tai, a leading Chinese bioethicist has referred to the five classical virtues in Asian culture[12]: *Compassion* as a basic human virtue in all situations, *Righteousness* in doing things right and doing the right things, *Respect* for fellow humans in all social interactions, *Responsibility* in personal and professional actions, and *Ahimsa* as respect and reverence for life and non-violence. He recommends using the three classical Confucian parameters for applying values and virtues to concrete situations: Cheng, Li, and Fa. *Cheng* means that the action needs to be according to the situation, i.e. each and every instance of applied ethics needs to be situational ethics. *Li* means reasonableness and propriety and asks whether or not an action, to be considered to be taken or to be reviewed, was or is reasonable and appropriate and does not violate stabled norms and expectation in society. *Fa*, lawfulness, in all situations of decision-making or reviewing is a principle of last resort, against which actions – past, present or future – need to be checked, as in morally extreme situations, lawyers might have the final word. Tai has developed a Basic Checklist which could be used in Asian cultures in mixed committees of health care professionals; it represents an open checklist similar to the Bochum Questionnaire and calls for patient-oriented treatment and care: 1. Identify the issue. – 2. Speak with nurse

[12] Tai MC 2008 The Way of Asian Bioethics. Taiwan: Princeton Intern. Publ. Co., p. 122-125.

and family if request comes from physician or vice versa. – 3. See the patient and allow the patient to speak without interruption. – 4. Ask open-ended question. – 5. Talk with the physician. – 6. Prepare an ethical analysis. – 7. Provide recommendations. – *Questions*: Do you think that this checklist can or should only be used in Asian countries? Use this checklist in your own institution or in clinical ethics consultation, whether in Asia or elsewhere, as an exercise in clinical practice. Apply this checklist to cases you have encountered in your professional life or have dealt with in consultation; will the outcome be different to using other questionnaires? Review other cases of cross-cultural conflict, including your own and those already discussed! Discuss the following cases using either checklist or your own.

In a Singapore hospital a Hindu woman of 35 weeks' pregnancy requests an elective Caesarian section so that birth will occur on a good auspicious and lucky day in the Hindu calendar. There were no medical complications with this pregnancy and the hospital had great experience with premature babies born at 35 weeks gestation; so they followed the woman's autonomous request. Unfortunately, the child developed severe respiratory distress which resulted in costly and distressful intensive respiratory care. Both, the parents and the pediatric team, regretted the decision later. [reported by Roy Joseph MD, Singapore]

A Muslim couple needed emergency surgery because of an impending rupture of the uterus requiring urgent cesarean section. The couple however requested that the intervention be performed by female staff only including the person pushing the trolley in and out of the operating room. During lengthy counseling the husband stuck very strongly to their demand, while the woman did not say anything but seem to be supportive of her husband's demands. The hospital did not want to bow down to the request and made contacts to send them to a private hospital. At that other hospital the intervention finally was performed by an all-female team under the leadership of a junior obstetric trainee; fortunately, the intervention was successful and mother and baby survived [reported by Joseph][13]*. Questions: Which of the hospitals made the correct decision? How should you or your team have decided? Think about similar situations in your field of professional responsibility; present and discuss facts and conflicting values!*

An 80-year old man suffered from cerebral hemorrhage and his Glasgow Coma Scale was down to 3. Previously he had clearly stated that in such cases without full recovery he would wish to pass on peacefully. The family in this case and his 73-year old widow nevertheless requested medical treatment and the old man was kept alive for the 'sake of his family' [reported by Michael Cheng-tek Tai PhD, Taiwan].

---

[13] Joseph R 2011 A Clinical View of Western and Eastern Principles in Global Bioethics, in: Asian Bioethics Review 3(1)3-13

A Taiwanese medical scientist had collected tissue from volunteers in an aboriginal village with consent of those involved. But the leaders of the community requested that the samples be destroyed because any research benefiting the community must be approved by the community and not only by individual volunteers [reported by Tai]. – Questions and suggestions: What are your experiences with personal, religious or cultural disagreements in the hospital setting? How were they resolved? Where you happy with the solution found? What would be major issues in your local setting? Discuss the interactive relation between universal values and specific cultural traditions.

A 4 years-old girl remained in a coma three weeks after brain surgery for a very severe traumatic hemorrhage. Since she was refused treatment by a well-equipped Taipei City Municipal Hospital she was transferred to a smaller hospital 100 miles south of Taipei where she was operated upon; public opinion was most sympathetic to her and supportive to apply all efforts to rescue her. When a brain death was declared, her parents refused to give up and demanded continuous treatment. Because of the pressure from the public, the health team continued treating her and promised that they would try their best to keep her alive hoping for a miracle [reported by Tai]. – Questions related to this case: What is autonomy in pediatric care? Who should the prime decision maker be? Should the decision be based only on individual or family wishes? How far should family wishes be taken into account with medical and nursing decisions? When health professionals know that the patient is still treatable, yet the family or the patient decides to forgo treatment, should health professionals go along and respect family's or patient's autonomy? When treatment is futile according to physician's knowledge and experience yet the patient or his surrogate insists upon continuing treatment, should patient's autonomy be respected? What role do cultural differences play in caring for others, such as young children or demented adults? – Test and develop other checklists such as those proposed by Tai, using 'compassion, righteousness, respect, responsibility, do not harm (a-himsa)' or other principles and virtues as landmark principles.

12.5. Preparing for yet Unknown Situations

There are two sets of situations for which advance reflection and pre-emptive training in decision making is essential for success. Case studies and interactive role playing have been used for routine business training and for in various emergency preparedness situations politics and public health. I use the two scenarios to explain the role of advance planning: (a) preparing a personal Advance Directive, and (b) group preparation for unexpected future emergencies.

(a) Preparing for a personal Advance Directive. Case studies discuss the role of individual experts and of groups in integrating special expertise in collective responsibility and success, but they also may prepare individuals to become familiar with situations they had not been exposed to before[14]. We have used stories in association with a checklist to help lay people who have not much or limited or extreme experiences with end-of-life decisions before establishing an Advance Directive for themselves[15]. Issues include the naming of a surrogate decision maker, full or partial or no detailed information about the disease and its most likely course, and refusal of treatment which may considered futile or uncomfortable. Here are three narratives out of seven, which we have used to familiarize citizens with situations before they execute an Advance Directives: 'Who shall decide? *Mr. C., 79 years-old and dependent on others. He seems to have lost all interest in life. At times he is confused and does not recognize others, even close family members or nurses. He has pain in his legs and can only walk short distances because of poor blood supply to his legs, which is caused by previous smoking. Blood vessel surgery might improve his mobility and reduce pain, also make nursing care easier, thus improving his quality of life. Mr. C. does not understand the issue and cannot make his preferences clear; he had not executed an Advance Directive when he was better off in earlier days. One of his sons and a daughter and the nurses favor surgery while his daughter is opposed. – (1) If you would be in a similar situation as Mr. B. unable to make decisions for yourself, who should decide on your behalf, the doctor, which one of your children or all together, your partner or who else; who should not be burdened with such a decision? (2) I someone previously has voiced opinions about the acceptance or refusal of certain interventions, should physicians and family feel bound to such suggestions? (3) If you would be in Mr. B.'s situation which decision would you make? (4) Rewrite the story of Mr. B. based on your visions, values and expectations. –*

Cancer and truth telling: *Mrs. M, 38 years-old, had her left breast removed 5 years ago because she had breast cancer. Now she has increasing pain in her lower back, and her physicians have determined that the cancer has metastasized to her bones. They recommend chemotherapy to reduce pain and to prevent or slow down the spread of cancer. Mrs. M. undergoes chemotherapy with uncomfortable side effects. Her pain increases and is not treated adequately. The physicians do not tell the 'full truth', that chemotherapy will not kill the cancer*

[14] For different approaches in medical and clinical ethics training, see Drane J 1998 Decision-making in Clinical Ethics, in: Consensus Formation in Healthcare Ethics, Ten Have H and Sass HM eds, Dordrecht: Kluwer, 143-157.

[15] Kielstein R, Sass HM 1993 Using Stories to assess Values and establish Medical Directives, in: Kennedy Institute of Ethics J 3:303-325; Sass HM 1998 Appendix, in: Advance Directives and Surrogate Decision Making. Baltimore: Johns Hopkins U Press, 224-278; original German version Kielstein R, Sass HM 2001 Die persönliche Patientenverfuegung. Ein Arbeitsbuch zur Vorbereitung mit Bausteinen und Modellen. Münster: Lit, 2nd ed.; Spanish version Kielstein , Mainetti JA, Manzini JL, Roubicek M, Sass HM, Viefhues H 2002 Directivas Anticipadas. La Historia clinica orientada a Valores. Muenster: Lit.; an English version in Kimura R, Sass HM, Veatch RM 1998 Advance Directives and Surrogate Decision Making. Baltimore: Johns Hopkins Press, 269f

but might prolong her life. Mrs. M. dies in the hospital 8 months later, not as she had wished, at home. Without chemotherapy she might have died a few months earlier. – (1) Would you want that physicians always fully inform you about your diagnosis and also if successful therapy will not be possible? (2) Would you accept full treatment of pain, also when such palliative care might compromise your alertness? (3) Would you accept a treatment which would reduce your pain and suffering and only prolong your life for a limited time? (4) Rewrite the story of Mrs. M. based on your visions, values and expectations! – 'Refusing medical treatment: *Mr. D., a 44 years-old diabetes patient, has been blind for 4 years now. Two years ago, he became a patient in the neighborhood dialysis center. After first refusing dialysis treatment, he finally accepted it. A year ago, his right leg had to be amputated; he consented because he wanted to live long enough to witness the wedding of his daughter and the birth and baptism of his first grandchild, both of which he enjoyed very much. Now, lifesaving amputation of his left arm is mandated. He refuses the surgery and also dialysis treatment, stays at home, glides into a coma and dies, as he had wished, 10 days after his last dialysis treatment. – (1) How would you have decided? (2) Do you think that you would get used to the progression of disease and suffering, as many fellow humans do; which impairments would you not accept? (3) Would you want to accept pain and suffering in anticipation of a special event? (4) Rewrite the story of Mr. D. based on your visions, values and expectations!'* The option to rewrite a story puts the reader closer to the issue and allows for a very personal response without discussing feelings, wishes and expectations in abstract terms.

Only after confronting the readers with those seven narratives, we gave them the following questionnaire to evaluate their actual and potentially future response to a serious of statements, which would help him/her in executing a personal Advance Directive. Actually such a questionnaire already could in the absence of an Advance Directive, to allow caretakers to interpret those responses as guides for certain interventions and omissions[16]: *'I want to be treated as a respected person. The visions, values, and beliefs that have formed my attitudes, preferences, and wishes as well as my personal understanding of the quality an meaning of life are to be respected by those who will care for me in situations in which I will be unable to communicate my preferences and directives ... Being aware of the risk of expressing preferences for future situations, I have tried to document how my self-determination for future situations could vary from preferences for actual situations.*

PRESENT SELF-EVALUATION: 1. Very important; 2. Important; 3. Not important; 4. I cannot decide; 5. No –

[16] Kimura R, Sass HM, Veatch RM 1998 Advance Directives and Surrogate Decision Making. Baltimore: Johns Hopkins Press, p 269f

FUTURE SELF-EVALUATION: A. very important; B. important; C. depending on the situation; 4. I cannot decide; E. no.

1. I want to live as long as possible	
- if I am in good health	*1,2,3,4,5 – A,B,C,D,E*
- if I am ill but recovery is expected	*1,2,3,4,5 – A,B,C,D,E*
- if I am permanently unconscious	*1,2,3,4,5 – A,B,C,D,E*
- if I am mentally incompetent	*1,2,3,4,5 – A,B,C,D,E*
- if I am terminally ill	*1,2,3,4,5 – A,B,C,D,E*
2. I want to be without pain	
- even if clear thinking is compromised	*1,2,3,4,5 – A,B,C,D,E*
- even if I become drowsy or sleepy	*1,2,3,4,5 – A,B,C,D,E*
3. When time has come, I prefer to die	
- at home	*1,2,3,4,5 – A,B,C,D,E*
- in the hospital	*1,2,3,4,5 – A,B,C,D,E*
- with loving people around	*1,2,3,4,5 – A,B,C,D,E*
- being left alone	*1,2,3,4,5 – A,B,C,D,E*
4. I want a comfortable dying process	
- even at the cost of heavy sedation	*1,2,3,4,5 – A,B,C,D,E*
- even if it means 'active euthanasia'	*1,2,3,4,5 – A,B,C,D,E*
5. If my prognosis is terminal	
- I want full disclosure	*1,2,3,4,5 – A,B,C,D,E*
- my proxy must be told	*1,2,3,4,5 – A,B,C,D,E*
- my family must be told	*1,2,3,4,5 – A,B,C,D,E*
- my family physician must be told	*1,2,3,4,5 – A,B,C,D,E*
- ……… must be told	*1,2,3,4,5 – A,B,C,D,E*
6. I do not want to be a burden	
- to my family	*1,2,3,4,5 – A,B,C,D,E*
- to the financial resources of my family	*1,2,3,4,5 – A,B,C,D,E*
- to health care professionals	*1,2,3,4,5 – A,B,C,D,E*
- to society	*1,2,3,4,5 – A,B,C,D,E*
7. I want my values govern my treatment	*1,2,3,4,5 – A,B,C,D,E*

***(b) Group Preparation for Unexpected Future Emergencies**:* Using narratives of other people in preparation for yet unexperienced personal situations can also be applied in preparing for extreme situations of public emergency. I have used the following scenario of emergency planning in meetings of hospital leadership and public officials for epidemic preparedness planning. We discussed various initiatives by different agencies and plans for coordination and raising public awareness. During the meeting I had someone come in with a handwritten message that major parts of the province were without electricity because workers had not shown up for work due to being infected or just being afraid to become infected. We had already assumed that a number of doctor's offices, of supermarkets and drug stores had not opened and that the supply line because of similar man power problems. I did not provide any leading questions, but immediately due to the (fabricated) story the awareness level was raised and other 'not expected' issues came up, including suggestions for localization and decentralization of intervention, closing of facilities including hospitals to protect those inside from infection, also issues of how to handle civil unrest and a breakdown of public services and powers including communication in a scenario without digital networks. Without the made-up story about the loss of electricity and subsequently of most digital networks, the meeting would not have been as serious as it finally was. It turned out that in similar situations of severely limited public powers, to sequester and preferentially protect certain groups such as emergency personnel and institutions alike hospital and nursing homes can become a priority over 'equal rights for all'.

12.6. Conflicts unsolvable in Training and Discourse

Finally, some 'hard case' situations are discussed in the bioethics literature that unfortunately occur again and again in real-life. But they cannot be solved or adequately prepared for in academic or professional discourse taking place outside of the 'real situation.' I mention just four: (1) Investigational torture of terrorists to gain information that could save hundreds, thousands, or millions from attack and death; (2) killing fellow humans out of compassion and mercy; (3) saving the life of an enemy in situations of limited resources; and (4) knowing that a government is lying to start a war.

Investigational torture: *A person is captured who very likely has information on the whereabouts of other members of his superiors and team, as well as on plans for an immediate attack on a large number of people. The captors ask you to assist and consult as a medical expert in torture as a means of last resort to save many innocent people who are in immediate danger His mother, wife, and 4-year-old child have also been captured. Would you torture the terrorist to get life-saving information? Would you preserve him and establish an audiovisual link to another room or bring him directly to the place where his family members are being tortured one by one? What else would/could you do? Would you assist in either one of these scenarios to extract the names of superiors and locations or only in the perceived immediate danger of a large number of innocent people being killed?* Possible benefits are evident, including saving many innocent people, establishing a disincentive for potential criminals, and the possible capture of other criminals. One of the prime ethical principles in all cultures of medical ethics is 'do no harm.' Torture harms people tremendously, and they may say anything to have it stopped, even if they lack the information the torturer wants. Yet if severe harm or even death to thousands of people can be prevented, would that be a higher principle in extraordinary situations? Would it justify all means, including severe harm and pain to one individual? An Israeli court justified interrogative torture in extreme situations of necessity.[17] In 1982 and again in 2004, the World Health Organization passed a resolution that 'medical ethics during armed conflict are identical to those in peacetime'[18] (i.e., no extraordinary rules are allowed). The moral options are as follows: treating one potentially criminal person according to civilized ethics and accepting the potential or real death of a great number of people, or possibly saving a great number of people by violating moral norms for normal times. This is an 'unsolvable' issue for the academic classroom and for interdisciplinary discourse, not to mention for the person who has to make such a decision in a crucial situation.

Mercy killing: *After a car accident, a triage situation develops, and the most severely hurt cannot be treated. They scream in agony, and some ask to be killed. They and everyone else know that they cannot be saved and that all of them will die a painful death. Would you kill those who plead to be killed? Would you also kill the others who are in similar agony but can only scream or can't even scream anymore?* Situations like this have been reported from battlefields where wounded soldiers were screaming between enemy lines with no hope of rescue. In some cases their soldier friends shot them; in others they listened to the screams of their comrades for hours. Mercy killing does not occur in warlike situations only; it is an everyday issue in treating terminal patients who are suffering. Professional codes of conduct in medicine vehemently refuse the active killing of a fellow human as being contrary to the obligations of physicians and to the rules of ethics and nature. Situations arise, however, in which compassionate health care professionals and family members resort to killing patients or loved ones out of mercy and compassion. The bioethics literature discusses those normative issues under the term *euthanasia*.

Special health care for an enemy: *United States Special Forces capture a combatant in Eastern Afghanistan, only to find out that he needs dialysis treatment. The prisoner refuses, saying he would rather be dead than be debriefed and in the hands of the enemy. Doctors are reluctant to treat him without informed consent. Two days later, the U.S. Secretary of Defense orders dialysis, arguing that the prisoner is a high-level operator and certainly has valuable information on other terrorists and on planned attacks. What would you have done?*[19] The Geneva Convention on treating prisoners of war requires equal and fair treatment to all, prohibits medical experiments on prisoners if they are against the prisoner's interests, and requests informed consent. But this captive

[17] Los Angeles Times, June 13, 2004.

[18] Moreno J ed. 2003 In the Wake of Terror. Medicine and Morality in a Time of Crisis. Cambridge MIT Press.

[19] Zupan D, Solis G, Schoonhoven R 2004 Dialysis for Prisoner of War, in: Hastings Center Report 34(6): 11-22, with comment by George Annas, p. 12; Gross M 2004 Bioethics and Armed Conflict, in: Hasting Center Report 34(6)22-30; WHO 1983 Regulations in Time of War and Armed Conflict. Venice (Italy), Oct 19838;1;5.

seems to be of high military value, so the military leadership decides to keep him alive against his will.

A government deceiving their citizens and public opinion: *A government suddenly starts an aggressive war against other country under the pretext it has chemical and nuclear weapons and intends to use those soon on one or more other states. You have reliable information and documentation indicating that the government is lying. What can/will you do?*

There are more than these four cases to which an answer is not easily found and in regard to which bioethicists, health care professionals, public officials, and each one of us might have different opinions. Research literature in bioethics documents and reflects these different opinions. Hard cases can rarely be solved in the classroom and should not be solved there by instructional recipes such as in a cookbook or for standard treatment in medical care. But in classroom teaching and discussion, good arguments can be proven and checked for different moral options. When it comes to real-life decisions, cases of a very personal matter exist in which ethical and medical analysis is not enough of a basis on which to make decisions or to criticize them.

The moral agent who should make those decisions is the *person in the actual situation* deciding on the basis of *situational ethics*, taking moral principles and special situational factors into account. Only an actual situation, with its combination of expertise and ethics, can be the final test for professional, compassionate behavior based in personal responsibility. Decisions may be right or wrong; one might regret making a certain decision at a later date. One might regret refusing to be involved in interrogational torture because it later became evident that 1,000 lives could have been saved. But the memory of torturing a fellow human being will be with the torturer for the rest of his or her life. In such cases of extreme challenges in situational ethics, the criteria for justifying extraordinary means, such as those in a just as compared to an unjustified war, can and must also be applied. Classroom teaching and academic discourse go only so far in describing the challenges and underlining the rules developed over time that express the civilized and moral behavior of not torturing, killing, or treating someone against their will. The person in the situation of making tough decisions between life and death, potentially saving a high number of lives, relieving fellow humans from severe pain and misery, and saving life against the will of the refuser, will often be alone in that decision. He or she may be educated and better prepared for such decisions by knowing the normal rules and the literature, and by having been involved in academic discussions about those exceptional moral situations and challenges.

In the European tradition, Machiavelli[20] praises immoral behavior by the ruler for the benefit of protecting the land and the community. Jewish tradition reported with applause that Judith volunteered to have sex with Assyrian king and

[20] Machiavelli N 1532 Il Principe.

occupying general Holofernes, subsequently cutting off his head when he was drunk.[21] The Lao Zi differentiates between war and peace: 'You rule the land with justice, you fight a war with surprise, you win a country with effortless action.'[22] Would 'surprise' include the violation of normal rules and values, and would the purpose of the war as a 'just war' be relevant? But who would define a war as 'just' and from which perspective? Sun Zi[23] calls the 'Art of War of vital importance for the State' and requests that the commander have the 'virtues of wisdom, sincerity, benevolence, courage, and strictness.' Does 'courage' supported by wisdom and the other virtues include torture and other violations of human and civil rights? How would you define 'extraordinary emergency'? How could/should responsible citizens and/or the legal or political establishment of a nation or of the international community react to 'good intention' resulting in violations of human and civil rights, in killing, torture, and lying?

A CASE OF PROFESSIONALLY UNSUCCESSFUL SERVICE

Mr. T., 28 years-old, married Turkish patient of a German doctor in Germany suffers from low sperm count. The couple wants to have children. The doctor prescribes a mild prescription drug based on pig pancreas and explains to the patient that stronger medicines would be available if this one does not work. A week later the young Turk storms into the doctor's office, throwing the pills at the doctor and shouting 'You are a pig. Who does give a man pills from pig to make son. Doctor, you are a pig![24]' This doctor's treatment was unsuccessful, because the patient refused to take the adequate medicine for religious reasons. It is widely accepted in Jewish and Muslim traditions that the body is a gift from God, which we are charged to take good care of. Specific rules may be overrun if life is at stake, such as saving a cat from being drowned on a holy day or drinking and eating during Ramadan fasting, which definitely would include taking pills during Ramadan days and using prescriptions. Only the most extreme religious fractions would confuse pills containing pig pancreas with a delicious pork roast. - Is it always responsible to start with the least invasive therapy even when non-medical factors such as culture or religion or even unacceptable and crazy ideas would suggest otherwise? Would you have explained to the patient that eating pork and using medicine based on pig tissue by many Muslim (and Jewish) scholars has been defined as to be different and that in Muslim ethics

---

[21] Book of Judith, now in the Roman Catholic and Orthodox bibles only, not in the Protestant ones anymore; cf. Nelson M ed. 1991 Judith, Juliana, and Elene: Three Fighting Saints. New York: Lang.

[22] Dao Te Ching 57.

[23] Sun Zi (2012) The Art of War. Zhonghua Book Company: Classical Pocket Book Series of China: 'Sun Zi said: the Art of War is of vital importance to the State. It is matter of life and death, a road either to safety or ruin. Hence it is a subject of inquiry which can on no account be neglected.'

[24] Reported by Ilhan Ilkilic MD PhD

and medical ethics the protection of life supersedes other religious laws such as fasting? Would you in such a situation direct her/him to see another doctor or not? – Do you know cases from your own field of professional expertise where discussing values and ethics with the customer/provider/client would be good and healthy for successful business and the promotion of harmony and solidarity in society?

V. BIOPOLITICS AND COLLECTIVE BIOS

13. Companies and Corporations are Living Beings

CORPORATIONS ARE COMPLEX ADAPTABLE SYSTEMS OF BIOS

'Complex adaptive systems are often nested in broader systems. A population is a CAS [complex adaptive system] nested in a naturel ecosystem, which in itself is nested in the broader biological environment. A company is a CAS nested in a business ecosystem, which is nested in the broad societal environment. Complexity therefore exists at multiple levels, not just within the organizational boundaries; and at each level there is tension between what is good for an individual agent and what is good for the larger system.'[1]

13.1. Corporate Bios in integrated Biotopes

A *company* is formed by *companions,* who may be individuals, groups or other living beings and who share mutual interests and common goals; companies may or may not be registered in various legal forms in various districts. *Corporations* have a *corpus*, but the legal corpus of an incorporated company does not fully represent the whole corporations such as a skeleton does not represent a living human person. There are more non-vertebra forms of bios which do not have a skeleton such as we have. *Associations* are formed by associates for various purposes and thus share common visions and goals. Companies, corporations, and other forms of associations have different life plans and visions: to make profit, to provide charity, play a role in culture, politics, and society. Corporations, companies and other collective persons have diverse bodies, depending on legal liability, taxation, and purpose, and they have their specific *corporate biotope* and ecosystem. Some have a local neighborhood base, while others are also or only based in cyberspace. Some are vertically in tegrated as the big companies in early 20th century were and Apple and Tesla today; others concentrate on what they do best and outsource everything else[2]. Even today companies own other businesses which do not belong to their core expertise; cruise companies have bought Caribbean islands, Ikea, a Swedish furniture company, bought over 100.000 acres of woodland to secure wood supply, and General Motors and other big companies own their own financial businesses. Either way, companies such as individuals need to have and cultivate stable and secure environments and networks for their prospering and survival. Companies, like other species in the worlds of bios, can be understood as *complex and adaptive forms of living bios* in interaction and exchange with other individual and collective living beings in their specific territory, shaping their territory and being shaped by it as well. I use the term *corporation* in a general way as being synonymous with partnership, association, enterprise, organiza-

---

[1] Reeves M, Levin S, Ueda D 2016 The Biology of Corporate Survival. Natural Ecosystems hold surprising Lessons for Business, in: Harvard Business Review (Jan/Febr) 49.

[2] Peters T 2003 Re-Imagine. Business Excellence in a Disruptive Age. London: DK

tion, conglomerate and company, all of which constitute a *corpus, body* in one way or another, but all are different from each other at the same time.

From microbial integrated territories and biotopes to smaller and larger ecosystems of rainforests, multiple different human clans and communities, stock markets, companies and corporations, to the adaptive mechanisms of the seasons and the universe, – all these different shapes and shades of bios are interacting, modifying and surviving with more or less harmony and more or less success in cooperation and competition within their specific geographic and cyberspace rooms. *Robustness and survivability* of all of these different forms of bios are different, species-specific and depending on individual properties as well. Businesses, charities, associations, companies, corporations are part of this great and sometimes decreasing and sometimes expanding integrated world of bios. As individual bios, they must expect a limited lifespan, struggle for life and success, being ready for adaptation and modification. Reeves and others[3] suggest that business leaders look beyond the smaller world of their own into the interacting benefits and risk for their own survival; they describe the broader environment for corporate bios. For business, as for all other species of integrated CAS's, the rules of survival, interaction and happiness are the same: for a symphony orchestra, a law form, a supermarket, a restaurant, a hotel, a religious association or church, a website, a conglomerate. Company survival and good social interaction is essential for the corporate bios as it is for individual people, for colonies of ants and bees, and for all other biotopes, none of which is non-complex, all of which depend on robustness and connectedness. Good calculation based on well done contemplation of business options may lead to innovations which will increase life expectancy of the corporation in a changing biotope; Verganti gives this advice[4] in regard to provider-customer interaction: 'Identify fundamental changes in society and technology that might alter what customers will value. Then develop a new direction your company could take. To create this screen for assuming ideas, employ an inside-out process that relies on the art of criticism, not ideation.'

A successful stable emotional culture is also important for sustainability of a robust internal structure and of successful recognition and appreciation within the corporate biotope[5]. Different to ants and bees, human biological properties are not as hard wired and need to be trained and cultivated for human-specific complex adaptation and mutual success; but similar to ants and bees we need stable and robust ecosystems for individual and collective life. Important as competence and competition are for individual and corporate success, emotional communication and cooperation are the glue which keeps people together inside

[3] Reeves et al. 2016, l.c.

[4] Verganti R 2016 The innovative Power of Criticism: Judgment, not Ideation is the Key to Breakthroughs, in: Harvard Business Review 2016 (Jan/Febr) 91.

[5] Russel Hochschild A 2012 (first edition 1983) The Managed Heart. Commercialization of Human Feeling. Berkeley: U California Press.

and outside the company. Barade and O'Neill argue: 'Decades of research demonstrate the importance of organizational culture, yet most of it has focused on the cognitive component … Organizations also have an emotional pulse and managers must track it closely to motivate their teams and reach their goals. Emotional culture is shaped by how all employees – from the highest echelons to the front lines – comport themselves day in and day out. But it is up to senior leaders to establish which emotions will help the organization thrive, model these emotions, and reward others for doing the same. Companies in which they do this have a lot to gain'[6].

13.2. The many Faces and Personalities of Corporate Bios

Corporate and partnership bios has many faces and personalities, just as individual people and other living being. They have body parts and organs which will have to work well together in order to be successful and to have a long and good life. They are integrated and interacting with their respective environment, with partners, friends, competitors, foes. They have to struggle for life, be competitive and competent in what they do. They age and rejuvenate; they can become weak and sick; they can die or live a long and healthy life. They as individual people are good or bad neighbours, are loved or hated or ignored. They are a part of ecosystems and neighbourhoods in smaller or larger geographical surroundings and also exist in professional, personal, cultural and political communities in geographical and in cyberspace based ecosystems. They share biotopes and fields of interaction with individuals, other companies and association and other natural, cultural and social biotopes. In everyday life, we speak of *the corporate person, the corporate profile, the corporate mission, the corporate ethics, the corporate culture, corporate recognition, the corporate climate, the corporate market, the corporate market player.*

Similar to individuals, corporations and other collective persons need to be viable and depend on recognition and on cooperation and competition in their specific ecosytem; they need nutrition and profits, recognition as well as a valuable and hopefully also somewhat indispensable corporate person. They have to take care of their health, their internal metabolism and their muscle powers and brain powers, their partnerships and friendships, their own dynamics and the dynamics of their environments in geography and cyberspace. They need to be prepared for potential disasters, such as every one of us, and for sudden changes in their respective biotopes. As all other living beings they have to cultivate their skills to adapt flexibly to changing biotopes or migrate into other territories. We use the case of a health care provider to demonstrate the many interactions a

---

[6] Basarde S, O'Neill O 2016 Manage your emotional Culture, in: Harvard Business Review. Febr. 2016, 58-66: 'Every organization has an emotional culture, even if it's one of suppression', 63.

company or a corporate person can and must develop to become a valued and indispensable good neighbour with good survival and good reputation.

Similar to individual persons, corporate persons have an inner life and a life in interaction with others. Some corporations, such as those formed by individual lawyers or law firms or landlords, just wear protective armour akin to that of a mediaeval knight, but that outside body does not represent the person and the mission. Churches and other spiritual communities have an outside skin which might include real property, bank accounts and legal frames and skeletons, but the true personality is not in those external parts, rather in the spirituality and mission of the religious community and brotherhood/sisterhood. Charitable bodies such as the Red Cross, the Rotary Club, the Lions Club, and the Salvation Army represent their personality, competence and compassion in their deeds, while at the same time enjoy and cultivate internal networks and friendship among their individual members. Just as individual people, corporate persons have to make good use of the eight C's in order to live successfully and happy and to be well integrated in their respective biotope.

Similar to individuals, corporations may *choose between good and bad, between me and us, between me and the others, between short-term and long-term success*, between exploitation and domination on one side and long-term survival, mutual aid and benefit and cooperation on the other. Mafiosi clans operate similar to corporate bodies. Well respected companies exploit trust and good corporate profile for immoral deeds: for a number of years Volkswagen AG knowingly produced software to deceive public inspectors in emission tests, betraying customers and oversight bodies, and hurting the environment. Bernie Madoff[7] and his New York Investment Company stole billions of dollars from trusting clients and friends in a Ponzi scheme, mostly likely with knowledge or help of major banks, using his and his firm's prestige among his Jewish friends and in rich circles. Transplantation centres were involved in falsifying documents to give patients waiting for organ transplantation a preferred place in the waiting list. A nurse deliberately hurt a patient in order to prove his skills in reanimation; other hospital employees killed patients which became too burdensome. Banks use their insight in trading and markets to 'front-running' or other unfair tactics to enrich themselves, and if they are considered to be 'too big to fail', governments will bail them out without anyone going to jail or banks going into bankruptcy. Vacation websites and other companies advertising on the web give incomplete or totally wrong information in order to attract customers; apothecaries advertising on the web might deliver wrong, or inefficacious or dangerous medicines. This list includes only a few examples and could be extended much longer any time.

Recent comparative research on common challenges and properties of individual and collective biological and corporate bios has identified diversity and

[7] The Huffington Post 07-29-2016 (Reuters 02-20-2014; Investing Answers 12-06-2011).

complexity of self-interested bodies, interaction with other agents, and competitive selection processes as the prime powers making *complex adaptable systems* (CAS's) successful and robust survivors in healthy ecosystems and biotopes[8]. *Heterogeneity* and diversity among people, ideas, innovations and endeavours are essential properties for survival in biological and corporate life; but changes in the ecosystem or in the biological or corporate body may render the business model obsolete. *Modularity* within the body breaks down barriers and allows for the exchange of communication and cooperation within the body; but shocks in one part may travel to other parts and result in risk of contagion. Similar to buffering shock absorbers, *redundancy* duplicates the robustness of the body, which still will be exposed to uncontrollable outside risks of natural or political disasters such as terrorism. On the managerial level, CAS's require *reduction of uncertainty* by developing early detection signals and patterns of change, in particular changes in technologies or markets. Also, the development and care for *feedback loops and adaptive mechanisms* from across the corporation will be helpful, inside the corporation but also in interactive involvement with the ecosystem.

Finally, *trust and reciprocity* must be cultured through the corporation and within its ecosystem, and this requirement can be generalized to society and all biotopes as CAS's: 'In society, complex adaptive systems require cooperation in order to be robust; direct control of system participants is rarely possible. Individual interests often conflict, and when individuals pursue their own selfish interests, the system overall becomes weaker and everyone suffers. This is the quandary of the so-called collective action problems: individuals lack incentives to act in ways that benefit the overall system unless they benefit in immediate ways themselves. Trust and the enforcement of reciprocity combine to provide a mechanism for organizations to overcome this quandary'[9]. Those properties mentioned by Reeves, Levin and Ueda can easily be integrated in our own 8 C model to understand and to support happy and healthy living bios and biotopes of all sorts. Below, I use the clinic as one type of a corporate person among other health care organizations and within the social geographical ecosystem to discuss some specifics of ethics of corporate bios.

13.3. Clinics and Health Care Institutions as Living Beings

Clinics are as different from each other as individual persons and collective or corporate persons are; some provide highly specialized research and treatment of rare diseases, others are specialized in the broadest range possible as a general hospital; others care to the elderly and citizens with dementia, other concentrate on all or very special forms of cancer. The more specialized clinics

[8] Reeves at al., 2016 l.c.; Levin S 1999 Fragile Dominion, Complexity and the Commons. Cambridge: Perseus.

[9] Reeves et al., 2016: 55.

probably provide their information and service as well in cyberspace to make the best use of their expertise.

Clinics that provide a wide range of services also will be able to become global leaders in all these fields by providing easy to understand health education, information and advice in simple issues in lifestyle improvement and modification, physical exercise and nutrition, or everyday health risks such as diarrhoea, constipation, running nose, sour throat, headache, fever or stress. But not all clinics, nursing homes, and other services providers in the care for health might want to become global players, preferring to concentrate in serving their local community. Some might form affiliations or networks of finance, management, and research, if they share similar or equal religious or humanitarian commitment and vision. We as individuals have different faces and bodies, why should all corporate or institutional bodies in the health care sector be identical and uniform? Of course, there are other corporate persons in the modern world of caring for health such as insurance companies, and medical and pharmacological research facilities; there are drug companies, public health offices and service agencies, who cooperate with clinics, individuals and other corporate persons. They all have individual persons and teams as their body parts. It is always a give-and-take between all sorts of individual and corporate persons, biotopes and communities as in each and every interaction, which will give them a competitive edge[10]. To provide the professionally possible service in the care for health is in the best self-interest of the corporate person. Of course, self-cultivation is a pre-condition for cultivating one's biotope, as Confucian doctor Sun Simiao requested from a great physician, '*nurture one's own nature*' (yang xing 養性)[11]; the same can and must be said for the corporate person, not just in the field of providing service in the health care sector, but everywhere else. Moral distress on the part of nurses and doctors has been reported, and that is an indication of an unhealthy corporate body.

The various parts of a corporate person are not naturally tied together as the parts of our individual bodies; corporations in order to survive and to live a happy, healthy and successful life, corporations have to take good care of their integration and coherence. Only when the corporate person is fully integrated

---

[10] Fritz Jahr elaborated on the close integration of doing good for myself and doing good for others; the same can be said for companies and corporations as well as for all other living beings: 'We have to take into account the principle of struggle for life and existence, a principle which in some way also modifies our obligations towards fellow humans, even if we might feel unhappy about it. Our entire life and activity in politics, in business, in administration, in the laboratory, in the workshop, in the fields ... is in its reasoning and goals not focusing on love in the first place, quite often rather focused on struggle for life with some sort of fellow competitor. Quite often we don't recognize it, as long as such a struggle is without hate and in an open and legally accepted way', Jahr l.c., 2013 (1928), 39.

[11] Ni Peimin 1999 Confucian Virtues and Personal Health, in: Confucian Bioethics, Fan R ed., London: Kluwer, 31.

and functional, she will serve her own self-interest and become a strong and well respected neighbour as well. There is the old Roman story about the organs of a human body being angry towards the stomach which they thought was lazy and only receiving and consuming. They stopped feeding him, but very soon recognized that they became weaker and less efficient because they all were part of one integrated entity. A strategy of devising, implementing and cultivating a full rounded corporate profile serves both, the community and the corporate person. Such an interaction of self-cultivation and self-interest with the interest of society and with individual fellow humans as patients, partners, and competitors was a wise insight of the great physicians of the past. It again can and should become a leading tool in developing the clinic of the future. Doctor Sun Simiao of Tang Dynasty required that the 'great physician' (da yi 大醫) should cultivate and 'nurture one's own nature' and, of course, subsequently be of great service to his patients and the community. Such a request is as valid today in the 21th century as it was 1400 years ago valid for the individual health care expert as well as for corporate person in the field of caring for health. It is in the best personal interest of a great health care person, whether individual or corporate, '*to be skilled at nurturing one's nature is to treat disease before it arises*': 'If a person's virtue in actions is not abundant, even if they constantly take elixirs of jade and pills of gold, they will be unable to extend their longevity'. In general, a cultivated person lives modestly and obeys regularity in lifestyle and nutrition, avoids extremes of physical or emotional excesses, lives in harmony with his/her natural and social environment.

What Doctor Sun recommended for the cultivated and competent individual expert can also be said for the corporate person: 'The ancients, in their knowledge of the Dao, followed the pattern of yin and yang, were in harmony with skills and calculations, were moderate in their food and drink and regular in their living habits, and did not recklessly overexert themselves. Therefore, they were able to keep their body and spirit complete and live out their heavenly years to the fullest, only leaving after a hundred years had passed'. Sun Simiao was not an intellectual thinking abstractly; his books detail over 1000 essential prescriptions and procedures, and they give evidence that he knew the most up-to-date details of medical expertise and personalized treatment as is requested from modern individual and corporate experts as '*great physician*' of our times. Faden and others have started to discuss reforms in medical research and care by recognizing health care systems as learning bodies[12]. We will discuss in detail how he might be a guiding master for building the modern clinic with 21th century knowledge as a good corporate person in the service of healthy people and a healthy community.

[12] Faden R, Kass N, Goodman SN, Pronovost P, Tunis S, Beauchamp TL 2013 An Ethical Framework for a Learning Health Care System, in: Hastings Center Report 43(1):S16-27.

13.4. Building Healthy and Happy Corporate Bodies

Clinics today have many problem, among them financial and conceptual ones. They are squeezed by bureaucratic regulations, long working hours and shifts for staff, financial restrictions and the lack of incentives. So called quality norms require that individual patients be treated according to standardized disease classification norms. Inflexible financial reimbursement schemes keep clinics of today barely afloat. Bureaucratic regulation of medicinal drugs approves only 'one size fits all' remedies does not recognize well documented individual differences in drug metabolism. These and other inflexible bureaucratic generalizations originally might have been well intended to protect citizens and patients, but they have become obsolete in the 21th century as they do not take into account the traditional and necessarily future role of a partnership-in-trust between providers and recipients of health care. Compassion is often missing and staff burnout is high; there are not many incentives or even opportunities to change things for the better. Clinical routine for providers and recipients is dictated by numbers; but people are neither numbers nor cases, they are individuals as we all are, different in age, gender, hopes, angst, expectations and competencies.

How do we recover the treasures of the past in winning the future? Will citizens and patients or regulators, politicians or insurers lead the way out of dead-ends of norms and regulations? Clinics have to make the first in modifying themselves from being health repair shops to becoming great health care centers. In doing so, they will become better corporate citizens, improve their neighborhoods and their recognition as trustworthy partners in all fields of caring for the health of all individuals, all ages, all natural and social environments. Not unrelated to the success of modern medical science, the knowledge gap between the layperson and the expert and among experts is much larger than it had been over the centuries. I suggest a few preliminary steps that can be taken by clinics in the change for healthy health care[13]. The following list of suggestions may help a clinic polish its corporate profile and enhance corporate profit in a competitive market of nurturing and caring for health: provide competent and compassionate medical treatment, nursing care, and guest services: integrate stationary and ambulatory services, integrate the medical status and the value status of the patient in diagnosis, prediction, therapy and prevention; provide advice and support for lifestyle, nutrition and stress management to your community; provide services in health education and care not only to your geographic neighborhood but also to a wider community in cyberspace; nurture and cultivate your own corporate body and all of its parts for a better internal functioning and for better public recognition and appreciation as a great corporate neighbor.

[13] Sass HM 1995 Das Krankenhaus als Gesundheitszentrum der Zukunft, in Total Quality Management. Forderungen an Gesundheitseinrichtungen, Spoerkel H et al eds, Berlin: Quintessenz: 39-53

Of course, clinics as all other corporate persons are as different as we as individual persons. They have grown by their own eight-C properties and by the challenges and requcsts from their particular social ecosystem. They provide different services in rural and in urban communities; some of them are great ex-experts in rare diseases, others specialize in care for the general health of people and families; others have established a reputation for being the best in special fields of oncology, geriatric, pediatrics, gynecology or surgery of various kinds. Every individual and corporate person has to build on his or her capacities and meet the challenges to become a respected person in a well integrated community and in a competitive market of services.

(1) The clinic, the nursing home, and the small ambulatory medical practice are corporate persons. They can be hated or loved; they may have special character traits, being somewhat strange or fitting well into the service requirements and social environment. This corporate person is part of a living neighborhood; it should be known for a special expertise and a competent service; it needs to be respected as a good neighbor in order to be successful, to have a good life and survive as a living entity. As such it needs a corporate profile and identity which includes its very special corporate ethics as a leading tool for being recognized in the neighborhood and for internal education, training, treatment and care.

(2) Various wards or teams may provide different services to the neighborhood or internally, such as ambulatory or stationary treatment and care in areas as diverse as oncology, surgery, gynecology, pediatrics, psychiatry, gerontology. Each service requires a different and very specific competence and compassion, as do internal services such as accounting, kitchen, cleaning, and leadership, without which the corporate person would not be strong and capable of surviving, of being productive and successful.

(3) There are the individual persons, differing in profession, age, temperament, character, experience and compassion who need to work together. And there are also patients of different wishes and visions and with their specific genetic and health risk profile.

(4) There are the patients who seek relief from pain and suffering, the restoration of health, and preventive and life-style advice. Together with the families and the surrounding neighborhood, all of these individual organs make up the clinic as a well integrated and respected person the same way as individual organs have to be integrated and working in harmony in an individual person, animal or plant.

(5) Because corporate persons as well as individual persons need to integrate well into their social and professional territory, they should also be present as good and helpful competent and compassionate neighbors in the new environments of cyberspace. It would be a great service of the clinic in my neighborhood, if I could go there via the internet for normal and non life threa-

tening issues such as constipation, diarrhea, sore throat, sunburn, stress management and anger control, sleeplessness, lifestyle modification and advice on physical and mental activity at my preferred time. Their online presence would not only help individuals and families in the neighborhood; it would contribute positively to their public character profile and to the self-understanding of the people and the various branches and organs inside the clinic.

(6) Other institutions need to have a comparable corporate character profile to be valuable and respected neighbors providing good civilized service. As far as health care is concerned, public health services, insurance services, and society in general have to develop an integrated and harmonious approach in the care for healthy people, neighborhoods and environments.

(7) Extremely important and still neglected is the promotion and cultivation of health education and health competence for individuals, families and neighborhoods. Clinics can and should play a leadership role in promoting health literacy.

(8) Clinics should also contribute their share and establish together or individually easy to understand e-health website as one of their services as good corporate neighbor. In the old days of Hippocrates and Dr. Gong it was only the doctor and patient were partners, now treatment and care are provided in much wider environments and in modern corporate settings. Therefore, clinical bioethics has to reconstruct itself in all its organs, integrating them well and becoming not only an academic tool in research and teaching, but also a character profile in the ecosystem of caring for health. Tai quotes the Dean of the Taiwan University Medical College in regard to medical education: 'Medical education is to pass on a humanized medicine so that medical students may understand, experience and grasp the humanistic philosophy of medicine and thus establish their own value theory, ethical standard and eventually their own life philosophy. Only when we reach this goal can we say our education has succeeded'[14]. I would apply the same educational and developmental goal for clinics and other corporate bodies in the interest of their own success, survival and social recognition and appreciation. Similarly, we may say the same for the ecosystems of producing, driving, and repairing cars, of planting, processing, selling and consuming foodstuffs and many other areas of integrated activity and success.The rules for the survival and the good and respected life of a Clinic are the same as for all other living entities. The better they are interconnected with their social and natural environment, the more stable and harmonious and productive is their life.

The new construction of clinical bioethics as a truly, fully living being and as a productive integrated part of the social, political and cultural environment goes far beyond the actual European and American models of principle-and-autonomy. In further developing, integrating and applying clinical bioethics we

[14] Tai MC l.c. 144f

may use the eight-C virtues and principles 'communication and cooperation, competence and competition, contemplation and calculation, compassion and cultivation'. While being neutral to various competing religious and ideational visions and practices, they are at the same time fully open towards different religions and philosophies. It actually can be demonstrated empirically that these eight qualities had been an integral part of all successful religions and human endeavors for millennia. As they are 'universals' in the Aristotelian sense, they have been and in the future will be indispensible for each and every successful human activity, for better and healthier lives, and for harmonious connectedness and living-together. The reconstruction of bioethics cannot be the domain of one single school of contemporary bioethics; it is a common and integrating enterprise and should be recognized as such.

We need *integrated efforts* by all stakeholders in promoting good personal and public health and health care: *citizens of all stages in health and age, experts and expert teams, and corporate persons*. Of course, each of these three groups cannot do its job independently from each other; thus the reconstruction of clinical bioethics becomes an issue in self-cultivation and co-cultivation for all involved. Of particular importance are *central organs* such as clinical ethics committees for setting strategy, consultation, and education[15]. In chapter 9 we discussed interactive action guides for *citizens and experts*; here we add related action guides for *corporate and political bodies* as stakeholders in the same ecosystem of promoting health, justice, happiness, and harmony. Political bodies, social bodies, and companies in geo-/cyber-space are not just preconditions of expert–lay interactions; they are living bios within the dynamic balancing act of human cultures. Such Individual life, corporate life, communal life, cultural life, and political life are all interconnected and adjusting, challenging and supporting each other in complex interaction. Thus, *Action Guides* for the Clinic as a corporate person in interaction with citizens and experts may provide guidance for developing similar Action Guides for other corporations, companies, collectives, charities, and churches:

[15] Cf Gruetzmann T 2016 Interkulturelle Kompetenz in der klinischen Praxis. Kultursensible Ansätze zum Umgang mit interkulturellen Situationen im klinischen Alltag. Münster: Lit.

ACTION GUIDES FOR CORPORATE AND POLITICAL BODIES: THE CLINIC

For Corporate Bodies

1. *Treat citizens and staff as persons, not just as parts of a corporate system.*
2. *Set priorities in responsibility-based preventive and acute medicine and in personalized health care information.*
3. *Encourage individualized advice and treatment based on the integration of health status and value status.*
4. *Encourage your clients and patients to have advance directives and designated surrogate decision makers.*
5. *Expect your clients and patients to educate themselves in health care matters and offer health care training and education.*
6. *Be competitive with other providers in care, service, management, and financing.*
7. *Be aware of limits in organization and planning and include the neighborhood in setting priorities and in developing your corporate profile.*
8. *Use all options to decentralize and explain your services for the benefit of the citizens.*
9. *Integrate ethics and expertise to reduce or prevent organizational and administrative risk.*
10. *Support personal responsibility and act responsibly in the use of communal health care funds.*

For Political and Regulatory Bodies

1. *Provide a sound framework for literacy, responsibility, solidarity, and subsidiarity in health care policy and insurance.*
2. *Provide and guarantee individualized health care service and advice.*
3. *Support and assure basic services based on individual needs.*
4. *Support and assure reliability and quality in a market of additional services.*
5. *Promote improvements in quality of treatment and care based on progress in prediction, prevention, treatment, and care.*
6. *Guarantee the self-determination and responsibility of citizens in health care matters, including the right and duty to have advance directives.*
7. *Be aware of political and regulatory limits in the care for health and give service providers and citizens room for individualized decision making.*
8. *Use all possible options to support citizens' self-determination in issues of quality of life and health risk awareness.*
9. *Provide and protect an open market for all partners.*
10. *Support personal responsibility and act responsibly in the use of communal health care funds.*

14. DIVERSITY AND SURVIVABILITY OF POLITICAL BODIES

PROMOTING GREAT HARMONY

'Rule the land with justice, fight a war with surprise, and win a country with harmonious action (wuwei). How do I know that this? - The more prohibitions we have, the more rebellious the people will be. The sharper the weapons are under the people, the more turbulent the land will be. The shrewder the people, the more abnormal things occur. The more laws there are, the more thieves and robbers will be there. Therefore, the wise person says: When I am not greedy, the people will become rich by themselves. When I act with harmony, the people will change by themselves. When I refrain from imposing, the people will do justice by themselves. When I refrain from craving, the people will get rid of their cravings.'[1]

14.1. Political Bodies, Similar but not Identical

Political bodies are of similar living material as individual bodies, but they are not equal, in the words of Confucius '*similar but not identical.* The same can be said for societies and states of humans as for biotopes of microbes, states of bees and ants, natural and cultivated environments, and the myriads of microbiomes. Biotopes and individual bios are in permanent transition from one point in life to the next, changing themselves and changing their sceneries as well. Transition and interacting adaptation is part of life and the rule of life. Those rules are similar for the body politic as for bodies of individual people. In 1407 Christine de Pizan, a poet and writer at the Court of Charles V and considered one of the first feminists, published *Livre du Corps Policie*, describing the state as a corporate body, a *body of political nature.*[2] The front cover engraving on Hobbes *Leviathan or the Matter, Former and Power of a Common Wealth Ecclesiastical and Civil* by Abraham Bosse presents an demanding human body consisting of a multitude of citizens, surmounted by a super royal person, holding a sword and a spiritual stick as symbols of united physical and spiritual powers; the title is surrounded by images of a castle, a tank, a farming landscape, a house, a meeting place and other symbols of the political bios[3].

---

[1] Lao Zi, Guodian text: B 29-32; Dao te Ching 57.

[2] De Pizan c 1407 Livre du Corps Politic; cf Langdon Forhan K 2002 The political Theory of Christine de Pizan. Burlington VT: Ashgate; for the term body politic cf. Oxford English Dictionary: 'a nation regarded as a corporate entity'.

[3] Hobbes T 1651 Leviathan or the Matter, Former and Power of Common Wealth Ecclesiasical and Civil. Hamburg; the impressive engraving of Abraham Bosse at the title page displays the biological, bioethical, and biopolitical power of an oversized person symbolizing the body politic waving a sword in one hand and a rulers crosier in the other, governing the lands, his body formed by a large number of diverse individual people; for 'images' of Leviathan and Behemoth see the internet.

Internal metabolism and interaction with other political bodies depends on good internal and external communication and cooperation. Competence in managing internal and external affair and internal competition and competition with other societies and states keeps the body politics fit and strong. Calculating adequately the best way to keep the body healthy and from time to time contemplating and reviewing internal and external risks and affairs promotes harmony and cultivates political bodies together with their surrounding political territories. The *integrating matter* may be a king or emperor or head of state or, in Confucian reasoning the 'son of heaven', or even a spiritual continuity 'by God's grace" within or outside of the blood-line of the actual head of state and representing wholeness and continuity of the political body.

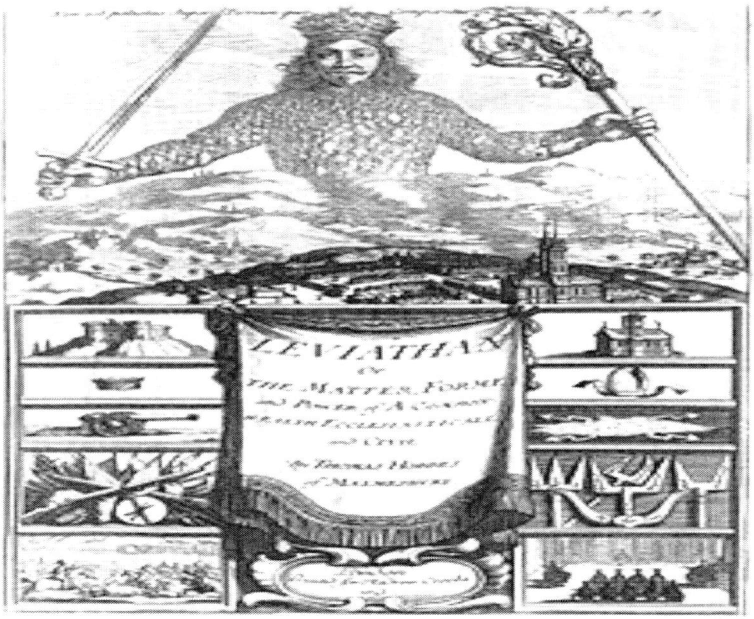

Modern societies are symbiotic complex and adoptable living beings of natural persons, natural communities such as families, clans and villages or neighborhoods, and economic and legal persons such as enterprises, institutions, bureaucracies, and of cyberspace based persons, communities, and powers as well. They all want to live well, to grow, and to sustain their lives and networks; this might lead to cooperation and support, network building, favoritism, mutual aid and help, also to corruption and exploitation in the interest of survival and protecting and even expanding one's biotope and influence. These tendencies of different players can and do lead to dysfunctional bodies and biotopes[4]. Other species exist in the same geographical spaces as we humans, but they recognize and live their and our worlds differently; bios is pluripotent and pluriperspective life all the time. As far as our human species is concerned, it seems 'that the evolution of our species privileged group survival over personal survival'[5]. Bees live in complex and highly structured social and biological communities, but sometimes they suddenly abandon their hives, a phenomenon described as 'colony collapse disorder'[6]; humans on and off destroy their complex political, cultural, social and economic communities as we these days in some Arab and Muslim countries and elsewhere in the world, a phenomenon for which we may describe as '*culture collapse disorder*', based on discontent, hate, extreme ideology, terror, exploitation, and just widespread unhappiness and the loss of mutual trust and mutual aid. In the coming age of globalization and the internet, national or regional states are going to share their integrating power and matter with other social, cultural, communal, and political bodies. Loyalties of citizens might be divided not in traditional ways such as between church and nation state. But in much more complicated and changing ways.

Individual bodies are more integrated as political ones; but political bodies may come in even more shapes and shades than individual bodies. Some body parts such as Mafiosi, dictators, and leaders of good or bad dominating economic, religious or social groups might be happy and healthy while the rest of the political and social body suffers, in disorder and sick because of negligence or exploitation. Political bodies strive on the same 8 C biological properties. We also find the 3 F's – *foods, funs, faiths* – as good constituents for long and happy lives of political bodies. *Food* in form of foodstuffs, other materials for individual and collective living such as housing, police, military, and hospitals is the basis for living together. *Fun* and satisfaction is essential for harmony and happiness of the various cells and parts of the political body; it includes festivals, good entertainment, and good housing, symphony orchestras and libraries, radio and television, enjoyment in having friends and families and making babies. *Faith* may be religious faith, but in a wider sense faith and trust in solidarity and camaraderie, in equal or relatively equal civil and human rights, in the sustaina-

4 Fukuyama F 2014 'The Sources of Political Dysfunktion' Foreign Affairs Sept/Oct 2014:5-26.

5 Lawler PA 2013 Moderately socially conservative Darwinism, in: The New Atlantis 38 (Winter/Spring) 155; he dolds, in quoting Haidt J 2012 'Why good People are divided by Politics and Religion' holds 'We are, as Haidt puts it, both "sociocentric" and "individualistic", but we find home, place, significance, and happiness in the sociocentric mode, being "full of emotions finally tuned for loving, befriending, helping, sharing, and otherwise intertwining our lives with others". So we find happiness not in autonomously pursuing it as a right but satisfying our natural social desires to belong', l.c..

6 Lu C, Warchol KM, Callahan KA 2014 Sub-lethal exposure to neonicotinoids impaired honey bees winterization before proceeding to colony collapse disorder, in: Bulletin of Insectology 67(1)125-130.

bility and even improvement of existing social, political and cultivated biotopes, of course for some also faith in a higher order of harmony created and promised by Gods, a spiritual togetherness and brotherhood in human bios and culture, of the Dao or Mother Nature as all-encompassing bios.

14.2 Diversity and Adaptability of Political Bodies

Public things and beings, in comparison to individual and private things and beings, have been called *res publica*; from there the term republic derives; other political bodies are called kingdom, empire, democracy, aristocracy, and meritocracy. Similar to individual bodies and other forms of bios, one size does not fit all. Aristotle[7] already had described different bodies of political bios and their advantages and disadvantages, suggesting a harmonious blend of meritocracy and individual virtue. Oligarchic and democratic bodies can deteriorate into totalitarian and anarchic bios, but neither power nor commerce is the life purpose of the body politic, rather happiness and body healthy. Healthy families and clans are the basic living matter out of which healthy, strong and happy political bodies are formed; this comes close to the Confucian model of the state being one large family in the wide world of bios consisting out of smaller families. Hobbes[8], in assuming that people naturally are egoistic and self-centered – *homo homini lupus*, one human is the other's wolf –, called for a strong powerful state to prevent killings and wars and to enforce harmony. Spinoza[9] had a most modern understanding of the political bios as a highly adaptable complex form of life and argued that the elimination of freedom and peace would as well eliminate the state as a healthy body.

Long lasting states and societies seem to have a rather modular body of more or less loosely integrated or interacting parts which allowed for transformations and modifications once one or the other part became weak, distressed, sclerotic, cancerous, or otherwise threatening the others or the entire body. Vast political bodies with relatively long lives were not run on a short dominant leash. The empire of Dschingis Khan was a superbody over multiple more or less independent bodies enjoying freedom of religion and internal affairs. Charlemagne run his European empire with only a few hundred people at the center, among them a few dozen riding messengers carrying mail to his various relatively independent fortresses. The more successful emperors of China ruled the provinces and instructed the mandarins by royal letters and only in most dangerous situations had to seek solutions and protect the body politics by war.

---

[7] Aristotle: Politeia

[8] Hobbes T 1651 l.c.

[9] Spinoza B 1670 Tractatus Theologico-Politicus contingens dissertationes aliquot, quibus ostenditur Libertatem philosophandi non tantum falva Pietate and Reipublicae Pace posse concendi; sed candem nisi com Pace Reipublicae, ipsaque Pietate tolli non posse. Hamburg.

The multi-centered 1000 years of the Holy Roman Empire[10] were marked by various interacting power bodies of kings, princes, dukes, bishops, and free cities in a decentralized manner, also by relatively autonomous rural peasant communes owning most lands and having their own rules and traditions on how to work the lands together as a commune or allocate o certain families. None of these political bodies were nation states, as they have developed during the last 200 years and might not last for another 200. The power of survival for political bodies seems to be quire similar as to those, which we already described for corporate bodies in chapter 12.

For millennia, important settlements were protected by walls; rivers were the connecting roads of choice; capitals and rulers quite often were far away. Today, I can fly in eight or ten hours from Beijing or New Delhi to other capitals in Europe and the Americas. Today, I can travel from Beijing to Shanghai by comfortable rapid train in four hours, and in at about the same time from Paris to London. How much longer than four months each way would Confucius have needed by ox wagon or donkey to travel from his family place close to Jinan, Shandong Province, which is halfway between Beijing and Shanghai to either one of these cities? How long did it take to get messages by riding messengers or sailboats from Paris to London or New York before telegraph cables were laid 150 years ago?[11] Today I can reach nearly every marketplace and person in no-time via internet and skype around the clock. How will our social and political bodies change and adopt to those new territories and yet unfinished ecosystems.

14.3. Social Bios Changing and Adapting

We humans over the course of the last tens of thousands of years have built houses and homes for us, our families and communities. The Westphalian single family farmhouse is different from small rural communities sharing a large amount of productive lands in communal ownership; people are the same but their social cultures have shaped them differently. City people have been somewhat different from rural people in all traditional cultures. Human settlements were and are as different as our individual and collective cultures have been and will be, interactively our homes and settlements shaping each of us and in turn we shaping those communities. The political body is not formed by individuals separated from each other; it is built upon families, clans, associations, neighborhoods, individual persons and collective persons and the way they live and socialize with each other Take the case of recent modifications in Chinese

---

[10] Wilson PH 2016 The Holy Roman Empire. A 1000 Years of Europe's History. Pinguin Books.

[11] Sass HM 2014 An Early Hegelian Vision of the Internet. Ernst Kapp's 1845 Philosophy of Cultivating Space and Time, in: Jahrb für Hegelforschung. St Augustin: Academia, 15/17:11-34.

mega-cities from traditional hutongs with private, semi-private and public spaces for rarely more than 20 to 100 families towards mushrooming high-rise buildings of 20 or more floors and many hundreds of 'neighbors' with no or minimal semi-private or shared social spaces.

A socially, economically, and culturally based diversity and modularity, respecting private and semi-private spaces and providing public places for markets of goods and gatherings for festivals and fun, has made human settlements strong segments of the body politic. Will new models of settlements develop different and stable models of neighborly bios integrating people in high-rises and Mega-cities by small modules of neighborhood activities from festivities with local flavor to special interest groups of music, dancing, card games, and discussion groups of all sorts, some offered by neighborhood associations, others more spontaneous. Will people in rental apartments or condos of large buildings develop similar neighborhood characteristics as small villages or hutongs in the past, will they have regular o irregular potluck or other neighborly activities additional to the in-house fitness club, coffee room, and green plant space or rooftop garden for developing a strong and stable neighborhood? Will city planners become aware of the importance of good neighborhoods for the health and happiness of the people first and for the city and the larger political body? Will they require architects to provide building space for the development of stable, happy and healthy neighborhoods? In former times highly centralized living conditions might have been used to silo poor people who could not afford better housing, but today luxury high-rises demonstrate that the rich and wealthy as well are attracted to new biotopes of civilized social and cultural living.

New cyber-territories allow the individual to escape from a local neighborhood in which she or he does not feel to be integrated or does not want to be active part of. But such conditions will not make a strong and stable local community on which the lager body politic can rest. Of course, individuals will not and should not become indistinguishable from their local neighborhood as this also would weaken the local community because good modular and adaptive forces within houses and neighborhoods would be missing and thus reduce the health and flexibility of the neighborhood bios. Good interaction with geographical and cyberspace territories will only strengthen the survivability of those new neighborhoods and high-rises and mega-cities by making them fit to adapt flexibly to new modifications of the ever changing political, social and cultural bodies.

14.4. Diseases and Disorders of Political Bodies

Czar Nikolas I in 1852 used biomedical terminology to describe the weakening Ottoman Empire as '*the sick man at the Bosporus*'. After 1000 years of good health and periods of great cultural and political success the empire had lost the vigor of life by arthritis and sclerosis of the body and by infections from the outside such as from the colonial powers of France and Britain. Dormant rivalries between Shiite and Sunnite denominations together with new tribal conflicts using extreme interpretations of Muslim traditions have and still mark the demise of a formerly great political body. US American meddling and military and political intervention devoid of any understanding of prevailing basic cultures of personal and tribal loyalty added to further metabolic and anxiety disorders of the successor bodies, so do geopolitical squabbles about influence peddling around the destructed or already cadaveric remains. Metastasizing cancerous diseases in the families of sick political offsprings of the former Ottoman Empire extend into Europe, challenged by anxiety disorder caused by too many refugees not familiar with traditional body functioning in pluralistic Western societies and themselves being within walls of despair and fear. Old social and political bodies such as Irak and Syria are disintegrating, infected by some sort of 'cancer' or 'auto-immune disorder'. Societies unwilling or incapable to modify into the modern world have been called 'sclerotic'; there are other coronary or infectious diseases, dementia, hypertension, diabetes, arteriosclerosis in many modern societies and cultures, in businesses, corporations and communities, some related to the rapidly changing half-time of social change. But there is also '*preventive health care*', democratic fitness training and body building, and the support of happiness in the cultural and social biotopes of economy and politics, in clans, communities, healthy and growing countries and societies.

In which biomedical terms should we describe the various biopolitical stages of good or mediocre health, of various diseases or disorders in the Chinese political body from the times of the Yellow Emperor to the demise of the Manchu Dynasty 100 years ago, after the Boxer Rebellion, corruption, hypocrisy, ignorance, other societal diseases in combination with sickening infections and invaders coming from the outside, reformulating the role of the 'son of heaven' by Mao and various ways by his successors and the Chinese people? Was the Cultural Revolution a necessary and healthy body cleaning or another disorder of a body politic in transition to find back to his old or to newer forms of health for such a large body? Did the Leninist evolution in Russia follow the blueprint of Marx 1848 Communist Manifesto[12] or was it a more complex and painful way to transform Mother Russia and later the larger Soviet Bloc, which included a quite diverse group of political bodies, into the modern age? Does Russian and China still have strong skeletons of Boyar or Mandarin heritage in their modern bodies and will they keep those amid strong powers of global integration? What happened to the various political bodies following the falling-apart of the Yugoslavian political body after Tito; did the various new bodies have lost their skills to develop harmonious and long-lasting healthy bodies after

[12] Marx did not expect that Russia would ever have a proletarian revolution, because it was lacking large numbers of exploited proletarians in comparison to Germany and England, as he explained in his letter to Russian nihilist Vera Sassulitch; cf. Sass HM 1983 The Transition from Feuerbach to Marx, in: Studies in Soviet Thought 26:123-142.

centuries of Habsburg or Ottoman rule and the Tito experiment of a relatively integrated communist body without Soviet domination?

Do parliamentarians in contemporary democracies, who are voted into office by their respective citizen constituency, really represent those citizens or is their primary power base to lobby for special interest groups, which in turn finance their lifestyle and the funds for election campaigns. Is this widely existing form of a mixture of oligarchy, plutocracy, and democracy the modern version of a mixed form of structure of the political body, as Aristotle has discussed. Will it survive diverse local and supra-local or even global rebellions of the *99% against the 1%* supported by the new powers of protest and revolt formed in cyberspace bodies but executing real power in geographic territories. Are these revolts a healthy fitness initiative to get the body politic healthy again or are they an endangering and progressive disorder for a not so well functioning political body? Can we use the model of *biocoenose*, as discussed by Moebius[13] for long-term survivability in multi-species ponds or other models of bioethical diagnosis for preventive health care of political bodies?

Yesterday the bios of culture was threatened by foreign invaders, corrupt officials, individual bad people in my community or even family; today and even more tomorrow the bios of culture and community can be threatened by individuals and groups far away destroying cyberspace environments and the basic technology based structure of our culture and life. The colossal body of the behemoth of our modern highly sophisticated and integrated bios stands on weak feet of clay and may collapse anytime; most of these scenarios we have not yet discussed publicly in a multidisciplinary and public debate at all. *Bioculturology* must become a new and influential interdisciplinary field of research and policy development[14]. So, despite great achievements in modern sciences we lack the knowledge which is beneficial – and lifesaving- for us and out cultures. Here is a hadith by Al-Tirmidhi from the oral Muslim tradition: ‘God, His angels and all those in Heavens and on Earth, even ants in their hills and fish in the water, call down blessings on those who instruct others in beneficial knowledge’; we may add the bloggers, and twitters in cyberspace and many of us who call down those blessings on providers of beneficial knowledge in medi-

---

[13] For Moebius and other models and strategies in bio-ethics, see chapter 1. - Successful biocoenose can occur in a small pond of fish, plant, and algae, but also in large socio-cultural lakes or oceans of people, cultures, and politics. Using the terminologies of biology, biocoenose, or biomedicine thus might help us to better understand social and political developments of and in living cultural, social and political bodies, business corporations, local clans and cyberspace communities; see also chapter 1 above.

[14] Bioculturology can be a new methodological and conceptual approach for the 21th century, very much needed and hopefully successful in looking at important things in way it was not done before; cf Sass HM 2014 What is Bios and how to protect and promote its Cultivation?, in: Proceedings of the International Symposium on Bioculturology. Guangdong Life Culture Association and Guangdong Medical College, Dongguan 2014:1-12.

cine, politics, social affairs and ethics. Another hadith by Bukhari answers the question of what actions are beneficial and excellent in the support of bioculture: 'What actions are most excellent? To gladden the heart of human beings, to feed the hungry, to help the afflicted, to lighten the sorrow of the sorrowful, and to remove the sufferings of the injured'.[15] We have similar biocultural wisdom and call for action in most other religions and traditions. If we would follow those, our survival knowledge might be regained, which has disappeared incredibly today as compared to the early industrial times and even more so since the Stone Age epochs[16].

The new world has gotten smaller, everyone and everything is interconnected nearly to everyone and everything. The geographical location of a capital or another important part of the body politic becomes irrelevant when compared to the power of the connectivity bios[17]. Fiber optics, networks of things, networks of commerce, instant global communication, cooperation, competition, and research have supplemented and soon might replace local trade and local competence. Material resources, expertise, capital, data and knowledge have lost their geographical base. At the same time, alternative cultures and rebellious groups find footholds in previously relatively harmonious or ungoverned geographies; the Arab Spring, blogging groups on the right and left of the political body, '*Occupy Wallstreet*' in the US, '*Nuit Debout*' in French cities, and the '*Alternative fuer Deutschland*' in Germany are early manifestations of modification of traditional political bodies, when many people lose their feeling-at-home and become discontent in their geographical territory. Where do I find my new neighbors, friends, compatriots, around the corner in my neighborhood or in cyberspace? What happens when ever more of the *traditional complex integrated supply lines for identification and cooperation* collapse? Are we seeing new '*walls of fear*' being erected by European political bodies for the protection from Muslim immigrants who are bringing their own '*walls of inflexibility*' into European territories, which are new to them?

Will we see a new *localism*[18] or even a narrow-minded provincialism as a form of geographical patriotism in a complex adaptation and modification based on discontent in our cultural and political bios or will powerful adaptive body politics eat up and integrate these newly developed alternative nerve systems into their body? *Whole Community Recovery,* a project by the Royal Society of

---

[15] Hadiths by Al-Tirmidhi (422) and Bukhari

[16] Dartnell L 2014 The Knowledge. How to rebuild Civilization in the Aftermath of a Cataclysm. Pinguin Books.

[17] Khanna P 2016 Connectography. Mapping the Future of Global Civilization. NY: Random House

[18] Moore MM 2014 (5th ed) Localism. A Philosophy of Government. Ridge Enterprise Publ; Schuhmacher EF 1973 Small is Beautiful. Economics as if People Matter. NY: Harper

Arts in London[19], for some time now has explored the role of social networks, connected communities, sustainability and whole person happiness and satisfaction in biopolitical perspective for similar communities in deterioration and people in discontent despite already established special services for the addicted, the poor and the sick. Future decentralization tendencies and movements most likely need to be seen as a positive contribution towards sustaining or regaining modularity which has demonstrated to be a central property in the survival of complex adaptive systems such as political bios should want to be. Highly centralized and not very modular national and international political bodies have less opportunities to recognize and implement health and happiness supporting initiatives from one of their organs or from grass-root levels and thus are threatened to sudden political failure and losing the sparks of individual and communal creativity, competition and innovation for modifying their body bios and its living body parts. New localism might or might not be multicultural. but it would be stronger and healthier if it would allow for cultural and social modularity.

It is only natural that the enormously expanding bios of integrated geography and cyberspace overwhelms many individuals and communities as information overflow and confusing new options for flexible adaption into new territories are too powerful. *Reduction of complexity* then is one of the strategies to cope with new information and options by protecting or regaining individual identity and self-respect by finding integration in hopefully harmonious and less confusing healthier interactive biotopes which offer solidarity and camaraderie, friendship and a new personal identity in such groups or movements in new and simple territories of local geography and supportive and attractive cyberspace[20]. Bu such a reduction of complexity and modularity can become dangerous for the life of the *corps politie* and *corps sociale* and does not seem to be the healthiest way of cultivating self-identity within the larger social and political body.

14.5. Political Struggles and Gross Happiness Products (GHP's)

Success and health of political bodies routinely is measured in economic terms by Gross National Product (GNP) and GNP has become an important infor-

---

[19] Pascoe S, Robson J (Royal Society of Arts, Action and Research Center) 2015 Whole Community Recovery. The Value of People, Place and Community. London: 'Three main principles from our work in West Sussex: Co-production is key for service users to own, and feel a valued part of their personal recovery process. A holistic whole person' approach enables services to encompass multiple dimensions of a person/s recovery, increasing the likelihood of a success I the short and longer term. Social connectedness – within the recovery community and wider local community – creates a network of support and opportunities for individuals, enhancing the sustainability of recovery', p. 37

[20] Lübbe H 1987 Politischer Moralisms. Der Triumph der Gesinnung über die Urteilskraft. Berlin: Siedler; Sass HM 2006 Differentialethik statt Moralismus, in: Sass HM. Differentialethik, Baumann E, Brink A, May AT. Münster: Lit, 3-17.

mation for political, economic, and social decision makers. In 1972 Jigme Singye Wangchuck, the King of Bhutan, introduced a *Gross National Happiness* (GNH) model for his country; the index includes issues of success in coherence, pride, satisfaction in culture, governance, knowledge and spirituality, physical and emotional health, harmony with the environment and a balanced use of personal time[21]. Since then, the Bhutan Gross National Happiness index is regularly reviewed and published; in 2015 8.4% were deeply happy, 35% extensively happy, 47.9% narrowly happy, 8.8% unhappy; this was a 1.8% improvement over the 2010 figures[22]. The 11th Five-Year-Plan for 2013-2018 details goals and estimates of cost in support of industry, transport and communication, internet and media, energy, trade, renewable natural resources, education, health, environment, governance, and vulnerable populations.[23] In 2012, the United Nations adopted the concept of Gross Happiness Product and defined the pursuit of happiness as a human right and a *fundamental human goal*[24]. GNH's and other GHP's are ideal instruments to measure the stability and health of a society or any political body; the slogan for the 2015 celebrations was 'your happiness is part of something bigger'; it has also been suggested that individuals on the Happiness Day celebration make their own 'Happiness Day Resolution' by choosing to cultivate one particular action supporting their happiness for the coming year[25].

The Gross Happiness initiative can be considered as a remarkable tool to measure and to promote the ethics towards bios into the wider population, to develop statistics for political and social decision makers and to alert people via festivities and celebrations that 'your happiness is part of something bigger than you', i.e. the health, happiness and sustainability of the body politic. Nian Zhong

---

[21] Policy Innovations, in: http://www.policyinnovations.org/ideas/briefings/data/000098/:pdf_printable.

[22] http://www.grossnationalhappiness.com/; men were happier than women, people living in residential areas happier than rural people, single and married people happier than widowed, divorced or separated, educated people were happier than others, farmers less happy than people in other occupations.

[23] Bhutan GNP, 11th Five-Year-Plan 2013-2018. Self-Reliance and Inclusive Green Socio-economic Development. GNH Foundation, XIX and 467 pages; internet 'Bhutan GNP' accessed 07-30-2016.

[24] 'The General Assembly ..., conscious that the pursuit of happiness is a fundamental human goal, ... recognizing also the need for a more inclusive, equitable and balanced approach to economic growth that promotes sustainable development, poverty eradication, happiness and the well-being of all peoples, decided to proclaim 20th of March the International Day of Happiness, invites all Member States of the UN system and other international and regional organizations and individuals, to observe the International Day of Happiness in an appropriate manner, including through education and public awareness-raising activities', in: Wikipedia: International Day of Happiness, accessed 03-0-2016; see also: http://www.illienglobal.com/ http://www.livehappy.com/practice/happiness-around-world; accessed 05-011-16

[25] 'Have you made your Happiness Day Resolution', in: inernationalhappinessday.net

has suggested to review classical Chinese concepts of family and family connectedness may serve as a model for new biocultures in the 21th century: 'Following the wisdom of Chinese people on family happiness could help to build a harmonious society in the world: draw on their empathy, putting themselves in others' shoes, addressing others' needs and concerns, showing love for one's nearest of kin, one's fellowmen and all living things'[26]. Ruiping Fan reminds us that cultural, social and political interconnectedness in the Confucian sense does not mean equal, but rather *differentiated and graded connectedness*: '1. One has moral obligations to take care of one's family members (such as one's parents, spouse, and children), than others in one's local or religious community (such as neighbors, friends, and acquaintances); 2. One has more moral obligations to take care of those in one's local or religious community than other citizens in the state; and 3. One has moral obligation to take care of one's fellow citizen in the state than other people in other states'.[27] A *Human Freedom Index* (HFI), published jointly by the Cato Institute, the Frazer Institute, and the Friedrich Ebert Foundation, measures personal, civil and economic freedom with Hong Kong, Switzerland, Finland, Denmark the first four and Saudi Arabia, Venezuela, Zimbabwe, Iran among the last of the 512 countries[28]. The HFI model covers 'rule of law, security and safety, movement, religion, civil society, expression, relationships, seize of government, legal system and property rights, access to sound money, freedom to trade internationally, regulation of credit, labor and business'.

At the end of a confrontational with Job, God boasts about his powers in creating all forms of bios on land and in the sea, the most powerful of them the gigantic land creature *Behemoth* and the most powerful sea dragon *Leviathan*.[29] The mythological animals of Behemoth and Leviathan had played a role already in the mythology of the Sumer dynasties, probably 7000 years ago in Mesopo-

---

[26] Zhong N 2014 The Concept of Family Happiness of Chinese People. A Perspective of Bioculturology, in: Proceedings of the International Symposium on Bioculturology. Guangdong Life Culture Association and Guangdong Medical College, Dongguan 152-159; 'Chinese people's idea of 'happiness for all people' could be used as a very important resource to enhance the happiness of all the people around the world', p. 152.

[27] Fan R 2016 Nonegalitarian Social Responsibilities for Health, in: Kennedy Inst of Ethics J 26(2) 204; Fan adds for a future contact with extraterrestrials as a 4th suggestion: 'one has more moral obligation to take care of one's fellow humans on earth than extraterrestrial aliens', p. 214.

[28] Vasquez I, Porcnik A eds 2015 The Human Freedom Index. Global Measurement of Personal, Civil and Economic Freedom, available on the internet; see also Lewis E, Cantor N eds.2016 Our Compelling Interests: The Value of Diversity for Democracy and a Prosperous Society. Princeton U Press, a publication sponsored by a project of the Carnegie Corporation.

[29] Job 40f; Book of Job, chapter 40f; cf. Schmitt C 1942 Land und Meer. Stuttgart: Klett; Sass HM 2015 An Early Hegelian Vision of the Internet. Ernst Kapp's 1845 Philosophy of Cultivating Space and Time, in: Jahrbuch für Hegelforschung. St. Augustin: Academia 15/17: 11-34.

tamia around Ur. The Gross Happiness Product of the future might have to be delivered by often bellicose, and rarely harmonious, interaction between these two powers. Euphrates and Tigris in Assyria, the Yangtzekiang in China, the Danube and Rhine in Europe, the Volga in Russia, the Mississippi in North America were the travel routes for material goods and for religions, philosophies and knowledge; the Mediterranean became the 'inland' water body for Phoenician, Greek, and Roman cultures. Then oceanic shipping routes were developed and railroads and autobahns formed wider and more stable networks of commerce and ideas; now it is the interplay between the geographic Behemoth giants and the cyberspace Leviathan dragons, which will decide the future of human civilization and culture. 300 years ago in 1716 the Ottoman Empire attacked the Christian Habsburg Empire, but was defeated by famous Price Eugen. Today in 2014 young German boys and girls in remote villages of the Westphalian province in Germany learn about Islam, become fanatic, travel in t-shirt and with backpack to Muslim countries in the Middle East and behead other Muslims. The first battle in 1716 was the fight between two Behemoths on land, the battle of today is the battle of the Leviathan against the Behemoths on land and in cyberspace. On September 11, 2001, the widely unknown little Leviathan Al Kaida attacked the most powerful Behemoth USA, and the Behemoth declared war against this ever growing Leviathan. Events in Syria, Irak and Libya over the last years have also Leviathanian feedbacks in European cities such as Hamburg, Paris and London, where Muslim Kurds and fanatic Sunnite Muslims fight each other in the streets of the European Behemoth countries, of which they are already a growing body part. Recently the liquid water dragon has conquered lands in Syria and Iraq and given birth to a new Behemoth of a radical Muslim Caliphate and exercised dominance on lands and people. Behemoth and Leviathan interact with each other. Thus, our dreams are of Leviathanian nature but they need to be embodied in the lands of the Behemoth for realized and lived happiness of people and communities. Individual human bodies and cultural and political bodies are different.

Hobbes gave the body politic, which was taming, dominating, and punishing, the name of the sea dragon Leviathan; he meant the geographic organization of robust human society. Today we may recognize the interacting and fighting powers of the land giant and the sea dragon symbolized in the powers of lands in cities, streets, police and military forces, factories and businesses, and the powers of the sea dragon in the fluidity of dreams and visions and the realities of internets of peoples and things, grapping more and more powers from the lands into the interconnected waters, streams, and lands as the new ecosystems. Many images display the struggle between the two beasts, symbolizing not only for us humans the eternal struggle for life and struggle[30], the *elan vital,* for all forms of bios. The Behemoth represents the strong lands and fortified cities, the armies of

---

[30] See the internet for 'Images of Leviathan and Behemoth'.

soldiers and military might; the Leviathan lived in the running streams and water bodies and nowadays in the liquid powers of the all invasive internet. This intermingling of both gigantic powers will more than ever before decide the future of human culture and human existence[31]. The narrative of the 'Little Town by the River' at the end of chapter 3 presents the vision of a future political body, who has succeeded in using the 8 C properties of our human individual and collective human bios to live in harmony, prosperity, and happiness, while constantly being aware of risks and dangers.

More than once we have mentioned, that Moses Mendelsohn in 1819 argued in regard to religious fighting: 'Brethren, if you want true peacefulness in God, let us not lie about consensus when plurality seemed to have been the plan and the goal of providence. No one among us reasons and feels precisely the same way the fellow human does. Why do we hide from each other in masquerades in the most important issues of our lives, as God not without reason has given each of us his/her own image and face'?[32] Given the quest for harmony and the diverse and often contrarian powers within social, cultural and political bodies, we may we rephrase Mendelsohn's insight into the diverse bios of individual humans, human communities, and political bodies into a bioethical suggestion:

SOCIETAL STRENGTH AND DIVERSITY IN POLITICAL BODIES

Brethren, citizens, politicians, and leaders, if you want peace and harmony in our political life, then let us not lie about uniformity when adaptability, complexity, plurality, and modality seems to have been the blueprint in the wisdom of bios. No one among the political bodies has a fully identical body structures and social interactions as compared to the others. Why do we hide from each other behind the masquerades of one-size-fits-all democracies or similar bodies, as the vital, interconnected, highly adaptable, diverse, and complex human bios has not without reason given us and our political bodies different shapes and shades?

---

[31] One of the messages of Jewish and Christians traditions is the narrative that on the 'last day of reckoning' God will end the struggle of life by killing the demonic serpentine, cf. Apocalypse 20:2ff; we find similar visions in Hinduism and Buddhism that finally in the state of nirvana will end all strive and struggle, pain and suffering.

[32] Mendelsohn M 1819 'Jerusalem oder über religiöse Macht und Judentum' Ofen: Burian, p. 201.

15. RISKS TO POLITICAL BODIES

RISKY ROADS, ROOMS AND TERRITORIES

Once upon a time, Mensch and his family left their biotope in the trees of African jungles and started walking around the globe, on foot, on horses and on camels. Lately, they also journeyed in trains, subways automobiles, ships, and aircrafts. They traveled the globe by digital networks and settled territories of social interaction, commerce, and information they had created in territories of geography and cyberspace. They illuminated the nights with electricity and built machines run by it. They assembled global enthusiasts to watch soccer or boxing broadcast in real time from a faraway continent. Facebook, books, interactive media, and commerce became digital and analog biotopes for communication and cooperation. Here they lived comfortably, successfully, and relatively safely. Sometimes they were in harmony and offered mutual aid; sometimes they were in conflict and hurt each other and their ecosystems.

Unfortunately, they were not aware that the grandiose, Leviathanian meta-organism of their bios stood on small, vulnerable feet of silicon and clay. One day a foot of that gigantic Leviathan broke away, and this magnificent social and cultural meta-organism of Mensch and his family's making fell down and broke into pieces, as did the Tower of Babylon some millennia earlier. Being of bios matter, some pieces started a new life on a much lower level. Other pieces did not survive, nor did most of Mensch's relatives, friends, and foes.

Some fellows, living in remote territories without electricity or internet roads and rooms outside of globalized networks, survived that huge catastrophe. When their offspring came across the deserted ruins of big cities generations later, as well as strange instruments and machines, they could not make much sense of them. They thought there must have been a catastrophe, but no one could find out whether it was caused by natural powers, by misdeeds of bad people, or by hardware or software running wild or engineered intentionally for wrongdoing. Bios still goes on today, but dinosaurs and mammoths are extinguished, but their distant relatives are still around. How will the family of Mensch survive? Will they ever again build cultural cathedrals as their mensch homes in new cultures of bios and bioethics territories?

15.1. Bios is not without Risk

Threats to individual bios and to collective, integrated biotopes occur naturally and are nothing new. The stream of integrated and integrating bios would not exist if not for the highly flexible, adaptive skills of non-human and human bios in adjusting to risks and threats in ever-changing ecosystems, thus avoiding hardship or even extinction. All individual and species bios is full of vital power, but it is also exposed to harm, suffering, disintegration, disease, and death. This is also true for the political and social bios and its various bodies: cultures, networks, societies, corporations, and institutions as communities located geographically or in cyberspace.

The operations of human societies, democracies, kingdoms, corporations, and companies are different from those of bees and ants, which are based on inflexible division of labor, hierarchical structures, and uncompromising service by the individual for 'the higher good.'[1] As part of human cultures, political bodies and corporations live for and should strive to reduce the tension between individual and collective interests. Human societies have been harmonious and disharmonious, tolerant and intolerant, tumultuous, rebellious, and despotic. As human individuals, clans, and cultures, we have developed our own skills and traditions in risk management and in surviving natural catastrophes by making good use of the species-specific eight-C properties. But those same biological capacities were also instrumental in causing self-inflicted injuries and catastrophes, such as destruction, torture, war, mishandling of machines, and various kinds of evil deeds.

Human bios has developed *bio-ethics* as one tool among many to use in reviewing social and ideational conditions, guiding harmonious coexistence, and avoiding catastrophes. The Greek term *kata-strophe* means downturn, fiasco, overturn. Catastrophes can be unexpected, expected, or expectable. Greek tragedy differentiates three stages of a fiasco: *protasis* as the introduction of the variables and persons in the scene, *catharsis* as the high point of development and potential catastrophe, and *epitasis* as the result and follow up. Today we face a new tension between two sets of powerful global bodies: 1) markets of values and valuables and of communication and cooperation on one side and 2) the priority of traditional political power based on the police, the military, and national law residing in geographic nation states on the other. Who are the new rulers and powerful players in modern analog–digital, integrated human biotopes? Can we still apply the old Daoist advice: 'The more prohibitions you have, the less virtuous the people will be. The more weapons you have, the less secure people will be. The more subsidies you have, the less self-reliant the people will be'[2]. How would we translate 'prohibitions,' 'security,' and 'self-reliance' situationally into our many different worlds of cultivated bios in the 21st century? Fellow humans of the Stone Age were subjected to catastrophes less often than we are because of their non-specialized survival skills, their higher risk awareness, their independence from cyberspace, and their geographical distances. They were more flexible in saving themselves and their communities in situations of natural or man-made crisis.

---

[1] In 'La Citta del Sole' (1602), Thomas Campanella (1568–1639) describes a society based on equal and mutual respect for human/civil rights and human dignity that features non-discrimination, common property, and jointly enjoyed exercises, and festivities. He bases the entire physical, biological, and spiritual world on the interaction of heaven and earth.

[2] Dao te Ching 57

Many crises in societies have come about as a result of static and inflexible decision-making and political rule. Examples include slave rebellions in ancient Rome, the 1776 storm on the Bastille by the hungry in Paris, and the call for a proletarian revolution by Marx resulting from social injustice amidst 19th-century European industrialization. In contrast, the same trends of industrialization and mechanization also offered hope that inequalities and exploitation could be overcome, such as the 1833 utopian vision of technology by John Etzler.[3] The most recent diagnostic model regarding technological progress and the rapidly reduced half-time of innovations has found a response in technical and cultural risk assessment alerting readers to the benefits and dangers of 'superintelligence.' The latter might be the next logical step in replacing human ingenuity and creativity with artificial, man-made intelligence,[4] introducing scenarios in which self-calculating, decision-making computers or integrated networks, developed and intended for serving only, are not necessarily 'human friendly' and make independent decisions regarding their own survival in the integrated struggle of bios and cultivation. As with all actions and interactions in the world of bios, such a scenario would not be a one-way street; it might fail in part, request a partial modification, or go totally wrong[5].

Viral and other infections have occurred on and off: some pandemics killed large populations, such as severe plagues in the Middle Ages or the Spanish Flu of 1918. Light and energy from the sun was never a threat; rather, it was the precondition for all life on earth, including human life. But modern cultures of microchip-based technology being central to most devices of everyday life are existentially threatened by electromagnetic pulses, occurring on and off. Only one generation ago, most people did not know about the dangers of severe gamma ray radiation and had no reason to care. The failure of machines has always been a threat to those who were close to them or who depended on their functioning correctly, but global systems of integrated, computerized trading of derivatives makes the 1630 breakdown of markets in Dutch tulip speculation look small. Because the value of derivatives is written on paper only and thus is based on good faith and the promise that they can eventually be exchanged for real things such as foods, goods, and services, unusual interruptions or problems

[3] John Etzler 1833 The Paradise Within Reach of All Men Without Labor by Powers of Nature and Machinery. Pittsburg PA: Etzler and Reinhold, 2 vol.; Marx actually had similar technological utopias such as his vision of men being free to go fishing in the morning and reading books in the afternoon; cf. also John Roebling's Hegelian argument that the Brooklyn Bridge, which he built, would dialectically integrate the different communities of Manhattan and Brooklyn, cf. Tolzmann DH 2007, John A. Roebling and His Suspension Bridges. Milford OH: Little Miami Publ; Sass HM 2014 An Early Hegelian Vision of the Internet. Ernst Kapp's 1845 Philosophy of Cultivating Space and Time, in: Jahrbuch für Hegelforschung 15-17:11-34.

[4] Butrom N 2014 Superintelligence. Paths, Dangers, Strategies. Oxford U Press.

[5] Wilson DH 2012 Robocalypse. New York: Vitage Books; Wilson DH 2013 Amped. New York: Virage Books.

in trading will cause panic and total loss of trust, reciprocity, and enforcement.[6] Markets of valuables and values are man-made of course, and our human biotopes rely on them more than ever in a globalized world. Rebellions and repressions are nothing new; they come from humans and have been with us for millennia of our history. But new, digitally based Internet connections enlarge the potential for both rebellion and repression enormously and may threaten peace and even the survival of humankind as we know it. While the biological risks of infection or gamma ray radiation can be blamed on Mother Nature, market risks and societal conflicts are the results of metabolic disharmonies in biotopes created by humans.

15.2. 21th Century Risk to Cultures of Human Bios

I select six scenarios to demonstrate specific risk features for the survival of modern biotopes of human cultures, societies and ecosystems: (1) a global pandemic killing millions or billions of people, (2) an electromagnetic pulse destroying the microchip-based infrastructures of modern societies, (3) a mushrooming loss of trust in a paper-and-promise global economy, (4) local or global potentials for revolts and repressions based in digital biotopes, (5) territorial mix-up risk of indivuduals and groups being confused about geographical and cyberspace realities, and (6) loss of control risk in vast complex and changing biotopes of integrated bios in geography and cyberspace.

Biological Risk: Two dozen people from around the globe attend a marriage in a small village of Southern China and unintentionally infect themselves with a virus similar to SARS, Ebola, or H5N1. Two weeks later, 20 have died and only four have survived. After traveling home, they had spread the virus, causing over a billion people to die worldwide. – *Electric Risk*: A strong electromagnetic pulse from the sun destroys microchips and causes a global meltdown of all electricity-based biotopes and the end of the world we know. – *Confidence Risk*: Non-market or market forces result in a severe loss of confidence in financial instruments based on paper-and-promise. They cause a halt in global trade and the life of commerce and production, with enormous consequences for everyone. – *Revolt and Repression Risk*: Fashionable trends or false prophets cause the revolt of vast numbers of unhappy people against dictators or strong economic forces, both sides using the same digital networks for either revolution or for repression or exploitation. – *Territorial Mix-up Risk*: Rules and customs in 'Second Life' are similar but not identical to customs and cultures in 'real life; this may cause severe confusion and traumata in individuals and cyberspace communities. – *Loss of Control Risk*: It does not seem to be impossible that bodies of integrated 'networks of things' will become crazy, sick, or will use their regulatory properties to manipulate their biotope in self-interest, by ac-

[6] The Bank for International Settlement records daily transactions of derivatives of $9.4 trillion U.S.; cf. Bird M 2016 For Derivates, London Is King, in: Wall Street J 07-29-16:C1f.

cident, or just because they become sick or infected. – There are many other risks in modern societies that can be exploited by disturbed or desperate individuals, by gangs, and by power-hungry, immoral leaders in politics and business.[7]

(1) Global Pandemics and Biological Warfare. We humans are integrated into a complex integrated bios and depend on its functioning. If for example, pollinating insects such as bees, will continue to disappear because of poisoning by herbicides or for other reasons, the entire food chain and the integrated ecosystems depending on pollination are threatened[8]. On and off, viral and bacterial infections break out naturally, mostly caused by naturally modified pathogens with different toxicities and lead times of incubation. But different from the innocent people who happen to be instruments of a worldwide pandemic as carriers of a new strain of the Hong Kong flu, bad people and bad governments may deliberately and strategically distribute debilitating or deadly microbes and even genetically manufacture viruses for different kind of warfare.[9]

Take the case of a group of lunatics or determined suicidal killers who infect themselves with a deadly virus of their own making and have a good lead time during which they can spread the disease before they die. They will use subways, buses, supermarkets, and airplanes strategically to infect fellow humans by dispersing the virus via exhalation or infecting surfaces touched by other people, who will serve as involuntary collaborators during their incubation time. Deposits of deadly or debilitating viruses under government control in many countries are easily available for those governments and, to a lesser extent, for individuals. But known pathogens such as those for Ebola or other microbes can also be collected in their natural biotope, reproduced in larger quantities, and even modified for better use as weapons. – Humankind's global integration makes biological combat a weapon of choice for desperate killers, who are ei-

---

[7] Casti J 2012 X-Events: The Collapse of Everything, New York: Harper Collins, lists 10 super-events that make our 'intricate, technology-dependent society … overcomplex and increasingly vulnerable to a sudden collapse … the flow of communication, transportation, electricity, finance, food, water, and medicine will cease … we will reenter the premodern world overnight.' He calls for 'adaptation, resilience and redundance' by systems and individuals: 'This means remaining adaptive and open to new possibilities, creating a life with as many degrees of freedom in it as possible by educating yourself to be as self-sufficient as you can,' p. 301f.

[8] Mohan G 2014 New Virus linked to Colony Collapse Disorder, in: Los Angeles Times, Jan 21.

[9] Sass HM 2009 Ethische Risiken und Prioritäten bei Pandemien. Bochum: ZME; cf. Sass HM 1987 Philosophical and Moral Aspects of Manipulation and Risk, in: Swiss Biotech 5 (2a):50-56; Sass HM 2006 'Crisis Management in Public Health Ethics' Chinese Medical Ethics 2006, 1:16-21 [in Chinese, transl. by Wang Chun-shi]; Sass HM 2006 Verantwortung im Notstand, in: Differentialethik. Anwendungen in Medizin, Wirtschaft und Politik, Baumann E, Brink A, May A eds., Berlin: Lit, 53-70; see also Hoffmann DR 2009 The Dead Hand. Doubleday.

ther suicidal or intend to infect others who are willing or unwilling to be messengers of death. In our integrated, modern world, it will be difficult to keep the spread under control. Biological warfare might endanger those criminal states and politicians as well, except they can initiate strict border controls after the attack and/or store an antidote to protect their own population. Microbes manufactured for warfare or mass control in unruly societies need not be lethal, as long as they help dictators or aggressors make military forces or entire populations incapable of resistance for a limited time by causing serious disorientation, pain, or discomfort.

In naturally occurring pandemics, deadly pathogens are the enemy; in biological warfare, the human aggressors are the enemies and the pathogens their weapons of choice. The very few acute and preventive weapons for defense include:
(1) complete, easy-to-understand public information and advice and (2) good public health infrastructures and pre-acute storage of remedies for easy distribution. Reducing freedom of mobility and other temporary restrictions in civil rights after the outbreak might become necessary as well. Official or voluntary quarantines in certain such as emergency offices, hospitals and nursing homes, and uninfected villages or provinces, as well as mandatory inoculations and other interventions are other extraordinary means necessary in winning the war. The goals of these extraordinary means need to be fully communicated before the outbreak. Preferably, independent, trusted individuals or groups of the civil society should simultaneously supervise such announcements.

When terrorists work alone in small cells, the best defense and prevention against all forms of terrorism and radical discontent in society is to support healthy cultural and ethical environments and to educate the populace to be risk competent and vigilant. Global high-tech networks of communication and travel allow good citizens as well as evildoers to work successfully in reaching their goals. Terrorists will most likely have direct or indirect support from one or more Mafia-type groups, even from governments and religious factions (like pirates had from official powers in the past). If this is the case, then those entities need to share the blame and punishment and must be exposed publicly. If biomedical killing of masses of innocent people is one of the options seriously contemplated by governments, the best defenses against this dangerous weapon are high levels of research and preparedness – and, unfortunately, a policy of threatening to retaliate similarly. During the Cold War, this approach was called the strategy of mutual assured destruction (MAD). The acronym MAD, when read as a word, means irate, imprudent, or senseless. It implies that the potential aggressor's calculation to win is too uncertain and suggests the probability of losing one's own population and power. For me, as an intellectual and academic ethicist without real responsibility and power in those situations, it is futile and irresponsible to even evaluate the arguments pro and con in analytical and ethical terminology. It will be the very personal responsibility of those in public office to make such decisions, which involve possibilities that are almost beyond human capacities to calculate, and to live with those decisions for the rest of his or her life.

It has been mentioned that the protection of certain high-tech biomedical research from patenting and public knowledge would be necessary to curb dual use or abuse of knowledge for terrorism or other immoral purposes – in particular, methods used to modify microbes to make them resistant to drugs. Such secrecy might be a means to slow down the distribution of knowledge, but centuries of technological development have shown that firewalls against double-use or spin-off technology rarely work in the long run. Of course, certain principles of governance to prevent potential abuse of biomedical knowledge are definitely warranted, as they are in scientific publication and patenting. But potential terrorists and mass killers need not develop their own weapons, for the arsenals of biomedical research are full of deadly pathogens. Also, pathogens such as dangerous forms of flu or other viruses will develop naturally, and evil-doers (in particular suicidal killers) will find ways to infect themselves and as many people as possible before they die. – Even in the most severe cases, the infrastructure of the technological society will remain intact, but it will be difficult to find competent people to use it. Non-human life will not be targeted, and a new form of integrated bios will prosper, with the participation of humans eliminated, severely changed, or diminished.

(2) Electric Risk and Electromagnetic Shock. Our sun emits various intensities of radiation constantly, from time to time it has been quite severe. In the past we did not care about it, however, and lacked the means to measure it.[10] Now we know that extremely strong lengths and kinds of radiation will interfere with our electric networks and may destroy hardware and software. But the same or similar radiation can also be initiated by states or by criminals using strong magnetic radiation as deliberate ammunition for destruction. If exploded in high altitude over Southern China or the East Coast of the United States (or fired from a harmless fishing trailer), a device similar to a hydrogen bomb that emits strong gamma radiation will render useless the digital infrastructure of the area encompassing Hong Kong, Shenzhen, and Guangdong or the Boston, New York, Philadelphia, Baltimore, Washington, D.C. corridor. The entire integrated electric grid will be affected, including microchips in phones, cars, supermarkets, and elevators, as well as all forms of digital communication and cooperation – also those of the police, military, rescue forces, and media.[11] People will die in

[10] On September 1 and 2, 1859, the biggest geomagnetic solar storm ever reported (called the Carrington Event after the British scientist who reported and documented it) destroyed many telegraph lines in Europe and North America and caused a number of fires; a similar storm today would render most infrastructure of electricity and communication useless; cf. Internet 'solar superstorm 1859.'

[11] A 2008, U.S. Congress Commission on EMPs estimated that 90% of the U.S. population would die within 12 months after a total loss of electricity from starvation, disease, or

their high-rise buildings and might kill each other over food and water. Cars will stop driving, and planes will fall out of the sky. People will be clueless as to what has caused the breakdown of civilization because the Internet and the media will not be functional. Attacks on utility infrastructures will have occurred and will likely occur again, destroying water dams, power grids, pumping stations, and all kinds of control systems. All sorts of private intellectual and real property will be stolen. A comfortable, civilized, highly complex, ultra-modern human bioculture reveals that it is literally built on sand, i.e. on silicon.

(3) Confidence Risk in Paper-and-Promise. Trade and commerce become more and integrated and thus are prey to unintentional or deliberate attacks on basic trust. We had an unintentional meltdown of markets in real estate and finance in 2004 and 2008, and only concerted efforts to rescue those who had caused this meltdown avoided an international catastrophe in the bios of economy and business. Today, individual computer hackers or state-supported criminals can create total havoc in the fully integrated commercial life of the planet. Because high-frequency trading (HFT) is already done primarily by artificial intelligence, glitches or technical inequality in the software of trading machines and not human competence in trading will result in winning or losing.[12] Hazardous legislation that is inept or corrupt still allows banks and other speculators to buy and manipulate commodities of all sorts; HFT has not proven to be economically necessary or beneficial; and governments print paper money uncontrolled. Unknown or undisclosed leverage of market players, predatory lending, deregulation, and computer-driven interconnection and trading cause fragile business architectures of proportions as yet unknown.[13] We have speed limits on autobahns and streets for you and me, but there are no speed limits on trading commodities or derivate products for the 'big players.' Central banks and government market players distort markets by unpredictable currency

societal breakdown (Woolsey RJ, Pry PV 2014 'The Growing Threat from an EMP Attack', in: Wall Street Week, August 13:A13); cf. Pry PV 2013 'Electric Armageddon,' CreateSpace; Metatech Corporation for Oak Ridge National Laboratory, January 2010 'Report Meta-R-320: The Early-Time (E1) High-Altitude Electromagnetic Pulse (HEMP) and Its Impact on the U.S. Power Grid' (Appendix: E1 HEMP Myths).

[12] Clark S 2016 Libyan Fund Cites Goldman Sachs Email, in: Wall Street J 07-29-16:C3, describes the controversy over whether or not people or computers on Wall Street were superior to those in Libya, when Libya lost enormous funds in dealing with Goldman Sachs. Banks considered to be 'too big to fail' include Citybank, Goldman Sachs, Bank of America, and Morgan Stanley. All of them have at about 25 times more exposure to trillions of derivatives than they have dollar assets.

[13] Ingham G 2005 The Nature of Money. Cambridge Policy Press; Roeder M 2011 The Big Mo: Why Momentum Now Rules our World. Virgin Books; Wray LR 2012 Modern Money Theory. Palgrave Macmillan; Barth JR, Caprio G, Levine R, 2012 Guardians of Finance. Making Regulators Work for Us. MIT Press; Calomiris CW, Haber SH 2014 Fragile by Design: The Political Origins of Banking Crises and Scarce Credit, Princeton U Press; Wolf M 2014 Shaping Globalization. In: Finance and Development, Sept [IMF], 22-25.

moves creating 'trade anxiety'; currency trading maneuvers by big banks and governments reach $4.9 trillion per day and make price predictions for manufacture and commerce impossible[14]. Central banks also enjoy the liberty of printing as much 'promise on paper' money as they wish. Their most recent cynical strategy is to reduce the value of the paper money to initiate inflation and thus cause more inefficiencies in markets that have already been proven to be inefficient because of bubbles in real estate and stock market valuations created by those central banks.

But central banks don't or can't assess the interplay of their *ad hoc* intervention with currency relations, job markets, job skills, productivity standstills, and tons of regulations by non-market polities. Market manipulations have been done by central banks in a race to reduce their own currency against other currencies to make their products more attractive in world markets. One thing that will be achieved by such arbitrary and inefficient interventions into national and international markets is the reduction in value of government bonds and of paper money for retirement pensions by employees. These and other governmental interventions and regulations have made the self-healing and adjusting market forces inefficient. They came into place after the gold standard was replaced by promise-on-paper bills only and certain other regulations guaranteed the survival of 'too big to fail' market players. On the other hand, reaction by other central banks in changing their own national interest rates results in developing market changes that will influence employment and profit, no matter what the other central bank expects from lowering or rising national interest rates and money supply. What happens, if national economies and central banks turn out to be 'too big to fail' and turn to 'self rescue'? Wouldn't it be better to encourage complex markets to build new territories of business and life beyond the imaginations of politicians and bureaucrats by prudent minimal legislation and issue regulations only with 'sunset clauses' naming the date of expiration? Existing regulations, of course, would be subject to review as well, the time of which can be determined by lottery over a period of 10 years.

I am not aware of tough, convincing proactive measures by states and businesses to avoid a global catastrophe that would render digital- or paper-based assets worthless. Take this case: A crazy person, a group, or a government throws a three-figure billion of U.S. Treasury bills on the European markets. The seller requests to be paid not in contracts or in futures, but to be paid and delivered immediately in real-value assets such as gold, silver, diamonds, land, corn, cotton, or even dollar notes. Once those billions are offered, European markets will suffer a shock. Little trading occurs, and the markets shut down in no time. U.S. markets do not even open, nor do the Asian bourses. If such a sale is prepared or accompanied by well-placed rumors, the disaster will be even

[14] Shelton J 2016 Trump's Contribution to Sound Money, in: The Wallstreet J 08-11-16, A11; cf. Shelton J 1998 Money Meltdown. New York: Macmillan.

bigger. Scared people will run to their banks for paper money. Having no paper money anymore, my local bank closes the next day, and my neighborhood ATM machine is empty. Gas stations and supermarkets decline my credit cards, occasionally accepting promise-on-paper money or bartering goods or services. This super colossus of paper-promise was not made of gold or even bronze. It was constructed of cheap paper and based on trust, and a kick to its feet made it fall apart. Because trust can easily be destroyed, even well-placed rumors for experts and the public might have already done the job of exposing the empty promises behind the signatures on paper money.[15] Civil discontent towards promise-on-paper will lead to civil disobedience and disorder and result in sick political bodies.

(4) Revolt and Repression Risk. When Karl Marx searched in 1848 for huge human masses as a powerful force for changing unfair social and political environments, he identified the exploited proletarians of the early European industrial revolution. Today he would identify the unhappy and frustrated segments of populations in transition from traditional to modern societies. These include youth in the so-called Arab Spring and its counterrevolutions, global fashion modes of rebellion against traditions, and reactionary revolts against the fast-moving developments of global integration and the loss of traditional points of orientation in religion and culture. These losses have led to uncertainty and disorientation on the part of many young people, resulting in a rebirth of religious and cultural extremism and backward-oriented narrowness. Many studies have examined discontent in cultures and the changes, destruction, and reconstruction brought about by rebellion.[16] The new century provides different reasons for confusion, exploding into rebellion and discontent and many new forms of protest. At the same time, political dictators or strong social or business forces may use the same new communication and cooperation technologies for microscopic invasions of privacy, for indoctrination and introjection, or for promoting their own selfish interest.[17] A new 'political class', comparable to the

---

[15] U.S. dollar bills present two signatures of government officials and the words 'legal tender'; but into what will the bill be tendered if not into paper of the same sort? More promising for some might be the slogan 'in God we trust' on the other side of the bill, but that has nothing to do with the economic value and health of the currency market, nor does it tell who the 'we' are, the two bureaucrats who signed the bill or 'the people of the USA'. The Paper Euro gives a signature of a European official without a title, just the name 'Draghi' – no explanation why that name is on the bill for other than ornamental reasons.

[16] Freud S 2005 Civilization and Its Discontents (Unbehagen in der Kultur, 1930) uses the psychoanalytical methods and principles, Freud had developed earlier to diagnose diseases in individual persons, to analyze the success and default of cultures and states.

[17] In his famous lectures on 'Biopower' at the College de France in 1978, Michel Foucault discussed the use of information and indoctrination methodology by nation states in Europe since the 18th century: 'when discipline is the technology deployed to make individuals behave, to be productive workers, biopolitics is deployed to manage population; for example to ensure a healthy workforce' (Foucault M 1903 'Society must be defended,' 239-

feudal circles of yesterday and including networks of political officials and business leaders, conducts their own business, which is based on self-interest and class power. New environments of information, communication, and cooperation based in cyberspace can work both ways, in favor of further liberation and the development of civil societies or in favor of state-controlled or business-controlled masses; in favor of better transparency or in favor of even more successful corruption and exploitation — similar to the double-purpose or spin-off use of old technology for doing good or doing bad.

(5) Territorial Mix-Up Risk: In the old days, communities always had eremites, who left the 'real' world in order to emigrate into close communication and integration with non-geographical spiritual powers; they might, however, still been indirectly related to the 'real' world by praying for peace and divine intervention. Nowadays, emigrants from the 'real' world become famous citizens in 'Second Life' or other internet territories as celebrated orchestra conductors or famous singers, football stars and boxing stars, inventors and savers of humankind, while at the same time they are 'nobodies' living unknown and not socially integrated or even recognized in their private quarters.

(6) Loss of Control Risk: Much is talked about the threat from artificial intelligence, turning against the existing balance of interaction and interdependence among the wide modern world of bios. Not much is known yet precisely about systems of mad and aggressive artificial intelligence turning outside of their sphere, running rampage in taking control of local or global automation, destroying all or some integrated forms of the world of modern human bios, such as mad and aggressive individuals today cause destruction by killing fellow humans with traditional explosives or deadly infectious microbes[18].

Well-functioning digital and microbial infrastructures and more or less harmonious biological, economic, social and political bodies are essential for the survival of the bios of our modern culture, but they have made the new complex adaptable and integrated of collective and political bios more vulnerable in many new dimensions. All in all, these six sets of scenarios demonstrate the not yet widely enough discussed risk of the impressive colossus of the modern global and integrated political body with its vulnerable cultural, social, and economic organs.

---

264). He traces the model of biopolitics back to the Greco-Roman and medieval emperors and kings; nowadays he might recognize the power of radio, television, and the Internet for even more successful forms of domination and indoctrination and their avoidance.

[18] For a detailed discussion of risk to social and political bodies from environmental destruction and complex integrated and programmed artificial intelligence see Diamond J 2006 Collapse. How Societies choose to Fail or Succeed. New York: Viking; Wilson DH 2012 Amped. New York: Vintage Books; Wilson DH 2012 Robocalype. New York: Vintage Books; different scenarios of self-reprogramming and self-adjusting machines artificial intelligence are discussed in other science fiction movies and novels.

15.3. Open Future for Human Biocultures and Political Bodies

As already mentioned, people lived for eons in farmhouses or small villages; now they live in high-rises with few semi-public or public spaces, yet they may share various cyberspaces both private and public. Most elderly people have experience with small communities both geographically and in cyberspace, but how will our children and our grandchildren be formed by complex ecosystems around them?[19] Modern societies are symbiotic, living creatures of natural persons (in natural communities such as families, clans, villages, and neighborhoods) and of economic and legal persons (such as enterprises, institutions, bureaucracies, and similar cyberspace-based persons, communities, and powers). They all want to live well, grow, and sustain their lives and networks. These desires might lead to cooperation and support, network building, favoritism, and mutual aid and help, as well as to corruption and exploitation in the interest of survival and of protecting and or expanding one's biotope and influence. These tendencies of different players can and do lead to dysfunctional bodies and biotopes.[20]

Mediterranean and European mythology has narrated a struggle between the land creature Behemoth and the water creature Leviathan. The land creature rules by walls, towers, armies, cities, and land; the water creature dominates the streams, lakes, ponds, reservoirs, and oceans by networks of information, commodities, monies, ideas, propaganda, and fashion. The global winner in the political and cultural life of the 21st century might be the Leviathan, jumping over walls of all kinds and great and small political, social, economic, and cultural mountains using the new, liquid bodies of audio and visual information, the Internet, and global travel and trade. Those entangled bodies politic of Behemoth and Leviathan are different from my body, in which organs such as the liver and lungs are fully integrated for a healthy, enjoyable life. Humans are social beings, but they are not just part of something bigger and more complete; as Nazi fascists used to say, 'you are nothing, your volk is everything.' Territorial borders are no longer a barrier for the wide breadth and long reach of the Leviathan. Karl Popper and Michel Foucault warned of the growing powers of the 'enemies' of an open society and the dominating power of the *corps état*. Much earlier, Edmund Burke and Arnold Ruge cautioned against the developing powers of socialism and nationalism in Europe.[21] They all reasoned primarily in terms of land, not water.

We have come a long way from the earliest information on the social life of civilized humans and animals some 20,000 years ago. For millennia, we were

---

[19] Sass HM 2014 l.c.; Sass HM 2012 l.c.

[20] Fukuyama F 2014 l.c.

[21] Popper K 1945 'The Open Society and Its Enemies'; Foucault M 1977 Le Bio Pouvoir'; Burke E 1790 'Reflections on the Revolution in France'; Ruge A 1846 'Zwei Jahre in Paris.'

quite familiar with traditional nature-based risks to bios and to the individual and social life of humans in particular. Social life happened circularly and was based on the seasons and the teachings of older generations. The wisdom of great-grandparents was also good for later generations. Since the 18th century, modern technologies and global interactions based on them – as well as the clashes and interactions of lifestyles and civilizations – have molded societies and cultures into progressive or regressive dynamics. These forces have developed new forms of interaction among individuals, communities, corporations, republics, and other political/social bodies in intertwined geospace/cyberspace territorial biotopes.[22] These new, amalgamated ecosystems caused new risks such as power struggles, wars, exploitation, and technical disasters. Some of these risks caused by humans could lead to severe catastrophes, such as the dependency of urban mega-life on electricity and digital communication/ cooperation. Those systems could be destroyed by terrorists or by state-based terror. System failure in medieval cities was related to such events as seasonal fluctuations, fire, and poor-harvests. System failure in modern mega-cities and in global commerce and trade will be based on infrastructure failure (e.g., electricity or digital technology).

As far as risks to the enjoyment and cultivation of life are concerned, human-based and -created life forms make us safer and more comfortable by building, heating, and cooling houses, providing safe and plentiful foodstuffs using agro-technology, and wiring the globe with electricity and radiation waves of various lengths for energy, light, communication, cooperation, and further cultivation of our lives. We humans are powerless to avoid nature-based risk entirely, being unable to influence the seasons, the sun and moon, or earthquakes and tsunamis. However, we have experience in protecting ourselves from some untoward events by avoiding the harshest environments, setting aside enough food in winter, wearing clothing appropriate to the season, and building safe, stable houses. Human-based risk, arising from such causes as war, social discontent, greed, error, and terror, has at times been successfully mitigated or avoided, however, by prudent bioethics and biopolitics. Developed over millennia, the instruments for the latter are still the previously mentioned eight-C forms of bios properties specific to humans, often called virtues, values, or principles.

15.4. Bioethics in Cultivating the Leviathan-Behemoth Struggles

Lao Zi once said: 'Cultivate the self and virtue will be true; cultivate the family and virtue will be complete; cultivate the village and virtue will grow; cultivate the country and virtue will be rich; cultivate the world and virtue will be wide.'[23] We can expand and translate Lao Zi's insight into a Bioethical Imperative for the 21st Century: 'Cultivate yourself and life and virtue becomes true; cultivate

---

[22] Cf. 'The Power to Create' in: Royal Society of Arts Journal, 2014, no. 2 [www.thersa.org].
[23] Dao te Ching 54.

individual and corporate persons and virtue will be great; cultivate social and natural environments and virtue will be full; cultivate communication and cooperation and life will grow; cultivate compassion and competence and life will be rich; cultivate life, and world and virtue will be wide.'

In regard to building corporations and institutions as well-respected, rich, and successful corporate persons practicing bioethics anywhere and everywhere in the world, we can say: 'Cultivate communication and cooperation and corporate persons and communities will be strong; cultivate competence and compassion and corporate persons and communities will be good; cultivate corporate persons and communities and the neighborhood will be healthy; cultivate the neighborhoods and the world will be healthy and happy.' From the old folks such as the Yellow Emperor, Confucius, Socrates, and Jesus to modern folks such as Edmund Burke, Michael Foucault, and Fritz Jahr, all could easily agree to such a modification and extension of Lao Zi's wisdom regarding the collective, complex and integrated virtue and happiness of persons, corporate persons, and environments. These guidelines apply to all fields of modern professional and corporate activity for the benefit of individuals, communities and environments, and all life.

We humans and our societies and cultures are an integrated part of the worlds of bios; therefore we need bioethics to protect and to improve what we have. Bioethics is vital for the following reasons: (1) because in comparison to other species we lack a firm and inflexible instinctive drive to 'do the right thing' at the right time; (2) because we have the freedom to either 'do right' or to 'do wrong' and potentially harm ourselves, our fellow humans, and our environment; and (3) because we want to be happy and healthy in sustainable, civilized, cultivated biotopes, whether geographical or non-geographical. As the history of human culture and ingenuity shows, the prudent use of our eight-C properties and virtues of communication and cooperation, competence and competition, contemplation and calculation, and compassion and cultivation has been a great success story. Using the words in the 'Last Will' of Van Rensselar Potter quoted earlier, we have no other biological means to advance bioculture and bioethics: 'Global Bioethics must evolve into a politically energized and socially concerned Bioethics Worldwide: Bioethics for the 21st century calls for Peoplecare with Healthcare and Earthcare with Animalcare.'[24]

The 21st century has already demonstrated that it will most likely see even more strength and power in the reign of the Leviathan via new fluidity in the globalization of all forms of bios and in the digital waters of the Internets of people and of things. Social networks vastly enlarge my options to meet people and make friends beyond my geographical village. Global emailing, blogging,

[24] Potter 2012 (2001) The intellectual 'Last Will' of the first global Bioethicist, in: Fritz Jahr and the Foundations of Global Bioethics: The Future of Integrative Bioethics, Muzur A, Sass HM eds., Zürich: Lit, p. 155.

and digital files outstrip the role of handwritten letters and printed books for communication and cooperation in science, culture, and information. Microbial bios, infections, and potential warfare travel by airwaves rather than traditional waterways. Old and new religious and spiritual traditions populate the minds of individuals and form fluid, non-geographical living communities and cultures, both small and large. Internet-based production and commerce compete with local markets of work, trade, and vision. Traditional armies, navies, and air forces are supplemented or even replaced by electromagnetic guns and mortars or by biological warfare. Unparalleled destructive powers hide unseen in the darkness of Leviathanian nuclear submarine 'dragons' that attack from underwater. Age-old ideologies, which might have been useful in protecting the lifestyles and territories of nomadic tribes in remote lands infiltrate unhappy people around the globe who search for guidance in the unchartered waters of oversupply in information, orientation, and guidance. The liquid powers of the Leviathan inflame the neural networks of individuals and communities and threaten the biological stability of the Behemoth in local governments and global cultures, in intolerant and tolerant communities alike. Cultures, communities, and individuals, thus, need to redefine their roles in the struggle between the Behemoth and the Leviathan in shorter and shorter half-lives of adjustment and alteration.

Philosophers and historians have debated whether human history is progressive, regressive, or a permanent power play between forward and backward. They all agree, however, that individual and political bios and the history of human bios all struggle among and within complex, adaptable, and cultivating ecosystems. In Hindu and Buddhist traditions, we also find visions of a final end to struggle that liquidates the stress and struggle of bios, replacing it with peaceful, endless Nirvana. We find this release as well in the Apocalypse of John, when God finally slaughters the huge Leviathan. In the meantime, the cultivating power of bios (the *élan vital*) might be given more options, despite previous and coming catastrophes. Human bios might be saved and continued in further cultivating and taming the powers of Behemoth and Leviathan.

TOWARDS A BIOETHICAL MANIFESTO?

Lao Zi, 2500 years ago during the Zhou Dynasty in China, discussing healthy and unhealthy human cultures, said 'We build rooms with windows and doors, but it is the inner space which makes the room livable'[25]*. Karl Marx, in the revolution year of 1848, who discussed workers exploitation in early industrialism in Europe in the 'Communist Manifesto', said 'Proletarians of all Nations unite!'*

Indeed, we humans build our own rooms: living rooms and sleeping rooms, hotel rooms and hospital rooms, operating rooms and hospice rooms, concert

[25] Dao te Ching, 11.

halls and town halls, factory halls and dancing halls, torture chambers and court chambers, office rooms and chatrooms, - what happens in these rooms depends on me and you. Also, these rooms themselves may not last forever and are threatened by arsonists, shortenings in cables of electricity or communication, by breaking doors and windows, by stealing values, by spreading rumors, by poisoning rooms in many other ways.

If we want, in recognition of our precious and more or less comfortable rooms, roads and territories, in the future successfully apply and cultivate our basic bios principles of communication and cooperation, competence and competition, contemplation and calculation, compassion and cultivation again in different shapes and shades, then we may rephrase Marx' plea into a 'Bioethics Manifesto: People of all cultures and countries unite!'

Index of Names

Abraham, Jewish Patriarch 123
Alexander the Great 94
Al-Tirmidhi 228f
Al Ghazali 87
Aristotle 107, 228
Azariah J 17
Bacon F 20
Basarde S 201
Beauchamp TL 16, 52, 150
Beecher HK 95
Behemoth 232ff, 246ff
Berkeley G 80
Bosse A 221f
Buddha 12, 30, 34
Burch RL 81
Burke E 246
Burckhardt J 50
Campanella T 236
Chang Tsai 35f
Charlemagne 224f
Childress JF 16, 150
Comenius A 107ff
Confucius 26, 31, 34, 43, 52, 187f, 225, 232, 247
Constantine, Emperor 34
Covic A 17
Dschingis Khan 224ff
Entralgo L 148f
Epiktet 50
Eisler R 12
Etzler J 2327
Eysenbach G 163ff
Fu Xi 45
Daedalus 71
Deng Xiao Peng 26, 31, 34
Engelhardt HT 154, 182
Faden R 215f
Fan Ruiping 125
Francesco Assisi 12
Freud S 244
Foucault M 18, 244, 246f
Galen C 129, 148, 178
Gehlen A 40
Giordano J 52
Gerard, Fra 181
Goethe JW 188
Gong Tingxian 144ff, 152f, 168, 178
Gostin L 131
Graff J 168
Hagar 123
Hanifa A 53
Hartmann E v 53
Hegel GWF 160
Heidegger M 48
Herder JG 13, 63
Hippocrates 150
Hobbes 221-224, 233
Hoffmann F 146f, 178
Ikarus 71
Ilkilic I 166ff
Isaac, son of Abraham 123
Ismael, son of Abraham 123
Ivy AC 94
Jacob, son of Isaac 59ff
Jahr F 11-14, 18, 21, 29, 35, 43f, 52, 62, 75f, 129, 178, 214, 247
Jean Paul II 30, 111
Jesus 25, 31, 33ff, 44, 160
Kant I 46
Kimura R 16

Kishore RR 151
Krause KCF 13, 63
Khroutski K 17
Koch R 88
Kropotkin A 29, 31
Lao Zi 31, 85, 182, 204, 221, 247f
Laban 59f
Lamassu 71
Landsteiner K 139
Leibniz GF 45
Lenoir N 18
Leopold A 20
Leviathan 221f, 231f, 235, 240ff
Levin S 209f
Lessing GE 33
Ligori SA 122
Lima N 70
Locke J 31
Lolas-Stepke F 148f
Machiavelli N 204
Macer D 22
Marx K 227, 237, 249
Marcel G 52
McCormick R 32
McNamee SP 75
Mencius 149
Mendelsohn M 31, 34, 53, 234
Möbius KA 19, 228
Mohamed, Prophet 53
Moreno J 203
Morus T 109
Mulla Sadra 48, 53
Muzur A 17f
Ni Peimin 97
Nicolaus I, Czar 226f
O'Neill O 211f
Orwell G 21
Otto R 46
Pellegrino ED 15, 18
Paulus, Apostle 27
Pizan C de 221
Pius IX 121, 173
Popper K 246
Potter VR 14, 24, 44, 248
Qiu Renzong 17
Rabelais F 110
Reeves M 209f
Reich W 15f
Rentdorff JD 16, 152
Roizen M 169
Rousseau JJ
Ruge A 246
Rumi 46
Russell WM 81
Sarah, wife of Abraham 123
Schleiermacher F 12
Schiller F 41ff
Schopenhauer A 12
Schroeder-Baeck P 133f, 162f
Seattle 50
Seneca 187
Shriver S 15
Singer P 21
Socrates 32ff, 247
Schweitzer A 22, 62, 77
Spinoza 31f, 182
Sun Simiao 145f, 178f, 214f
Sun Zi 205
Tai MC 17, 112, 126, 131, 137f, 140, 149, 151, 196f, 198, 218
Ten Have H 170
Tomasevic L 23
Thomas Aquinas 121

Ueda D 209f
Veganti R 210
Viefhues H 188ff
Voltaire 31
Wagner R 31
Wangchuck JS, King 231ff
Weizsäcker V 148f, 187f
Whitehouse P 20
Yang Chuan 91, 148, 150, 171
Zhai Xiaomei 16, 90, 98, 137

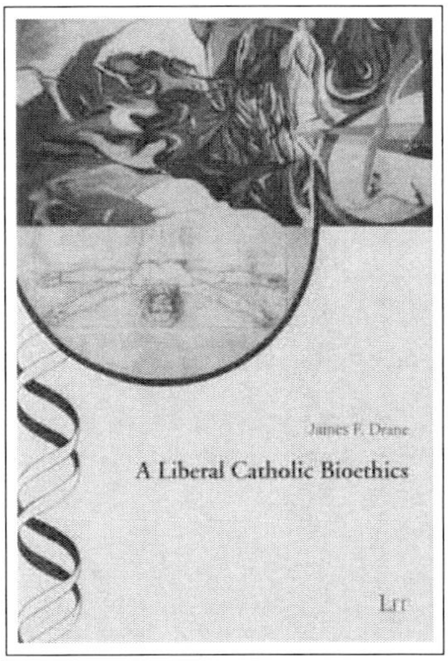

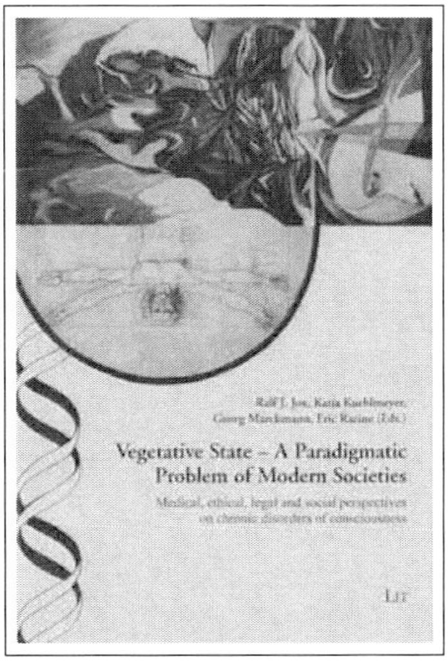

James F. Drane
A Liberal Catholic Bioethics
A Liberal Catholic Bioethics opens a new dialogue between Christian reasoning and belief and secular positions in bioethics. The well documented book covers in detail internal and external debates and positions of Roman Catholic theology and hierarchy: issues of contraception and abortion, palliative care and euthanasia, caring humanely for the demented, the use and abuse of modern technology in medicine. The doctrine of Papal infalliability is identified as a main reason in hindering and suppressing a dialogue within the church, with the faithful and with other religious and humanist positions. Were the Borgia Popes infalliable, was Pope Urban infalliabe when he condemned Gallileo, the author asks. He thus carries the debate far beyond specific bioethics issues towards a more humane medicine and culture.
Bd. 15, 2010, 296 S., 24,90 €, br.,
ISBN 978-3-8258-6877-2

Ralf Jox; Katja Kühlmeyer; Georg Marckmann; Eric Racine (Eds.)
Vegetative State – A Paradigmatic Problem of Modern Society
Ethical, legal, social and medical perspectives on chronic disorders of consciousness
Decision making for patients in the vegetative state is a complex issue and needs an interdisciplinary discourse that combines different perspectives. This book is based on an international neuroethics workshop for young academics and health care practitioners that took place in Munich and was funded by the German Ministry of Education and Research (BMBF). Various competitively selected participants from different countries describe their scientific contributions or their clinical experiences. Moreover experts from the field of medical ethics, neuroethics and neuroscience contribute their perspectives.
Bd. 36, 2012, 216 S., 34,90 €, br.,
ISBN 978-3-643-90097-5

Ethik in der Praxis/Practical Ethics

Materialien/Documentation

hrsg. von Prof. Dr. Hans-Martin Sass (Universität Bochum/Georgetown University Washington)

Schriftleitung: Dr. Arnd T. May

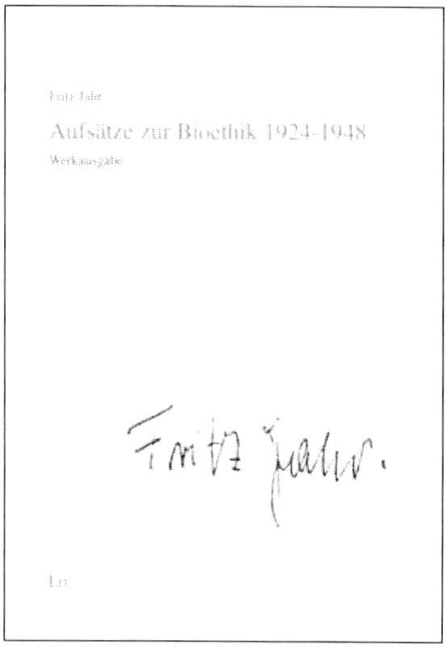

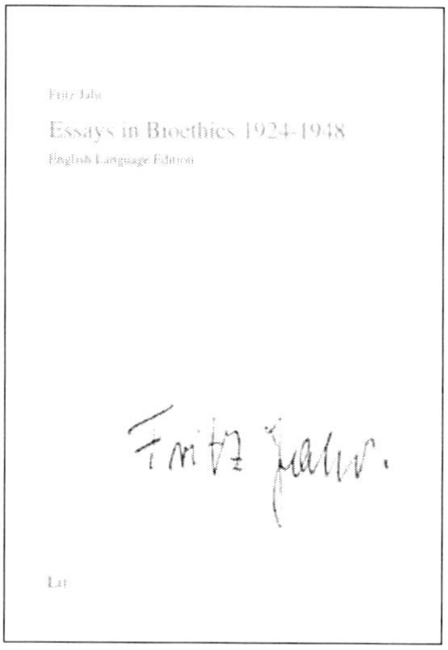

Fritz Jahr
Aufsätze zur Bioethik 1924 – 1948
Werkausgabe. Herausgegeben von Arnd T. May und Hans-Martin Sass

FRITZ JAHR (1895 – 1953), evangelischer Pastor in Halle an der Saale, prägt zuerst 1926 und dann prominenter 1927 den Begriff BIO-ETHIK in einem Leitartikel in der Zeitschrift „Kosmos" und formuliert als BIOETHISCHEN IMPERATIV: „Achte jedes Lebewesen grundsätzlich als einen Selbstzweck und behandle es nach Möglichkeit als solchen!" Er entwickelt damit in kritischer Auseinandersetzung mit dem Kategorischen Imperativ von Kant das Konzept einer situativen und abwägenden Ethik und den Rahmen für eine künftige integrative und globale Bioethik. Die Sammlung der zwischen 1924 und 1948 in verstreuten wissenschaftlichen, theologischen und ethischen Zeitschriften erschienenen Aufsätze von Fritz Jahr beleuchtet nicht nur die historische Entwicklung der Bioethik, sondern will auch zur Weiterentwicklung einer integrativen und globalen Bioethik beitragen.

Bd. 14, 2. Aufl. 2013, 160 S., 24,90 €, gb.,
ISBN 978-3-643-12137-0

Fritz Jahr
Essays in Bioethics 1924 – 1948
Edited and translated by Irene M. Miller and Hans-Martin Sass

FRITZ JAHR (1895-1953), a Protestant theologian in Halle an der Saale, Germany, coined the term BIOETHICS in 1926 and defined the BIOETHICAL IMPERATIVE:
"Respect every living being on principle as an end in itself and treat it, if possible, as such". In critical dialogue with Kant's Categorical Imperative he develops the concept of modern situational bioethics.
These 22 articles, written between 1924 and 1948, cover issues of ethics towards animals, plants and environments, also the ethics of social interactions with all forms of life.
The essays are of current and historical interest and serve as a guide to future global and integrated bioethics.

Bd. 15, 2013, 136 S., 29,90 €, gb.,
ISBN 978-3-643-90337-2

LIT Verlag Berlin – Münster – Wien – Zürich – London

Auslieferung Deutschland / Österreich / Schweiz: siehe Impressumsseite